Ergebnisse der Anatomie und Entwicklungsgeschichte
Advances in Anatomy, Embryology and Cell Biology
Revues d'anatomie et de morphologie expérimentale
Springer-Verlag Berlin Heidelberg New York

This journal publishes reviews and critical articles covering the entire field of normal anatomy (cytology, histology, cyto- and histochemistry, electron microscopy, macroscopy, experimental morphology and embryology and comparative anatomy). Papers dealing with anthropology and clinical morphology will also be accepted with the aim of encouraging co-operation between anatomy and related disciplines.

Papers, which may be in English, French or German, are normally commissioned, but original papers and communications may be submitted and will be considered so long as they deal with a subject comprehensively and meet the requirements of the Ergebnisse.

For speed of publication and breadth of distribution, this journal appears in single issues which can be purchased separately; 6 issues constitute one volume.

It is a fundamental condition that manuscripts submitted should not have been published elsewhere, in this or any other country, and the author must undertake not to publish elsewhere at a later date.

25 copies of each paper are supplied free of charge.

Les résultats publient des sommaires et des articles critiques concernant l'ensemble du domaine de l'anatomie normale (cytologie, histologie, cyto et histochimie, microscopie électronique, macroscopie, morphologie expérimentale, embryologie et anatomie comparée. Seront publiés en outre les articles traitant de l'anthropologie et de la morphologie clinique, en vue d'encourager la collaboration entre l'anatomie et les disciplines voisines.

Seront publiés en priorité les articles expressément demandés nous tiendrons toutefois compte des articles qui nous seront envoyés dans la mesure où ils traitent d'un sujet dans son ensemble et correspondent aux standards des «Résultats». Les publications seront faites en langues anglaise, allemande et française.

Dans l'intérêt d'une publication rapide et d'une large diffusion les travaux publiés paraitront dans des cahiers individuels, diffusés séparément: 6 cahiers forment un volume.

En principe, seuls les manuscrits qui n'ont encore été publiés ni dans le pays d'origine ni à l'étranger peuvent nous être soumis. L'auteur d'engage en outre à ne pas les publier ailleurs ultérieurement.

Les auteurs recevront 25 exemplaires gratuits de leur publication.

Die Ergebnisse dienen der Veröffentlichung zusammenfassender und kritischer Artikel aus dem Gesamtgebiet der normalen Anatomie (Cytologie, Histologie, Cyto- und Histochemie, Elektronenmikroskopie, Makroskopie, experimentelle Morphologie und Embryologie und vergleichende Anatomie). Aufgenommen werden ferner Arbeiten anthropologischen und morphologisch-klinischen Inhaltes, mit dem Ziel die Zusammenarbeit zwischen Anatomie und Nachbardisziplinen zu fördern.

Zur Veröffentlichung gelangen in erster Linie angeforderte Manuskripte, jedoch werden auch eingesandte Arbeiten und Originalmitteilungen berücksichtigt, sofern sie ein Gebiet umfassend abhandeln und den Anforderungen der „Ergebnisse" genügen. Die Veröffentlichungen erfolgen in englischer, deutscher oder französischer Sprache.

Die Arbeiten erscheinen im Interesse einer raschen Veröffentlichung und einer weiten Verbreitung als einzeln berechnete Hefte; je 6 Hefte bilden einen Band.

Grundsätzlich dürfen nur Manuskripte eingesandt werden, die vorher weder im Inland noch im Ausland veröffentlicht worden sind. Der Autor verpflichtet sich, sie auch nachträglich nicht an anderen Stellen zu publizieren.

Die Mitarbeiter erhalten von ihren Arbeiten zusammen 25 Freiexemplare.

Manuscripts should be addressed to/Envoyer les manuscrits à/Manuskripte sind zu senden an:

Prof. Dr. A. Brodal, Universitetet i Oslo, Anatomisk Institutt, Karl Johans Gate 47 (Domus Media), Oslo 1/Norwegen

Prof. W. Hild, Department of Anatomy, The University of Texas Medical Branch, Galveston, Texas 77550 (USA).

Prof. Dr. R. Ortmann, Anatomisches Institut der Universität, D-5000 Köln-Lindenthal, Lindenburg.

Prof. Dr. T. H. Schiebler, Anatomisches Institut der Universität, Koellikerstraße 6, D-8700 Würzburg

Prof. Dr. G. Töndury, Direktion der Anatomie, Gloriastraße 19, CH-8006 Zürich.

Prof. Dr. E. Wolff, Collège de France, Laboratoire d'Embryologie Expérimentale, 49 bis Avenue de la belle Gabrielle, Nogent-sur-Marne 49/France.

Ergebnisse der Anatomie und Entwicklungsgeschichte
Advances in Anatomy, Embryology and Cell Biology
Revues d'anatomie et de morphologie expérimentale

46·1

Radomír Čihák

Ontogenesis of the Skeleton
and Intrinsic Muscles
of the Human Hand and Foot

With 122 Figures

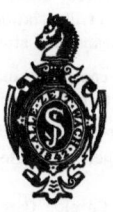

Springer-Verlag Berlin Heidelberg GmbH 1972

Dr. Radomír Čihák, DrSc.,
Department of Anatomy,
Charles University Medical Faculty, Prague

ISBN 978-3-540-05673-7   ISBN 978-3-662-09081-7 (eBook)
DOI 10.1007/978-3-662-09081-7

Contents

I. Introduction

The aim of the present publication is to summarize the results of studies of ontogenesis of the skeleton and muscles of the human hand and foot. Our primary interest in studying the muscles arose from observations of variations, in which a new form of the anomalous muscle in the popliteal fossa had been described (Čihák, 1954; Hněvkovský and Čihák, 1957) and in which changes of muscle forms in the congenitally malformed extremity had also been studied (Brůčková and Čihák, 1956). The desire to clarify muscle variations by means of the ontogenesis led to a study of ontogenesis of single muscles. During observation of the embryonic pectoralis major special muscle bundles were primarily observed, which could be homologised with the sphincter colli muscle of lower Mammals. Further observation revealed that this muscle (concordantly with its phylogenetic development) gradually develops in the course of human ontogenesis from a small primordium to its maximal extent and becomes reduced thereafter and finally disappears, still during the embryonic period (Čihák, 1957). This study was decisive for the further development of our theme, since it demonstrates, how consistently in the development of the locomotor apparatus the rule of recapitulation is asserted and how this can be employed in developmental studies of muscles. It was therefore presumed that the more complicated morphogenesis would be found in the course of the embryonic development of muscles undergoing more complicated changes of their external shape during phylogenetic development. For the subsequent developmental studies, therefore, the muscles have been selected according to the differences of their morphology in Mammals of various phylogenetic levels, e.g. some spinohumeral and thoracohumeral muscles. The studies brought about a number of results: five developmentally independent components of the pectoralis major were found in human ontogenesis, later fusing to form the typical pattern of this muscle (Čihák, 1959, 1960a); the typical ageneses of the pectoralis major were found to be mosaic-shaped defects occurring exactly according to single embryonic portions of muscle (Čihák and Popelka, 1961). The determination of five fundamental portions of the pectoralis major in human ontogenesis became the basis for the homologisation of the complicated pectoralis musculature in the comparative anatomy of various mammalian orders (Štěrba, 1967a, 1968a). The latissimus dorsi and its two components have similarly been studied (Čihák, 1960a, 1963a). In the course of the development of the latissimus dorsi also the dorsoepitrochlearis muscle was repeatedly found in young embryos (Čihák, 1961, 1963a). Contrary to this, the distinct portions of the trapezius muscle, which have been claimed to exist in adults, were never found in embryos and they appear as a secondary pattern (Čihák, 1960a); this view has been revised and supported from the comparative standpoint by Štěrba (1965, 1967b, 1968b) and by Štěrba and Berg (1963). In the development of the human deltoid muscle a similar result was obtained concerning its claviculo-acromial part by Hořejší (1968). The later description of the interesting muscular anomaly—the musculus sterno-cleidomandibularis—in man and an attempt at its developmental explanation also belongs to this group of studies (Hněvkovský and Čihák, 1967). In the lower limb a developmental independence of components of the quadriceps femoris was found (Čihák and Puzanová, 1960). The developmental recapitulation of changes in form in the deep portion of the masseter and in the corresponding region of the mandible was also encountered (Čihák and Vlček, 1962).

During this first step of our studies valuable experience was obtained, revealing the existence of changes of the external form of muscles in a relatively late foetal period. It was possible to employ the standpoints of the comparative anatomy and the findings in the teratology and to combine it with the information concerning the embryonic development of muscles, and to continue in this manner the fundamental embryological studies, which from the beginning of this century dealt mainly with the early development of muscles. We soon recognized the necessity to keep muscular components in view and to consider their independence according to the form of the neurovascular hila, as described by Brash (1955). On this basis it was possible to demonstrate that many muscles developed during ontogenesis by fusion of originally independent elements, such muscles being at first a group of fully separate individuals and later a system of relatively independent components which each have their own nerve. From this standpoint the anatomical nomenclatorial usage, expressing the individuality of the muscle also by its name, is not always in accordance with reality, and this is to be taken into account when homologies are considered. The detailed knowledge of muscle components permitted clinical applications: it was possible, also in adults, to separate such a developmentally independent and separately innervated component and to employ it for the replacement of a paralysed function of another muscle (Čihák and Eiselt, 1962; Čihák and Hněvkovský, 1963).

After the above mentioned experience in the studies of developing muscles and muscle components it was possible to start studying an interesting and complicated muscle group—the intrinsic hand muscles.

There has been up to now only a fragmentary knowledge of the ontogenesis of hand muscles, with many contradictory points between the embryology and the comparative anatomy. Therefore, we tried primarily to assess the typical layers of the intrinsic musculature and their homologies. It was also found that the first dorsal interosseus originates by fusion of two neighbouring components corresponding to the so-called flexores breves profundi muscles of lower Mammals (Čihák, 1960b). An attempt at explaining (in the same paper) the origin of the three other dorsal interossei by the same mechanism was, however, incorrect, and was revised in subsequent studies (Čihák, 1963b, c, 1967a), in which the homologies of deep layers of hand musculature primordia (giving rise to the interossei) were established. In addition, in the embryonic human hand a layer of muscular primordia was found corresponding to the four contrahentes muscles of lower Mammals (Čihák, 1963b, c). Later on, the origin, extent and a special type of extinction of a part of this layer was observed in the hand (Čihák, 1967a, b, 1968a, b) as well as in the foot (Čihák, 1969a, c). The above quoted observation of fusion of the first dorsal interosseus from the two parts permitted the surgical reconstruction of thumb opposition by means of intrinsic hand muscles (Čihák, Eiselt and Fleischmann, 1963).

The revision of the disposition of primordial layers in the hand enabled further collaborators to extend the studies to the development of further muscles, e.g. the flexor digitorum superficialis which in the embryo is originally a hand muscle (Dylevský, 1967, 1968a, c), to the development and the spacial relations of the palmaris longus muscle and the palmar aponeurosis (Dylevský, 1968b, 1969a, c). The pattern of the layer of contrahentes muscles and of their embryonic primordia was examined in the rat (Trnková and Dylevský, 1969); the embryonic primordia of the interossei in rats were studied and the dorsal components of the interossei, typical of many Mammals, were found in rats to disappear during the course of embryonic development (Dylevský and Trnková, 1969). The study of the intermetacarpal space in chick embryos revealed the constancy of development of typical muscular primordia (known in Mammals) even in the intermetacarpal space of the extremely specialized Sauropsid extremity (Dylevský, 1968d).

In the developing human hand, moreover, further muscular and connective tissue components were observed. The accessory primordia of the dorsal interossei were described (Čihák, 1963c, 1967a, 1969c) and their persistence in adults was observed (Chmelová, 1963). Also the differentiation of the retinaculum flexorum and its relations to the developing skeleton and thenar musculature were observed (Čihák, 1966b, 1969b, c), as well as the clinical significance of anomalous muscles on the dorsum manus (Lunda and Čihák, 1967) and the phylogenetically ancient pattern of tendons of the embryonic extensor digiti minimi (Kaneff and Čihák, 1970).

Many principial points of the studies quoted are summarized as a basis of the present publication. During studies of extremities a question arises concerning comparisons of the upper and lower limbs. The study of developing muscles of the foot and the comparison with the hand is, therefore, one of the main themes of this paper. The further, non-subsidiary theme concerns the development of the hand and foot skeleton and its relationship to the developing musculature, since preliminary observations suggest that the developing skeletal elements also bear many phylogenetically ancient features (similar to developing muscle primordia) which permit developmental explanations. In considering the development of skeletal elements of the hand and foot the problem of their comparison and homologues cannot be overlooked, since there are many contradictions concerning this point even in relatively recent literature.

The present publication therefore examines step by step the development of the skeleton and of single muscular groups in the human hand and foot. The extent of the chapters and the different partial subjects do not permit the employment of the conventional simple scheme of the paper, with the final discussion and conclusions regarding all points after all observations at the end of the paper. It is necessary, for the sake of clarity of this paper, to proceed according to thematic chapters and to provide each with the given question, its solution and conclusions. Single themes are supplemented by the comparison of corresponding pattern in the hand and foot.

II. Material and Methods

During the many years of work on this subject, 373 series of human embryonic hands and feet were collected. This material contains 270 histological series of hands of human embryos and foetuses from 10 to 100 mm in crown-rump length. Most of them are transversally sectioned; for control the remaining series were sectioned either sagittally or parallel to the palm. The further material contains 103 series of feet of human embryos and foetuses from 15 to 90 mm C-R length, sectioned again transversally, sagittally and parallel to the sole. A series of embryonic hands of various mammals was also employed for comparison. From this entire material partial collections of 50–80 series were picked out for studies of single problems. The selection for those single studies from the entire material was always performed individually so that basic comparable stages of development have been repeated in all single studies and, moreover, so that the maximal number of series employed has belonged to the time of maximal morphogenetic changes of studied pattern (according to the range of their C-R lengths). It was thus possible to study the detailed sequence of development. The material extends to foetuses of such a size that no further changes in external muscle forms and in skeletal pattern can be observed, where the basic ligamentous and fascial structures are also formed, hence where the foetal hand and foot are closely similar to those of the adult.

The choice of material for individual partial series will be referred to in the subsequent text, always in front of the respective chapters. The number of series employed in partial studies (50–80 series) has made a sufficiently detailed examination of the developmental process possible. It was, therefore, not necessary to imagine the course of developmental changes between two remote stages, as commonly done in the papers of previous authors. We note for orientation that Ruge (1878a) performed his study on four foetuses (23, 35, 40 and 100 mm in length) and Windle (1883) also on four foetuses (24, 50, 70 and 120 mm). Gräfenberg (1905/06) does not indicate the number of his specimens, but it could be deduced from his text that he had 1–2 foetuses per week, from the fifth to the thirteenth foetal week; however, his descriptions do not correspond with the respective weeks according to the degree of differentiation. Bardeen and Lewis (1901) had 13 embryos; from this number they reconstructed six embryos. McMurrich (1903) illustrated his conclusions by one foetus of 60 mm, where, however, the developmental changes concerned took place a long time previously. Really extensive embryonic material appeared first in papers by O'Rahilly (1954), O'Rahilly, Gray and Gardner (1957) and Gray et al. (1957).

Due to the fact that in the critical stages of morphogenesis the C-R lengths of our material increase by half of a millimetre or one by one millimetre and that there are mostly a number of specimens of the same size, the continuity of the C-R length sequence represents a simultaneous control. By comparison of successive stages it can be demonstrated that no deviation from the form sequence occurs such as would signalize an anomaly. Such certainty is also supported by the fact that most of our series were obtained from the termination of normal pregnancies. This material was of two kinds: in one part of it the C-R lengths were preserved and it was hence possible to measure the embryo exactly; in the second part of the material, the C-R length could not be measured. Therefore our collaborator Dr. Ivan Dylevský employing the collection of undamaged embryos worked out a method of estimating the C-R length by means of external dimensions of extremity parts or by means of skeletal stylopodial or zeugopodial dimensions (by measuring and correlating lengths of extremities with other body dimensions — Dylevský, 1965, 1969b). This method enables us to assess the C-R lengths of the incomplete material from terminations.

Preparations studied by means of the stereoscopic microscope were used very little in this work, only for controlling the comparative material of hands of the following Mammals: Ornithorhynchus, Didelphys, Erinaceus, Nycticebus, Galago, Lemur, Hapale, Macaca, Pan, Gorilla (foetus). Comparative data were also taken over from the literature.

During processing histological series the question of staining the slides arose. In embryonic material which had frequently been preserved in formol for many years before processing there were difficulties in differentiation of very early myoblasts by the usual staining methods. Held's molybden hematoxylin which has suitable qualities for the simultaneous staining of various tissues was therefore selected. Later on this stain was modified with respect to the

differentiation of muscle and connective tissue by applying the well soluble phosphomolybdic acid instead of the molybdic acid of Held's original formula (Čihák, 1963 b, c). Staining with the thus modified Held's hematoxylin was useful for the old formol preserved
material. The dye partly differentiated the early myoblasts in a dark violet to blackish tone
from surrounding mesenchymal cells, partly stained all cellular processes, all membranes
etc. in a very good and contrasting picture. In more advanced specimens the connective
tissue can also be distinguished by the stain. By employing phosphomolybdic acid we obtain
the components of connective tissue—especially if the collagen is already formed—in a red
tone, well differentiated from that of future muscle cells. Moreover, the described method
also stains the axons of peripheral nerves. This method was very suitable for the demarcation of early muscular blastemas in young developmental stages; on its basis the drawing
of slides for plastic reconstruction was easily possible. The method, however, is not completely suitable for cytological purposes because of the lack of clear contouring of intracellular
structures. We therefore changed this method later for staining with Ehrlich's hematoxylin,
alone or with eosin, and still later for staining with Weigert's hematoxylin and eosin. This
method yields the best results in the embryonic material, assuming that the material has
not been fixed in formol for too long a time.

   Some of the series were reconstructed. In two series of hands (embryo 15.5 and 21 mm
in C-R length) the muscle primordia with the skeleton were completely reconstructed; from
one series (embryo 28 mm in C-R length) the reconstruction of important parts of hand
skeleton has been performed. The method of Born was employed for the reconstructions.
The drawings were performed either by use of Abbe's apparatus, or from microphotographs
with simultaneous microscopic control of the specimens, or directly from the microscopic
slides projected on the paper. For the proper technic of reconstruction a plastic material
known by the name of Modelit (produced by the firm Rohoplast, Prague) was employed
in place of the wax normally used. This white material, based upon mixing pulverized PVC
with organic softeners of the phthalate group, is used in schools as material for modelling.
Modelled while cold, this material hardens without change of form and with only a slight
change of volume into a white ivory-like matter on heating to 100–120° C. We worked in
three steps:

   1. The mass was rolled to the calculated thickness in a normal manner by a roller warmed
to 40–50° C which made the mass smoother. While rolling the mass was dusted with talc
so that it did not stick to the base or to the roller.

   2. The rolled plates were warmed in the thermostat to 70° C for 5 minutes. After cooling
down the material became slightly firm of approximately rubber consistency and could be
well cut without adhering to the knife and without deformation. Drawings were copied on
plates so prepared and cut out.

   3. After mounting the reconstruction, and working its surface by apposition and subsequent modelling of fresh mass between the steps of reconstruction layers, the finished
reconstruction was heated in the thermostat to 100–120° C for about five minutes per centi-
metre of object thickness; then the reconstruction was cooled down slowly in the thermostat.

   There are several advantages of employing this new plastic material as compared with
wax: its minimal combustibility, working in the cold, cleaness of working, easy surface
modelling, hardness and durability of the reconstruction (Čihák, 1963c, 1966a). All these
advantages fully compensate for the rather tiresome rolling. Besides Born's method graphic
reconstructions have also been employed for detailed points of series. During studies of
muscular primordia the reconstructions served mainly for improved spatial comprehensions.
The reconstruction, at least a graphic one, was necessary for studies of the developing carpal
skeleton since only on its basis could the really independent or the fusing parts of primordia
be recognized.

   We are aware that slight inaccuracies may accrue especially from surface modelling;
the main contribution of the reconstruction, however, the plastic illustration of the observed
pattern and the exclusion of errors in continuity or discontinuity of elements observed in
histological series, fully counteracts the minute technical imperfection. We therefore avoided
figuring patterns on the object surface which cannot be exactly revealed by the reconstruction, e.g. the direction of muscle fibres, surface details etc. The reconstructions, worked

out minutely in this respect by Bardeen and Lewis (1901) and by Lewis (1901/02), carry significant traces of artificial modelling, based naturally upon adult muscle. This gives their reconstructions an appearance of structures more advanced than we find in our specimens, and than they are actually.

III. Ontogenesis and Homologies of Human Carpal and Tarsal Components

1. Problem of Development of the Carpus and Tarsus.
The Morphology of Carpal and Tarsal Elements

The question of the origin, derivation and homologies of carpal and tarsal components has been an onerous problem in developmental anatomy for more than a hundred years. Interest was evoked by the work of Gegenbaur (1865) where the structure of the tetrapod extremity was derived for the first time from the fin of elasmobranch fishes. In the course of the subsequent development of the problem this idea was gradually exactified and geometrised (Gegenbaur, 1870a, b, c, d). Less known in the history of the problem, but quite important for later views on the development of the extremities is Gegenbaur's consideration of the uniserial "archipterygium" as the elemental extremity type, presented in these early works. From the archipterygium he derived the five-toed extremity so that he at first located the main axis through the radius and the fifth finger and derived the remaining fingers as collateral rays (Fig. 1 A). Later on, influenced by Huxley's criticism (1873), Gegenbaur (1876) transposed the main extremity axis into the ulnar margin of the uniserial archipterygium and other fingers again were derived in the form of collateral rays.

In the meantime Gegenbaur (1873) established his famous, now already abandonned "theory of the archipterygium" where on the basis of Günther's (1871) he considered the pattern of the biserial Ceratodus fin, claimed this biserial archipterygium to be the initial form, derived the uniserial form from it and from this again by the above established process, the five-fingered extremity. From this original work of Gegenbaur, however, the questions of the comparison and homologies of carpal elements still remained topical and unsolved.

The basis for all subsequent considerations therefore became the pattern of the primitive carpus and the number of its elements as stated by Gegenbaur: three elements of the proximal row—the radiale, intermedium and the ulnare; two centralia—the radial and the ulnar one; five distal row elements, ossa carpi (distalia) I—V (Fig. 1A). These elements, declared by Gegenbaur to be constant, were then called by Braus (1906) canonic elements, to point out their distinction to additional accessory carpal components. (It will be pointed out later that much more constant elements were established subsequently.) According to Gegenbaur the elements in the primitive carpus are assembled symmetrically to the third digit; however, the line set through the autopodial margin represents the original main axis of the biserial and uniserial archipterygium.

At that time also in connection with Gegenbaur's general idea of extremities, carpus and tarsus, a series of works appeared applying or varying in detail this concept of carpal and tarsal elements in comparative anatomy and in embryology as well as in human anatomy and variability (Fürbringer, 1870; Wiedersheim,

1876, 1877, 1880; Born, 1876a, b, 1880; Bardeleben, 1883a, b, c, 1885a, b, c, 1894a, b; Baur, 1884, 1885a, b, c, 1886, 1889; Leboucq, 1884, 1886; Kollmann, 1888; Stieda, 1889, 1897; Emery, 1890, 1897a, c, d, 1898, 1901; Rosenberg, 1891/92; Pfitzner, 1893; Eisler, 1895; Sewertzoff, 1904; Schmalhausen, 1908).

Pursuing the geometrising derivation of the extremity from the archipterygium, Gegenbaur (1873) tended in the same geometrical manner to derive the origin of the entire (according to him, original) form of the biserial archipterygium from the pattern of rays of the branchial arch. Only later did this conception assume its definitive form together with the schematic picture (Gegenbaur, 1876) which then passed for years from one textbook to another, whether accepted as a fact, or as a history of the solution of the problem (Wiedersheim, 1893).

Meanwhile a new viewpoint occured (Balfour, 1876/77) deriving paired extremities from the continuous lateral fin fold. This theory, complemented and supported by further authors (Thacher, 1877/78, 1878; Mivart, 1879; Balfour, 1881a, b) and later propounded especially by Haswell (1883, 1884), Dohrn (1884) and Wiedersheim (1892, 1893), conflicted with and won against Gegenbaur's theory of the archipterygium derived from the branchial arch—though at that time Gegenbaur's view also found supporters (v. Davidoff, 1879, 1884). Although D'Arcy Thompson (1886) had already raised objections to Gegenbaur's concept, Gegenbaur still in 1894 insisted upon his unchanged idea of the archipterygium, of its development and of the origin of the pentadactyl extremity. On the contrary, the theory of the fin fold has been supported by further observations of fin development in various fish groups (Mollier, 1893, 1895, 1897; Harrison, 1895; Dean, 1896, 1907; Goodrich, 1906). The controversy of the archipterygium theory culminated at that time in Rabl's (1901) polemic against Gegenbaur and Fürbringer's (1902) against Rabl. The theory of the archipterygium was directly opposed by Dean (1896), Emery (1897b), Rabl (1901), until ultimately the fin fold theory was fully accepted (Wiedersheim, 1892, 1906, 1907; Osburn, 1907; Goodrich, 1930).

Gegenbaur's theory of the archipterygium and of the primitive carpus symmetrically constructed from it was not upheld, evidently due to its forced geometrical method. There appeared therefore new tendencies to derive the primitive extremity in another way or from another type of the fin. In this respect Emery (1887) considered the fin of Polypterus and Calamoichthys to be the interstage toward the extremity of a higher type. Klaatsch (1896), still influenced by the theory of archipterygium, then derived in detail the pattern of the tetrapod extremity from the fin of the Polypterus. The result of this attempt was not satisfactory because the assumption of development of carpal elements by splitting of the original medial plate (mesopterygium: Klaatsch, 1896; basale: Versluys, 1927) lacks any further support from the comparative anatomy and embryology. Inspired by Haswell (1883, 1884), Semon (1898) with hesitation and reservation modified Gegenbaur's derivation of the tetrapod hand from the biserial fin, constructing the symmetrical hand by means of the median axis of the original Ceratodus fin. His attempt was no more successful than that of Gegenbaur. The modification by Braus (1901), fully influenced by the archipterygium theory, accordingly also yielded unsatisfactory results. In this concept the extremity is constructed in an asymmetrical manner where only preaxial

rays of the biserial archipterygium are employed. Another manner of derivation
of the extremity was claimed by Emery, who in a series of papers (1890, 1897a,
b, c, d, 1898, 1901) took the rudimentary praepollex consistently into the scheme
of the primitive carpus and derived the extremity on an asymmetrical plan.
By this standpoint he only got ahead of his time. His homologisation was taken
over by Vialleton (1924). All these attempts at new modes of derivation and
homologisation of the extremity demonstrate the inadequacy of solutions presented hitherto. No contribution was made, of course, by Rabl's theory (1901,
1910), aimed against Gegenbaur, which originated, on the contrary, in the reduced
pincers-like hand of some Amphibians and from this deduced the evolution of
the five-toed extremity.

The deductions of the tetrapod extremity from the fins of recent Dipnoi
and Brachypterygii clearly failed. Soon afterwards, therefore, a new concept of
the development of the cheiropterygium arose, based upon the views of Broom
(1913) and Watson (1913, 1914). According to them the basic form of the cheiropterygium is represented by the pectoral fin of special pattern which occurs
in fossil fishes from the subclass Crossopterygii, order Rhipidistia, family Rhizo-
dontidae, genera Eusthenopteron and Sauripterus. Later on, their view was
approved by Gregory (1915), Gregory, Miner and Noble (1923), Gregory and
Raven (1941), Goodrich (1930), Westoll (1943), and is now commonly accepted
in paleontology and in comparative anatomy. The developmental line of the
extremity is led from fishes of the Eusthenopteron or Sauripterus type to fossil
Amphibians of the Eryops type. The extremity derived in this manner also
allows the inclusion of the praepollex and an increased number of central elements into the scheme of the primitive carpus. Comparative anatomy and
embryology indicates in fact that there can be more centralia than the two claimed
by Gegenbaur (Baur, 1885a, b, c, 1889; Bardeleben, 1894a; Emery, 1897a, c,
1901; Schauinsland, 1900, 1903; Schmalhausen, 1910).

The derivation of the extremity from the fin of the Eusthenopteron or Sauripterus type, the evidence of the primitive pattern in embryology, together with
homologies of carpal and tarsal elements then assumed a concrete form in two
groups of works based upon extensive comparative embryological material. These
are on the one hand, the work of Steiner and of Schmidt-Ehrenberg (Steiner,
1921, 1922a, b, 1934, 1935, 1942; Schmidt-Ehrenberg, 1942), on the other, the
work of Holmgren and Kindahl, similar in concept, different in many details
(Holmgren, 1933, 1939, 1949, 1952; Kindahl, 1941a, b, 1942a, b, 1944a, b, 1949).
In these papers Steiner demonstrated the recapitulation of form of the uniserial
archipterygium at the stage of the limb bud in the early mesenchymal blastema
of the extremity skeleton in various Tetrapods. Schmidt-Ehrenberg demonstrated
the pattern of the similarly shaped skeletal blastema during early ontogenesis
in Mammals also. During further development this blastema changes from the
simple form of the uniserial archipterygium into the form of the fin skeleton of
fishes of the Eusthenopteron or Sauripterus type, with the main axis passing
from the humerus through the ulna into the ulnar margin of the hand skeleton
(Steiner, 1935). According to Steiner the origin of cartilaginous anlagen inside
single sectors of this prochondral blastema demonstrates their connection with
the axial ray or with collateral rays and becomes the basis for their homologies.

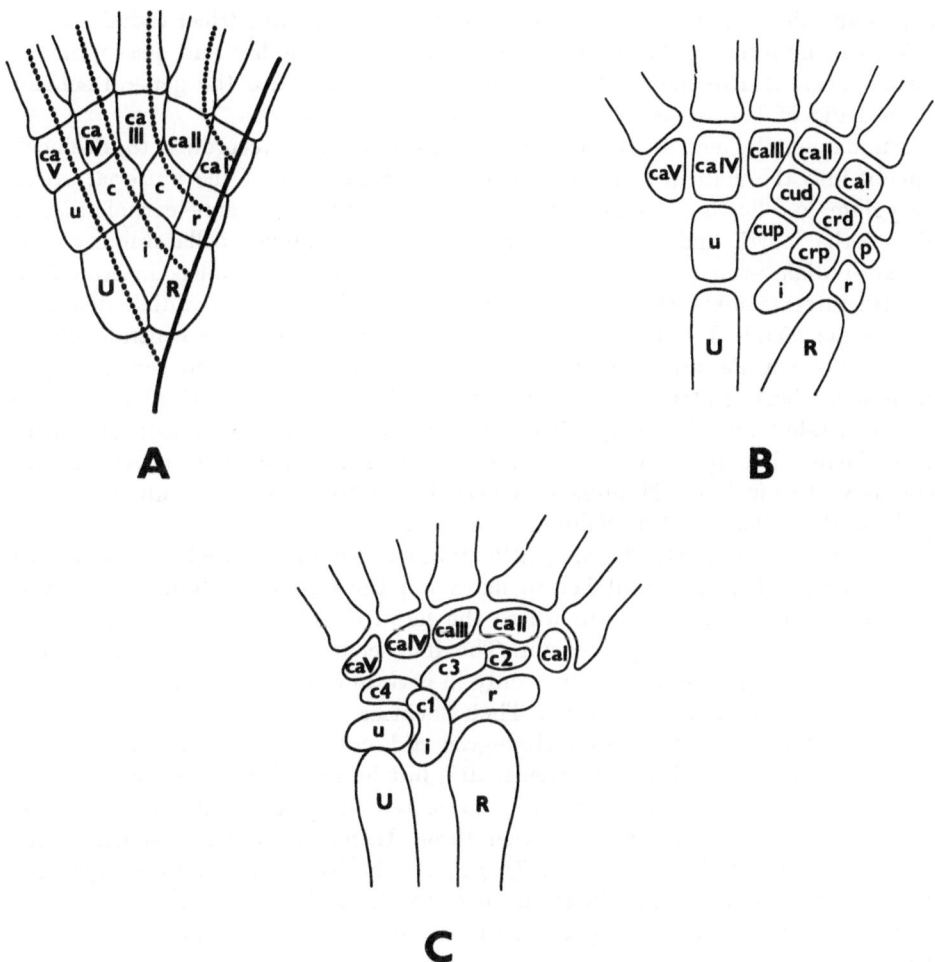

Fig. 1 A–C. Comparison of general schemes of the carpus and of its components in: A) Gegenbaur's scheme (1864, 1870b), B) Steiner's scheme (1942), C) Holmgren's (1933, 1952) and Kindahl's (1941–1949) scheme; *R* radius; *U* ulna; *r* radiale; *i* intermedium; *u* ulnare; *c, c 1–c 4* centralia; *crp* centrale radiale proximale; *crd* centrale radiale distale; *cup* centrale ulnare proximale; *cud* centrale ulnare distale; *p* prepollex; *ca I–V* carpalia distalia I–V

For this homologisation Steiner, as well as previous authors, proceeded essentially from Gegenbaur's scheme of the carpus and in conformity with Gegenbaur he distinguished the following elements in the carpus of primitive Tetrapods: the radiale, intermedium and the ulnare in the proximal row, five distal carpalia in the distal row; contrary to two centralia recognized by Gegenbaur, Steiner derived four centralia from the comparative embryology of the tetrapod hand, namely the centrale proximale radiale et ulnare, and the centrale distale radiale et ulnare. He also included the praepollicial ray into the scheme of the primitive carpus and derived the entire carpal skeleton in an asymmetrical radial scheme inside the uniserial archipterygium. Besides the praepollex and postminimus, the pisiforme is also included by Steiner (1935, 1942) into the general scheme of the hand of Tetrapods.

Fundamental elements of the carpus are arranged according to Steiner's concept into the main (axial) ray and the collateral rays of the uniserial archipterygium in following manner: the axial ray: the ulna—ulnare—carpale distale IV, V—the fourth and the fifth digit; the first (proximal) collateral ray: the radius—radiale—the praepollex; the second collateral, so-called intermediate ray: the intermedium—the centrale radiale proximale—centrale radiale distale—the carpale distale I—first digit; the third collateral ray: the centrale ulnare proximale—centrale ulnare distale—the carpale distale II—the second digit; the fourth, distal collateral ray: the carpale distale III—the third digit. The carpale distale V and the fifth digit stand as postaxial hand components (Fig. 1 B).

All included components may be considered as demonstrated in lower Tetrapods as well as in lower Mammals, at least in the form of embryonic primordia (Steiner, 1921, 1922a, 1934; Schmidt-Ehrenberg, 1942).

Holmgren's studies (1933, 1939, 1949, 1952) also demonstrated the occurrence of four central elements in all Tetrapods except the Urodeles. Holmgren derived the Urodeles as a special group where the hand developed in a manner other than from a biserial archipterygium. The four centralia, found by Holmgren, are visible as independent structures only in certain developmental stages during the ontogenesis of studied species. Their location also is given by Holmgren differently from Steiner's views. Holmgren did not derive the middle part of the hand from collateral rays as Steiner did, but he considered it as rays spreading out distally (Fig. 2). Accordingly he indicated the position of one of the centralia more proximal than that of other three. In his concept the centralia just spread out from the intermedium (Fig. 1 C, 2) distally in two or three rays and are numbered from the proximal one ($c1$) to the radial one ($c2$) towards the middle ($c3$) and the ulnar one ($c4$). The centrale 2, 3 and 4 are thus one row further distal than $c1$.

Steiner (1934) himself admitted that the regular arrangement of the central bones gets wiped out towards higher Tetrapods both in paired position and in parallel collateral rays. According to Kindahl (1941a) the situation of centralia differs from the paired arrangement demonstrated by Schmalhausen (1910) in Salamandrella. Holmgren's studies were followed by a series of papers by Kindahl (1941a, b, 1942a, b, 1944a, b, 1949). She tended to demonstrate the existence of all the centralia assumed by Holmgren and by Steiner in the ontogenesis of mammalian carpal elements. Her studies admitted the occurrence of four centralia during the ontogenesis of various Mammals though with the modification that two centralia fuse together ($c2$ and 3) and the other two remain independent. In her view the distribution of the centralia does not correspond to the paired arrangement given by Steiner, but she considered the situation of the centralia according to Holmgren's scheme (1933, 1939, 1952). Steiner's view on one hand, and Holmgren's on the other, differ both in concept as well as in nomenclature. By comparison of Steiner's with Holmgren's concept some inaccuracies arose in the literature. Although both these two standpoints originate

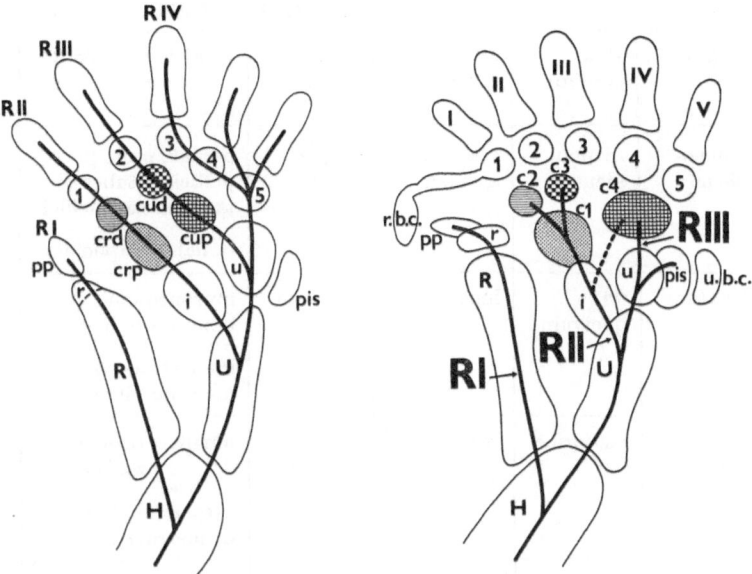

Fig. 2. Scheme of differences of Steiner's (1942) and Holmgren's (1933, 1949, 1952) concepts of pattern of the primitive carpus. Whilst Steiner derives the carpal components from the uniserial archipterygium according to the main axis and the collateral rays, Holmgren sees in the carpus a system of branching rays expressed by the positions of central elements. $R\ I$–IV supposed branches of the original fin; H humerus; R radius; U ulna; r radiale; i intermedium; u ulnare; pis pisiforme; pp prepollex; rbc radial sesamoid; ubc ulnar sesamoid; $c1$–4 the centralia 1–4; crp centrale radiale proximale; crd centrale radiale distale; cup centrale ulnare proximale; cud centrale ulnare distale; 1–5 the carpalia distalia 1–5; I–V the metacarpals. According to Holmgren (1952). The elements which we consider as corresponding in both concepts are accordingly shaded

from two different concepts of the phylogenetic development of the hand, the mutual comparison of the centralia is still possible. After comparing illustrations in Kindahl's papers with those by Holmgren, Steiner and Schmidt-Ehrenberg we take centrale 1 to be the centrale radiale proximale, centrale 2 as identical with the centrale radiale distale. Centrale 3 corresponds to the centrale ulnare distale and centrale 4 to the slightly shifted centrale ulnare proximale (also as compared by Westoll, 1943). This view is in disagreement with the interpretation of both nomenclatures found in Rajtová's paper (1967). The occurrence of an increased number of centralia is evidently constant in the mammalian carpus too. Slabý (1958a, 1962a, 1963a, b, 1964a, b, 1967a, b) demonstrated that even in a specialized carpus like that of Ungulates the elements may be interpreted in line with Steiner's and Holmgren's concepts, though during ontogenesis.

Still more contradictory views concern the homologies of carpal elements and their participation in definitive carpal bones. From Gegenbaur's considerations on carpal homologies onward the authors take into account various possibilities of fusion of the proximal row of carpalia with the centralia or of the centralia mutually in various interrelations; the differences are best visible in

Table 1. *Various views concerning the*

Canonic carpal elements in Tetrapods	Gegenbaur (1864)	Baur (1885c)	Baur (1889)	Bardeleben (1883)	Bardeleben (1885c)	Bardeleben (1894a)
Radiale	scaphoideum	scaphoideum	sesamoid element	scaphoideum	carpale prox. prae-pollicis = tuberositas ossis scaphoidei / radiale = scaphoideum	scaphoideum
Intermedium	lunatum	triquetrum	lunatum	lunatum	intermedium 1 = lunatum radiale / intermedium 2 = lunatum ulnare	lunatum
Ulnare	triquetrum	pisiforme	triquetrum	triquetrum	ulnare = triquetrum radiale / carpale prox. 5 = triquetrum ulnare	triquetrum
Pisiforme	pisiforme		pisiforme	pisiforme	pisiforme	pisiforme
Centrale	centrale	lunatum	c 1 rad. = scaphoideum / c 2 uln. = centrale	tuberositas ossis scaphoidei	c 1 = part of the scaphoideum / c 2 = caput ossis capitati / c 3 = proximal part of the hamatum	centrale
Carpale distale I	trapezium	sesamoid element	trapezium	trapezium	carpale dist. prae-pollicis = tuberositas ossis scaphoidei / carpale dist. I = trapezium	trapezium
Carpale distale II	trapezoideum	trapezium	trapezoideum	trapezoideum	trapezoideum	trapezoideum
Carpale distale III	capitatum	trapezoideum	capitatum	capitatum	distal part of the capitatum	capitatum
Carpale distale IV	hamatum	capitatum	hamatum	hamatum	hamatum	hamatum
Carpale distale V	hamatum	hamatum	hamatum	hamatum	hamatum	hamatum
					carpale distale VI = hamulus ossis hamati	

homologies of canonic carpal elements

Emery (1897)	Weber (1927)	Foster-Cooper (1940)	Holmgren (1952) Kindahl (1941–1949)	Steiner (1942) Schmidt-Ehrenberg (1942)	Slabý (1967 b, 1968)
proximal part of the scaphoideum	scapho-ideum	scapho-ideum	scaphoideum	processus styloideus radii	processus styloideus radii
lunatum	lunatum	tri-quetrum	part of the lunatum	lunatum	proximal part of the lunatum .... triangulare
triquetrum	tri-quetrum	pisiforme	processus styloideus ulnae	triquetrum	triquetrum
pisiforme	pisiforme		pisiforme	pisiforme	pisiforme
rad. {centrale or a part of the scapho-ideum .... uln. {proximal part of the capi-tatum	centrale .... extinct or fused with the capi-tatum	centrale .... lunatum	c 1 = part of the lunatum .... c 2 } c 3 } = centrale normale .... c 4 = triquetrum	proxim. }scapho-rad. .... }ideum distale } .... distale = centrale normale uln. .... proxim. = extinct	} = scapho-}ideum .... centrale normale .... distal part of the lunatum .... + a centrale in the prox. part of tri-quetrum
trapezium	tra-pezium	tra-pezium	trapezium	trapezium	trapezium
trapezoideum	trapezo-ideum	trapezo-ideum	trapezoideum	trapezoideum	trapezo-ideum
capitatum	capi-tatum	capi-tatum	capitatum	capitatum	capitatum
hamatum	hamatum	hamatum	hamatum	hamatum	hamatum .... part of the triquetrum

tabular form (Table 1). This table shows the various interpretations of homologies of canonic elements as well as of the centralia. They all arose in order to explain the homologies in a geometrical manner and without remnants.

The table also demonstrates that there are three points critical as for correct homologies in the carpus: 1. the homology of the radiale and the view of origin and homology of the scaphoid, joined to it; 2. the view of the homology of the ulnare and of the subsequent homologisation of the triquetrum; 3. the view of the fate of the carpale distale V. The decisive role in all these views on homology is played by the central elements.

Because our previous studies concerning the ontogenesis of hand muscles (Čihák, 1963b, c, 1967a, b, 1968a, b) have shown that on the basis of the recapitulation rule even very primitive structures and their pattern appeared during the ontogenesis, we decided to attempt to revise the developmental problems of the carpus and tarsus on the basis of human ontogenesis. The above quoted statements by Slabý of the recapitulation of the primitive pattern of the carpus during ontogenesis even in Mammals with a highly specialized adult carpus also support this concept of research. Moreover, even in adults the human hand retains many of the primitive developmental features.

The ontogenesis of human carpal elements was already followed by numerous authors in the nineteenth century. Henke and Reyher (1874) noted that the components of the carpal skeleton were formed sooner, in embryos of 18—20 mm, whilst other formations in the carpus (joint capsules, ligaments) developed later, first in the third embryonic month. Similarly Schulin (1879) established the presence of all carpal components from 27 mm of embryonic length onward. Retterer (1884) observed the presence of all carpal components and of their articulations in the foetus of 55 mm in length, with the same shape as in adults. At the same time Leboucq (1884) found that the carpalia and the metacarpalia differentiated as early as in an embryo of 12.5 mm in length. Thilenius (1896a) placed the definitive differentiation of form of carpal elements in the first half of the second prenatal month. In 1900 Hagen presented the first reconstruction of the hand skeleton in a 17 mm embryo; Bardeen and Lewis (1901) and Lewis (1901/02) studied the development of human musculature and skeleton and also reconstructed. Their oldest embryo (20 mm in C-R length) already had all carpal elements in typical disposition. Many works were concerned with the development of both the normal carpal elements and the supernumerary, temporary or persistent components. The findings of supernumerary elements in the human carpus are centred in two regions: in the region of the scaphoid, trapezium, trapezoideum and capitatum—that is the region of the central carpal bone, and in the area radial to the ulnar styloid process—i.e. the area of the triangular bone. Both areas were described in connection with the normal development of the carpus by a number of authors (Henke and Reyher, 1874; Rosenberg, 1876; Schulin, 1879; Leboucq, 1884, 1886; Thilenius, 1894, 1896a, b, 1897; Corner, 1898; Gräfenberg, 1905/06; Lucien, 1906, 1907; Henckel, 1931; Beau, Sommelet, and Cayotte, 1952; O'Rahilly, 1954; O'Rahilly, Gray, and Gardner, 1957; Gray, Gardner, and O'Rahilly, 1957; Slabý, 1958a, b, c). The course of carpal chondrification in accordance with single embryonic horizons was described by Senior (1929), Streeter (1951), O'Rahilly, Gray and Gardner (1957). The form of the embryonic carpus was reconstructed by Olivier (1962).

It may be seen from this review of basic publications that the development, the blastemas, chondrification and existence of the centralia etc. of carpal elements, have been described and controlled many times. It is hence unnecessary to focus our observations on these questions of an elementary descriptive character. On the contrary, the control of the ontogenetic occurrence, position and syntopic relations of single elements, aimed at establishing the morphogenetic participation of centralia in the carpus, is of importance. It is also important to consider the problem of the carpale distale V and to compare general aspects of morphogenesis of the carpus and tarsus known in the literature, with observations of the ontogenesis of the carpus and tarsus in man.

In connection with considerations on the development of the carpus and tarsus we shall also try to make more precise the interpretation of the elements by inducing more strict criteria for the independence of components. We will therefore consider the carpus and tarsus mostly according to the development of chondrified elements. As a proof of the independence of a certain component either its strictly separate existence at the prochondral stage or its occurrence in the form of a chondrified element will be recognized. The contingent temporary changes in the form of carpal elements, as far as they are conspicuous enough to permit a past characteristic process to be inferred must also be considered. We formed this postulation to assess the carpus only according to chondrified components because all elements, assumed by the authors, are so fixed from phylogenesis that their existence during ontogenesis must become evident in the form of a distinguishable cartilaginous anlage. The classification of single carpal components at the stage of the blastema before the origin of prochondral tissue leads inevitably to error. In chondrified elements their successive changes of form will be taken into account. The homologies of elements will then be deduced not only from their position and relation to single rays (as stated by Steiner), but also from their mutual spatial relations (changing during ontogenesis) and from similar relations in comparative morphology.

2. Material for Observations on the Ontogenesis of the Carpus

Histological series of 62 hands of human embryos and foetuses from 10 to 80 mm in C-R length were employed for the study of ontogenesis of carpal elements. The series were sectioned either parallel with the palm or transversely. Four sagittally sectioned series were also used for control.

Crown-rump lengths of embryos and foetuses employed were: 10 mm, 12, 13, 13.6, 14 (2 hands), 15 (3), 15.5, 16 (2), 16.5, 17, 17.5, 18 (2), 19 (4), 19.5, 20 (3), 20.5 (2), 21 (2), 21.5, 23 (2), 24, 25 (3), 26, 27, 28 (3), 30 (3), 33, 35 (2), 38, 40, 46, 47, 49, 51, 55, 60 (2), 65, 68, 70, 75, 78, 80 mm.

The series were stained either by Weigert's hematoxylin and eosin, or by the modification of Held's hematoxylin. One part of the series sectioned parallel with the palm was stained by hematoxylin and mucicarmine according to the work of Schmidt-Ehrenberg (1942). This dye distinguishes the cartilage really well already in very early stages of differentiation. Moreover, it was easier to compare the results with those of the quoted author.

Three plastic reconstructions of the carpal skeleton were also employed for this study: of the embryo 15.5 mm in C-R length, of the 21 mm embryo and of the embryo of C-R length 28 mm. The technic of reconstruction was described on page 11.

3. Changes in Carpal Elements during Ontogenesis

The process of chondrification of carpal elements in our material corresponds with the statements by Senior (1929), and O'Rahilly, Gray, and Gardner (1957). In our material also among the last chondrifications observed were those of the scaphoid and the centrale, then followed the chondrification of the lunate and the last was that of the pisiform. In our material not such a great range of embryo sizes in single stages of the process was found, as given by O'Rahilly, Gray, and Gardner (1957) in accordance with Streeter's horizons (Streeter, 1929, 1942, 1945, 1948, 1949, 1951). The chondrification process as seen in our material corresponds mostly to mean values of size ranges given by the above quoted authors for single horizons.

Except of a small formation at the styloid process of the radius we found no other blastema formed only by condensed mesenchyme or by the prochondral tissue without any signs of chondrification. If there was such a finding in our series it was always a sectioned perichondrium of a normal carpale which then appeared in the next sequence of the series. In the following description we shall try to present the image of sequence of form changes and of mutual relations of the already chondrified carpal elements. Some of them originate approximately in their definitive form and change neither their shape nor their location in the course of further development. These are: the trapezium, trapezoideum and the capitate. The others undergo changes in form and spatial interrelations. These include: the distal end of the radius, the scaphoideum, centrale, lunatum, triquetrum, the distal end of the ulna, hamatum and the basis of the 5th metacarpal.

The distal end of the radius has the typical form known in the radius of adults, in 14—16 mm long embryos, except that the styloid process is not so conspicuous. In its place there is an anlage of condensed darkly stained cells continuous with the distal end of the radius, into which the subsequent chondrification of the radius proceeds in the form of an increasing cap set on the distal end of radius. This dark blastema reaches far more distally than the chondrified radius, being here and there even separated (Fig. 3). This pattern of the distal radius end continues up to the C-R length of 19 mm. From this stage onward the dark anlage still persists and the chondrified radius tissue projects into it; however, the adjacent part of the radius gets swollen in an ovoid form (never observed in adult bone) with a convexity turned toward the carpus. The anlage of the scaphoid is attached to this convexity. Contact of the enlarged ovoid-shaped radius portion, adjacent to the future styloid process, with the scaphoideum occurs by the appearance of convexities in both adjacent elements; their contact occurs in a disto-ulnar direction (Fig. 4). At about 25 mm of embryo length a slightly different cell disposition appears in the distal radius part at various section levels demonstrating that this region is not completely continuous with the other anlage of the radius (Fig. 5). Distal to this region the condensed dark blastema is still present.

On comparing these findings with Steiner's concept of the carpus we must admit that the embryonic form changes of the radius end can really be considered as an indicated recapitulation of the taking of the carpale into the radius and connecting the scaphoideum in a new spatial relation. This new relation may be seen as proved by the mutual contact, incongruent at first by convexities of both components. The distal radius end remains in the described form up to 30 mm C-R length and gradually attains its definitive form. Its distal end still carries some differences in the course of chondrification, the peninsula-shaped passing of the chondrification into the future styloid process being especially striking. The definitive form of the radius is attained at about 70 mm C-R length after the radio-scaphoid articulation has reached its typical form and the joint capsules have been completely differentiated. The slight persisting incongruence of joint surfaces is removed by a discus (Gray, Gardner, and O'Rahilly, 1957; Čihák, 1969c) developed in the meantime, which enters the joint cavity from the radial side. [In human embryos similar disc has been observed by Lewis et al. (1970) between the triquetrum and the ulnar styloid process.]

The scaphoideum is found at the distal end of the radius during the beginning of its chondrification. The growth of both, the scaphoid and the radius, brings them together so that from 19 mm C-R length onward the scaphoid and the enlarged distal radius end are in contact by their convexities in a manner described above (Fig. 4). This first incongruent contact does not have the shape of the future articulation. This form is best visible in embryos from 20—25 mm in C-R length. Further development forms the congruent pattern of the contact line. During this development the scaphoideum elongates a little. Its definitive form is achieved by the fusion of the original scaphoid anlage with the os centrale (normale).

The centrale appears from the very beginning of chondrification as independent, situated at the distal end of the scaphoideum, between the trapezium, trapezoideum and the capitate (Fig. 6). It is a solid element; only in one of our cases did we find an exception in the embryo of 20 mm, that was a centrale divided by an insufficiently chondrified zone into the dorsal and palmar part. We do not assume that two carpalia are concerned here, because in the reconstruction also we find a normal centrale in the form of an hour-glass, compressed by its middle part among surrounding carpalia and widened on the dorsal and palmar sides. If blood vessels enter into the dorsal and palmar parts independently, there appears the so-called palmar centrale, commonly known in the literature (Thilenius, 1894, 1896; Pfitzner, 1900; Slabý, 1968). On the basis of the appearance of the centrale in human ontogenesis we do not consider the palmar centrale an independent, phylogenetically based structure, as interpreted e.g. by Schmidt-Ehrenberg (1942). The centrale, visible in all embryos up to 30 mm, corresponds to the so-called centrale normale, known in the literature. From 20 mm of C-R length onward the darkly stained interzone[1] between the scaphoideum and the centrale narrows and both elements gradually fuse together (Fig. 5). Because the fusion of these both already well chondrified elements occurs by the gradual chondrification of the condensed dark interzone, the process goes on for a long

---

1 This term was employed by O'Rahilly et al. (1957). The changes of this interzone are characteristic for the developmental stage of the joint. Therefore, a simple interzone and a three layered interzone are distinguished, the later with a loosened mesenchyme between two condensed layers already represents the joint anlage, its surfaces and the future joint cavity.

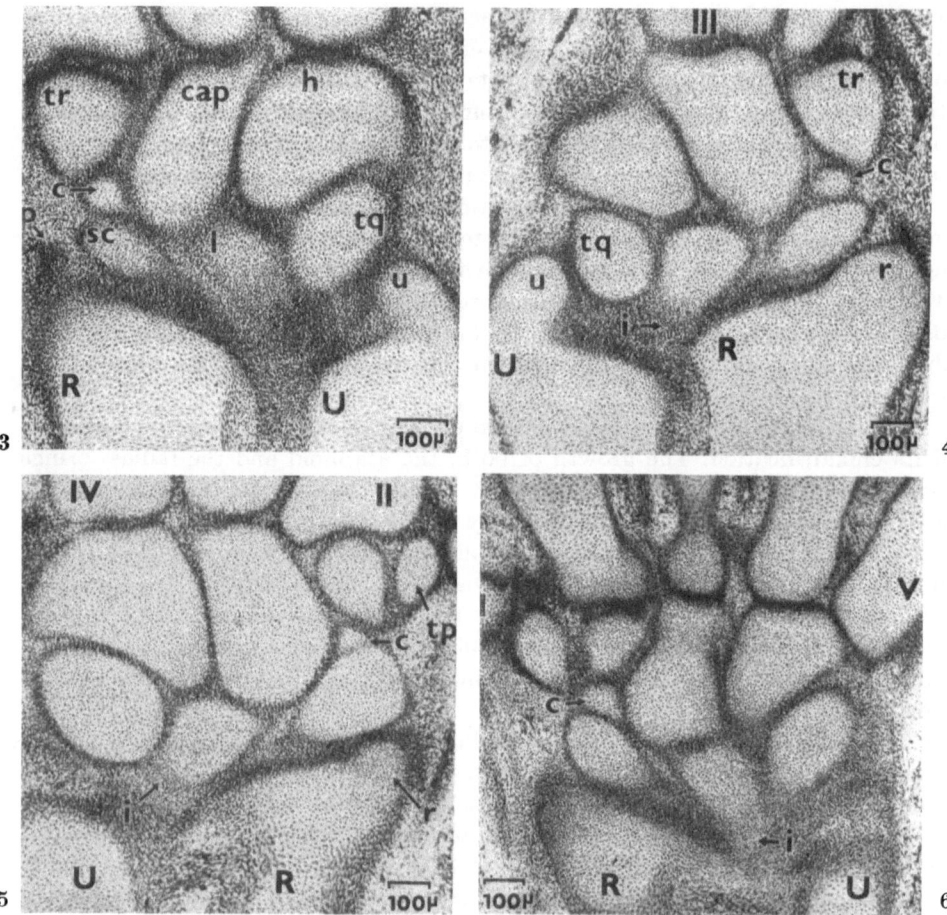

Fig. 3. The carpal primordia in the embryo of 16 mm C–R length, sectioned parallel to the palm; a condensation of prochondral tissue is seen in the site of the prepollex, the styloid process of the ulna visible in form of a large spherical element; between the primordia of the lunatum and the scaphoid is a strip of loosened mesenchyme; the centrale normale is well developed. Legend to all microphotographs in Figs. 3–12: *R* radius; *U* ulna; *r* radiale; *i* intermedium; *u* ulnare; *c* centrale (normale); *sc* scaphoid; *l* lunatum; *tq* triquetrum; *tp* trapezium; *tr* trapezoideum; *cap* capitatum; *h* hamatum, *I–V* metacarpals; *p* prepollex

Fig. 4. Carpal primordia of the embryo 25 mm in C–R length, sectioned parallel to the palm. The ulnare and the radiale contained in form of bulky ends of the radius and the ulna, characteristically shaped. The intermedium is less chondrified than the proper lunatum

Fig. 5. Carpal primordia in the embryo 25 mm C–R length, sectioned parallel to the palm, nearer to the palmar surface of the carpus; the centrale (normale) starts to join the main scaphoideum primordium, the intermedium separates from the lunate primordium; in the distal radius end a structure different from the remaining radius anlage is visible

Fig. 6. Carpal primordia of the embryo 16 mm in C–R length in the section parallel with the palm. All typical carpal elements with the centrale are visible. The intermedium is separated from the lunate

time and even after 30 mm in C-R length of the embryo the boundary between
the two components is still visible. The definitive joining where no trace of a
dividing line remains comes first after reaching 50 mm of embryo length. Inside
the definitive scaphoideum the centrale forms the part articulating with the
trapezium and trapezoideum (Fig. 14D).

After the pisiform, *the lunate* has the most prolonged start of chondrification.
As a slightly chondrifying element it reaches far more proximal between the radius
and the ulna than the definitive lunatum does (Fig. 6). The proximal part of
this primordium is well comparable with the intermedium of lower Tetrapods.
The primitive lunate is met in this form up to 19 mm C-R length of embryo
as a strip-like primordium fading out in the proximo-ulnar direction between
the two anlagen of the fore-arm bones. From 19 mm embryo length onward
the proximal, more loose part strikingly stagnates in its chondrification and
separates from the distal part (Fig. 7) which continues the chondrification process alone. Thus a doubled anlage, a proximal and a distal one appears in place
of the next lunate. The distal part represents the future definitive lunatum and
continues its development whilst the proximal part is retarded in its development and gradually disappears undergoing specific changes. In the 28 mm long
embryo this proximal part is still visible in its original loose form. It then diminishes (in relation to the surroundings) and appears temporarily as a very small
tissue islet (Fig. 8) which in older embryos joins the articular disc of the ulna
(after its differentiation) and is contiguous with it in the direction of the definitive
lunatum, being well visible and clearly defined. In the meantime its chondrification (stagnating at first) has been continuing, and the formation now appears
as a cartilaginous anlage of the so-called os triangulare (Fig. 9). By its proximal
situation between the fore-arm bones the proximal part of the original lunate
primordium evidently corresponds to the intermedium of canonic elements.
Therefore, the distal anlage is to be taken for an element of a further more distal
carpal row which has entered the radiocarpal articulation in place of the intermedium.

The os triangulare, if occurring as a variation in the adult, is hence by its
origin a rudiment of the intermedium. As a cartilaginous anlage it is adjacent
to and contiguous with the ulnar articular disc, which—as will be described
later—in embryos stands in close relation to the styloid process of the ulna.
After 60 mm in C-R length the cartilaginous anlage of the triangulare becomes
extinct. The distal (definitive) anlage of the lunate then evens the articular
line of the future radiocarpal articulation.

The Triquetrum and the Distal End of the Ulna. The development of these
two formations is directly connected. The triquetrum does not change very
much in form from the beginning of its chondrification. From its first appearance
as a chondrified element it is situated considerably more distal to the next
articular line which will be represented by the articular disc of the ulna. In small
embryos a large spherical styloid process already protrudes from the distal end
of the ulna towards the triquetrum. It extends gradually and after reaching
20 mm C-R length of embryo leans against the triquetrum (Figs. 3, 4). Their
contact looks precisely like that of the scaphoid and the styloid process of the
radius, i.e. it is effected by convexities of both. Up to 30 mm of embryo length

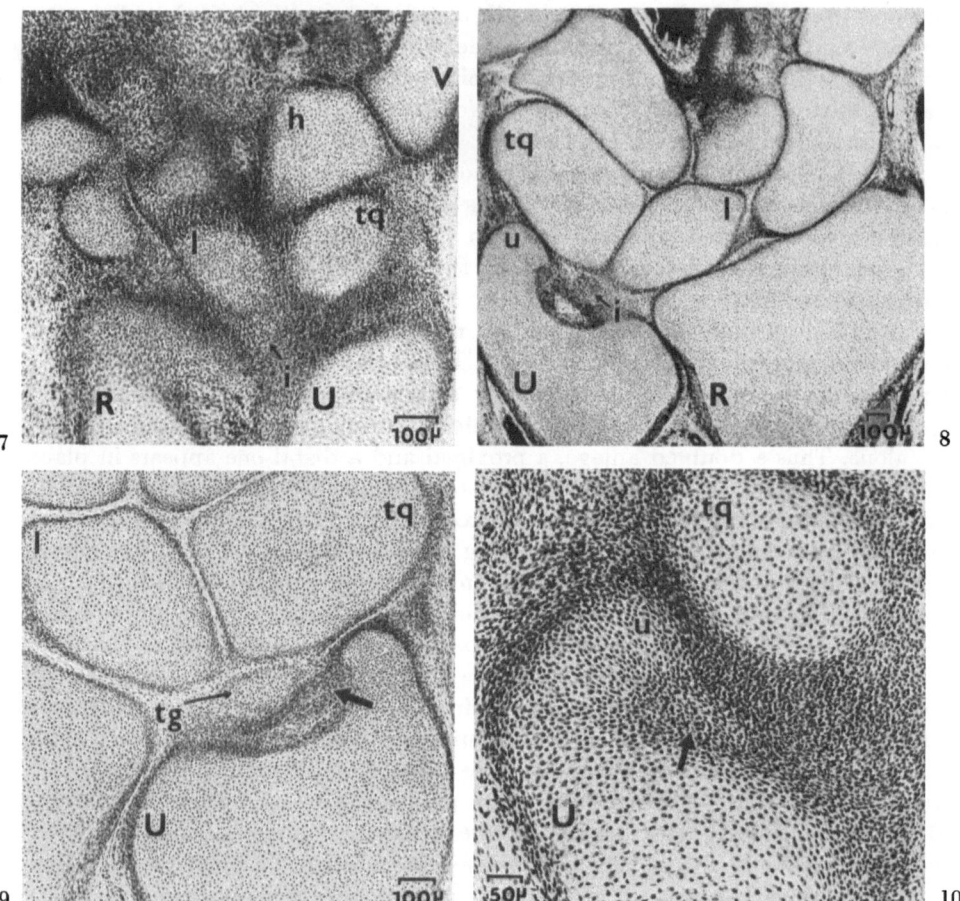

Fig. 7. Carpal primordia of the 19 mm embryo in the section parallel to the palm, nearer to
the palmar surface of the carpus; the intermedium is distinctly separated from the lunatum;
the 5th metacarpal reaches far proximal to the side of the hamatum. The centrale and some
further elements not sectioned

Fig. 8. Carpal primordia of the foetus 55 mm in C–R length, sectioned parallel to the palm.
The radiocarpal articulation obtained the congruent articular line, the styloid process of the
ulna remains in contact with the triquetrum; the intermedium remains in form of an islet of
condensed tissue (indicated by arrow) between the lunate, triquetrum and the ulnar articular
disc

Fig. 9. The ulnar region of the proximal carpal row in the section parallel to the palm in the
60 mm long foetus. The styloid process of the ulna remains in contact with the triquetrum; the
separated intermedium islet chondrifies as the anlage of the triangulare (tg). The arrow
indicates the simultaneous chondrification in the articular disc

Fig. 10. Ulnar part of the carpus in the 28 mm embryo, sectioned parallel to the palm. Close
by the large spherical styloid process of ulna the starting chondrification in the discus articularis (arrow)is seen. The directions of cell rows in the disc are in connection with the cell
rows in the styloid process. The whole chondrification in the disc and the styloid process
seems to be the rudiment of the original ulnare

a darkly stained large cellular zone remains between the two formations. On reaching 30 mm of C-R length this changes into a typical three-layered interzone as a joint anlage. The contact surfaces of the two formations are congruent and finally a joint cavity even appears (Figs. 8, 9). The processus styloideus ulnae grows distally (together with the adjacent triquetrum) and the distance between the triquetrum and the ulnar articular disc increases up to the stage of 50 mm. During subsequent development the styloid process becomes relatively smaller and in the 70 mm embryo a normal pattern of the styloid process and of the articular disc appears. The styloid process ceases to be in direct articulation with the triquetrum.

The continuity of the ulnar styloid process, especially of its spherical distal end, with the formation situated radially to it, is fully evident in younger stages (Fig. 10). The described developmental course and relations of the processus styloideus ulnae and the triquetrum, especially their form changes and contact by convexities, offer a striking similarity to developmental changes seen in the processus styloideus radii and the scaphoid. They are only more accentuated and the processus styloideus ulnae develops into a temporarily larger and more independent formation. In accordance with Kindahl (1941a, b, 1942a, b, 1944a, b, 1949) we therefore consider it to be the reduced and in the ulna absorbed original ulnare which is recapitulated during ontogenesis in this form, temporarily enlarged and then reduced. It seems also that the entire region of the ulnar articular disc belongs to the original material of the ulnare (Fig. 10). However, the triangulare anlage, situated between the disc and the lunate (Fig. 9) and traced back as a rudiment of the original intermedium, does not belong to the ulnare rudiments. Moreover, close to the "head" of the ulnar styloid process, inside the future discus region, there appears in young embryos a very similar chondrification (Fig. 9) in striking coherence with the styloid process (Fig. 10). We consider this chondrification a part of the original ulnare. It therefore seems possible that the triangular bone as a variation can be—though in the typical form and in almost the same position—of two possible origins, from either the intermedium or from the ulnare.

The hamatum and the base of the 5th metacarpal have a form differing from that in adults at the beginning of their differentiation in that the hamate in embryos is obliquely cut on its ulnar side. The 5th metacarpal joins this oblique surface from the ulnar side, set by its base far proximal at the level of the distal carpal row (Figs. 6, 7, 11).

In very young embryos of our material (13—15 mm C-R length) a small islet of starting chondrification appears on the side of the carpale distale IV situated between the 5th metacarpal and the distoulnar margin of the triquetrum (Fig. 11). This chondrification stands in definite relation to the primordia of the hamatum and of the 5th metacarpal, to those places of their surface where later an incompletely formed perichondrial layer is formed (Fig. 12). We did not observe any fusion of this small anlage with the hamatum or the triquetrum. This anlage, which we consider an originating carpale distale V, becomes extinct before the C-R length of 17 mm is attained by the embryo. The 5th metacarpal originally lies ulnar to the hamate. After extinction of the carpale V rudiment, the 5th metacarpal comes to lie closer to the hamatum and its base is transiently

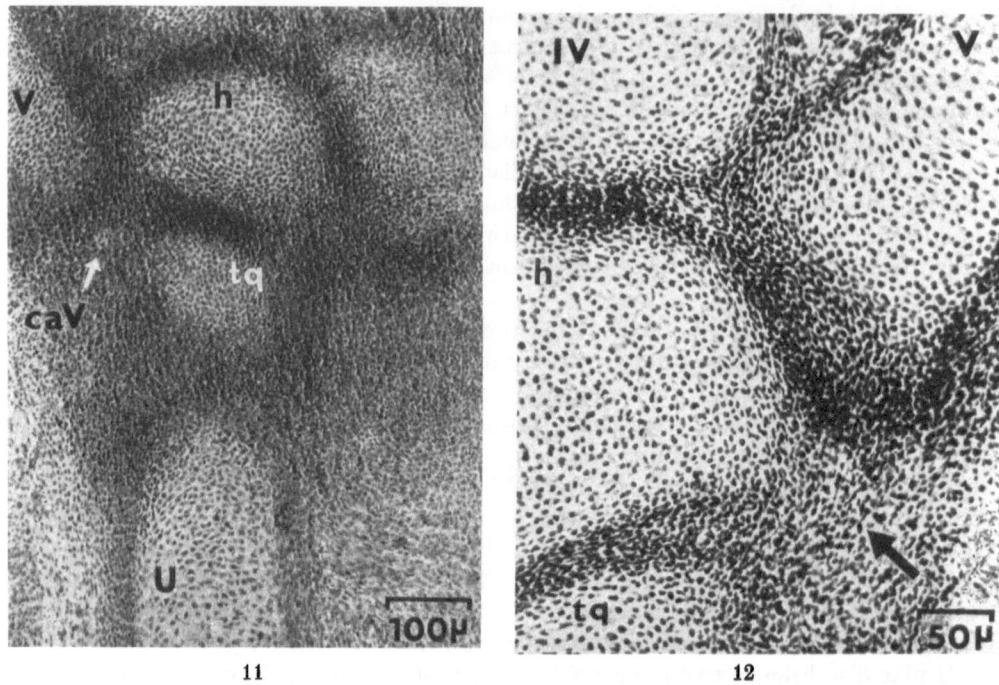

11   12

Fig. 11. Carpal primordia of the embryo 13 mm in C–R length, sectioned parallel to the palm. In addition to typical elements a small region of the early chondrification is visible between the triquetrum, hamatum and the 5th metacarpal (ca V), which can be considered to be the transiently appearing primordium of the carpale distale V. This area is stained by mucicarmine in the same manner as the surrounding carpal elements

Fig. 12. The basis of the 5th metacarpal and the adjacent region of the carpus in the 21 mm embryo, in the section parallel to the palm. The site of the disappeared carpale distale V indicated by arrow. The perichondrium of the hamate and the 5th metacarpal facing this region passes into the region of the disappeared element

enlarged. A part of the material of the fading out carpale V has evidently been taken into the base of the 5th metacarpal. The transient primordium of the carpale V corresponds according to its position to the typical os Vesalianum which, if formed as a variation, completes the form of the definitive 5th metacarpal proximally into the form of the embryonic 5th metacarpal (Fig. 13). On reaching 30 mm in embryo length, the form of the metacarpal changes; the proximal enlargement of its base becomes reduced so that the metacarpal gets more and more on the dorsal side of the hamatum, until finally both articular surfaces of the hamatum for the metacarpals are directly distally, in the same form as in the definitive bone. The articulations develop simultaneously with these form changes.

In the histological slides of the carpal region one more interesting point is seen: it is a triangle-shaped, slender, lightly stained formation situated in the section between the lunatum, scaphoideum and capitatum. In younger embryos

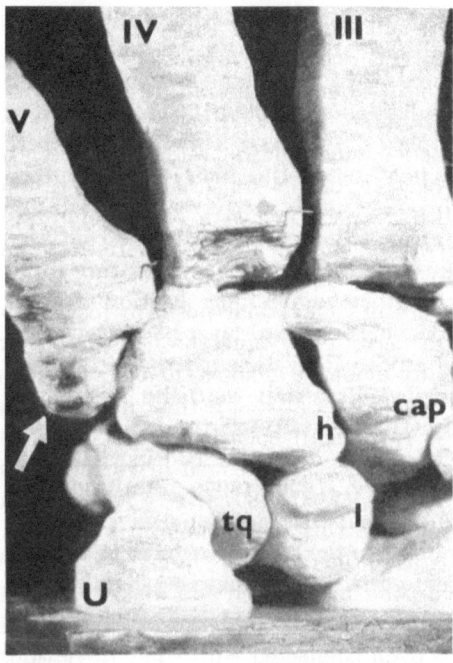

Fig. 13. Reconstruction of the carpal skeleton of the 21 mm embryo. The ulnar part of the carpus seen from dorsal. The form of the 5th metacarpal corresponds by its proximal elongation (arrow) to the form of the difinitive 5th metacarpal with the persisting os Vesalianum (var.)

it looks like an accessory central elements at the beginning of its chondrification. The detailed examinations of the tissue and of its staining affinity show, however, that it is not a chondrification and thus a carpal element, but that it is a loosening of the mesenchyme ascending—as seen in transverse section—from the palmar surface of the carpus. The arteria perforans is not found in this place, nor does the position of the formation suggest that it could be the foramen interosseum. After comparing the sections parallel with the palm with the transverse ones we consider this loosened space to be a trace left after the secondary distension of the scaphoid from the lunate. Both elements also expand into this loosened place during subsequent development. In the definitive form there is a small distodorsal process on the dorsal side of the radial margin of the lunatum.

4. Analysis of Observed Ontogenesis of the Human Carpus.
Discussion and Conclusions

The original concept of Gegenbaur (1864, 1870b, 1873, 1876) of the proximal carpal row composed universally in all Tetrapods of three primary canonic elements—the radiale, intermedium and the ulnare—and by the accessory pisiform has already been controversial for a long time. Single solutions appeared successively (Table 1) and demonstrate that the question is not clear and that its revision is desirable.

The radiale problem seems to be best solved by the work of Steiner (1921, 1922a, 1934, 1935, 1942) and Schmidt-Ehrenberg (1942). According to them the radiale is included in the distal end of the radius and to this part the praepollex is applied (Fig. 1B). Slabý (1958b, 1960, 1967b, 1968) is in agreement with their view. In the quoted papers Steiner and Schmidt-Ehrenberg convincingly demonstrate that the basic pattern of the uniserial archipterygium appears during early ontogenesis of all Tetrapods inclusive of the Mammals. In the course of ontogenesis the same typical elements always differentiate and are then situated inside the axial or the single collateral rays of this archipterygium. For their specification and homology not only their position inside the whole carpus but also their relevance to a certain ray must be considered. It is also impossible to find in our material any evidence against their statement (made on extensive comparative embryological material) that the radius, radiale and praepollex differentiate in the first (proximal) collateral ray. This coherence of the first collateral ray had likewise been acknowledged in various forms already by Baur (1885c, 1889) and by Emery (1890, 1897a, c, 1901). Because in our material a primordium well comparable with a praepollex rudiment is seen in the course of human ontogenesis distal to the radius, we have to look for the radiale proximal to this anlage, i.e. inside the most radial and distal part of the radius. According to our observations this radius part undergoes characteristic and, in the main, temporary form changes even connected with some deviations in cartilage structure and in the chondrification process. These changes permit us to assume that the radiale has really been taken into the distal radius end and that it there represents more than a mere styloid process. We suppose, however, that the process fusing the radiale with the distal radius end proceeded so far back in the phylogenetic past that its traces are hardly visible during ontogenesis. The observations of the temporary contact of the scaphoid with the radius in early ontogenesis by convexities of both and the gradual development of the congruent contact also support the idea that a phylogenetic rebuilding really occurred and that the scaphoideum therefore stands in a new position, with a secondary, during phylogenesis (and also during ontogenesis) newly obtained articulation. The temporary ovoid-shaped enlargement of the radial end of the radius up to the size of the other carpal components contributes to this concept. We are, therefore, convinced that the radiale in the human hand is comprised of the distal radius end and that the carpale adjacent to this distal end, i.e. the scaphoideum, is an element arising from a next carpal row, hence the centrale. According to the scheme by Steiner (1942) and Schmidt-Ehrenberg (1942) the scaphoideum is formed by two centralia of the second collateral ray, the centrale radiale proximale et distale. On the basis of the course of ontogenesis in the human we assume that from this second collateral ray only the centrale radiale distale is contained in the scaphoideum as its basal part; the second component of the scaphoideum which fuses with the basal part during ontogenesis is the so-called centrale normale, i.e. the centrale ulnare distale of Steiner's scheme. Otherwise, Baur (1889) already supposed that the scaphoid corresponded only to the central element while the original radiale had been shifted towards the carpal margin as a sesamoid. The view of the scaphoid as a central element was held also by Emery (1897a, c). It is hence evident that Steiner's view has arisen on the basis of the previously established direction of research and homologisation and that our observations and views follow in the same direction.

The problem of the ulnare and of its place in the mammalian carpus has been resolved, like the question of radiale development, by various authors in different manners. Whilst in Gegenbaur's scheme (1864) the ulnare is homologised with the triquetrum, Albrecht (1884) and Baur (1885 c) considered the ulnare as being homologous to the pisiform. Bardeleben (1894 a, b) returned again to the homology of the ulnare to the triquetrum. Steiner (1942) and Schmidt-Ehrenberg (1942) also attributed to the ulnare of the mammalian carpus an original position and the functional significance of the proximal row canonic element, and homology with the triquetrum. On the contrary, Kindahl (1941 a, b, 1942 a, b, 1944 a, b, 1949) and Holmgren (1952) considered the ulnare a homologue of the processus styloideus ulnae—a view similar to that of Steiner (1942) and Schmidt-Ehrenberg (1942) who thought the same of the radiale. Slabý (1958 b, c, 1959, 1967 b, 1968) held Holmgren's and Kindahl's view as important but he did not decide explicitly for it.

We assume that the two views—Steiner's on one side and Holmgren's on the other—are both one-sided to a certain extent and that both of them prove certain signs of a geometrizing approach to the carpus homology. Steiner starts in his homologisation from the ascertained relations of the radiale to the radius and praepollex inside of the first collateral ray. After employing the four centralia for the carpal scheme (one of them set as a rudimentary element) remains the ulnare for this concept as an unchanged element. Holmgren and Kindahl start similarly at the other side of the carpus. Having determined the ulnare as an element fusing with the ulna, they set the four centralia into the mammalian carpal scheme in place of the ulnare and in the following places; after the four centralia have been set into the carpus scheme, the radiale remains as an original unchanged element. We have already noted that our observations support Steiner's view of the radiale without bringing any proof against his concept. Our observations, however, confirm Holmgren's and Kindahl's views as well. The relatively large styloid process of the ulna, similar to a real carpale, fixed during human ontogenesis by a stalk to the ulna, supports Holmgren's conception. The independent ossification of the processus styloideus ulnae, described as a variant by Borovanský and Hněvkovský (1930) may be considered as further support of this view. From the two described standpoints the need arises to link both and to attempt to make a suitable homologisation of carpal elements. Both Holmgren's and Steiner's views seem to be well founded and difficult to refute; it is hence necessary to look for a solution. Slabý, 1967 b, is also aware of this fact and tends to find a compromise between the view of Steiner and of Holmgren's school on the question of the relations of the intermedium to the adjoined centrale.

Part of the ulnar articular disc develops in connection with the original ulnare besides the processus styloideus ulnae. Inside this disc blastema a contoured cartilaginous primordium may originate which was considered by Gray, Gardner, and O'Rahilly (1957) as a temporary anlage of the triangulare. We also observed the coherence of the processus styloideus ulnae with a part of the disc, especially the continuity of their early chondrification in young embryonic stages (Fig. 10).

It seems therefore that the original ulnare was larger than suggested by a bulky embryonic styloid process.

The Intermedium and its Relations to the Lunatum and Triangulare. We have already mentioned that the primordium situated in the position of the future lunate is very large and extends proximally between the two forearm bone primordia. It then soon becomes detached in young embryos into proximal and distal portions. The distal part chondrifies rapidly, becomes the definitive lunatum and takes its place in the line of the future radicoarpal articulation. Holmgren (1933, 1952) and Kindahl (1941a, b, 1942a, b, 1944a, b, 1949) supposed that in the lunate the intermedium is joined by one of the centralia (denoted as centrale 1). Slabý (1967b) partly agrees with their views considering that a part of the intermedium remains contained in the lunate but that most of it corresponds with the os triangulare (in Artiodactyls).

In our observations a distinct separation of two parts is visible inside the lunate primordium. We assume, therefore, that the lunate proper corresponds to only one centrale, and that the proximal primordium part represents the intermedium. Also the different rate of chondrification process of the two parts during early ontogenesis contributes to this view. We demonstrated in our observation that the retarded proximal part, i.e. the rudimentary proper intermedium also attains the chondrification stage and that it represents in this form a temporary triangulare primordium.

The triangulare has already been known for a long time both as a variation and as a rudimentary primordium occurring in the embryonal carpus (Henke and Reyher, 1874; Schulin, 1879; Leboucq, 1884, 1886; Thilenius, 1894, 1896a, b, 1897; Corner, 1898; Gräfenberg, 1905/06; Henckel, 1931; Beau, Sommelet, and Cayotte, 1952; Gray, Gardner, and O'Rahilly, 1957; Slabý, 1967b, 1968). Pfitzner (1900) considered the triangulare to be an independently ossified styloid process of the ulna. Beau, Sommelet, and Cayotte (1952) think that the triangulare primordium is a cartilage detached from the styloid process of the ulna. Gray, Gardner, and O'Rahilly (1957) consider this cartilaginous anlage inside the articular disc to be a primordium of the os triangulare. On the contrary Slabý (1967b), in accordance with Leboucq (1884, 1886), considers the triangulare to be the rudimentary intermedium and states that in Artiodactyls it joins the triquetrum.

In the course of ontogenesis in the human we have actually found the triangulare primordium developing in continuation with the disappearing intermedium. The intermedium, whose detachment from the lunate and ulnar shift are well visible, diminishes relatively during further development but its chondrification proceeds until reaching the stage of a cartilaginous anlage. Individual variability lets this process go on up to different degrees. This triangulare is then situated distal to the ulnar articular disc (Fig. 9), being adjacent to it but never inside. The cartilaginous primordium inside the disc, figured by Gray *et al.* (1957), can be observed together with the coincidentally occurring triangulare derived from the intermedium (Fig. 9). Consequently, there are obviously two possibilities of development of the triangulare primordium of similar position and shape, one from the intermedium rudiment, the other from the ulnare. The triangulare observed in our material disappears quickly after the chondrification stage. We did not observe its linking up with any of the surrounding formations.

It results from the above analysis that the entire proximal row of the original carpus scheme became extinct and replaced by central elements. The homologisation of these central elements must conform with the concept of Holmgren (1933, 1952) and Kindahl (1941a, b, 1942a, b, 1944a, b, 1949) on one side, and of Steiner (1942) and Schmidt-Ehrenberg (1942) on the other. The number of four centralia taking part in the carpus of Tetrapods was determined by these authors on the basis of extensive comparative embryological material. We assume therefore that it is unjustifiable to assume that there are more centralia, which is necessary if trying to complete Steiner's scheme by the $c4$ from the concept of Holmgren and Kindahl (Slabý, 1967b). We also consider that in the centralia homologies it is possible to overcome the differences of the two concepts, i.e., by fusion of those features of both views which we consider as right and which can also be supported by observations in human ontogenesis. From this standpoint the following homologies result:

The scaphoideum in the classical carpus concept is homologous with the radiale. This homology is attributed to the scaphoideum also in the papers of Holmgren and Kindahl. The mechanism we consider to have led to this homology has been quoted above. On the contrary, other authors consider the scaphoideum a formation resulting from the joining of at least two elements (Bardeleben, 1885b, c; Emery, 1897a; O'Rahilly, 1954). Steiner (1942) and Schmidt-Ehrenberg (1942) hold the scaphoideum to be the homologue of two fused centralia of the second collateral ray, the centrale radiale proximale and the centrale radiale distale. This view has also been supported by Slabý (1958b, 1967b, 1968). Rajtová (1967) demonstrated two scaphoideum primordia in the guinea-pig but claimed no homologies. O'Rahilly (1954) and Olivier (1962) observed the fusion of the centrale normale with the scaphoideum in the course of human ontogenesis. During ontogenesis we see the basal scaphoideum anlage always solid, without any suggestion of two parts. Starting from the previous consideration (v.s.) that the scaphoideum cannot correspond to the radiale, since the later is taken into the distal radius end contacted by the scaphoideum, we can only consider the homology of the scaphoid to be one of the centralia of the second collateral ray. We cannot homologise the basal scaphoideum with two centralia, as Steiner does, because no sign of duplicity of this basal anlage is found.

We therefore consider the basal part of scaphoideum as homologous with the centrale radiale distale of Steiner's scheme. According to Holmgren's and Kindahl's scheme this centrale could be denoted as centrale 2. During the subsequent course of development the fusion of this element with the proper centrale (i.e. with the centrale normale) is always seen. All authors agree that the so-called normal centrale (in the human carpus as well) is the most typical residuum of the central carpal region. Steiner (1942) and Schmidt-Ehrenberg (1942) denote it the centrale ulnare distale; according to Holmgren's and Kindahl's scheme it should be their centrale 3 (Holmgren, 1952; Kindahl, 1941a, b, 1942a, b, 1944a, b, 1949). Kindahl, however, claims this element in mammals to be fused with the centrale 2, which according to our observations corresponds to the basal (proximal) scaphoideum portion.

It may thus be concluded that also if viewed from the course of ontogenesis in the human carpus the scaphoideum appears as originating from two elements. Most authors agree that the scaphoideum has two components. We consider both as homologues with the ossa centralia of the primitive carpus of Tetrapods, i. e. with the centrale radiale distale (centrale 2) and the centrale ulnare distale (centrale 3). In the scaphoideum, which represents a developmentally new element, the centralia of two neighbouring collateral rays of the uniserial archipterygium scheme joined.

The lunatum originates in the course of carpus ontogenesis in the human from the distal part of a more extensive primordium. The proximal part of this primordium is substantially reduced. We demonstrated that from it the triangulare primordium arose, though chondrified, yet temporary and retarded in its development. The distal part of the primordium, the proper lunate, develops as rapidly as the surrounding carpal elements. Its formation, developmental rate and its early detachment from the proximal primordium part demonstrates that it is another element. If in view of its typical position between forearm-bone primordia the proximal primordium part is justifiably homologised with the intermedium of lower Tetrapods, the distal anlage then belongs to the central group. Because this element is the centrale that is attached to the intermedium on one side and on the other to the scaphoid (which we have homologised above with the centrale radiale distale), it must inevitably be the centrale radiale proximale of Steiner's scheme. The lunate, applied as a centrale to Holmgren's and Kindahl's scheme, represents the centrale 1 (Figs. 1, 2, 27).

Here we come into conflict with the homologies of Steiner, who holds the lunate to be the intermedium and considers the two radial centralia to be the components of the scaphoid. The homologies, stated here, are supported not only by the situation during the ontogenesis of the carpus in man but also by comparison of the carpal pattern in some Reptiles. In the carpus of Sphenodon (in four specimens) we found an element not described in the literature, standing at the radial side of the carpus close to the distally prolonged radius end (Fig. 14 B). This element could be homologised either with the rudimentary radiale or with the praepollex. If it is the praepollex, the radiale must be contained inside the distal radius end—supposing that the radius, radiale and praepollex develop in one row inside the first collateral ray. If it is the radiale, no further element can be the radiale. Whether this element is the radiale or the praepollex, the radiale cannot correspond to the elongated almost hour-glass-shaped element of the hatteria carpus that hence must be partially or completely homologous with the mammalian scaphoideum. In the carpus of Sphenodon there is a well formed intermedium; the element situated in place of the scaphoideum is hourglass in shape as if fused from two neighbouring elements. Günther (1867/68) described this element in Sphenodon as a double one; Schauinsland (1900, 1903) stated that two ossification centres develop inside. We can therefore homologise this formation with the two radial centralia as Steiner wanted to homologise the scaphoid in common. We then obtain a specific picture of the carpus in Sphenodon with an ulnar part of a typically primitive type, whilst, in the radial part, the process of fusion of the radius and the radiale is already finished and this carpal sector therefore bears certain mammalian features. This pattern can be applied not only to the carpus of the very primitive Sphenodon but also to the carpus in some closely related primitive Reptiles and is even not contradictory to the situation in the Theromorphs known in the literature (Romer and Price, 1940; Romer, 1956). From this situation two conclusions may be drawn: 1. After extinction of the intermedium (observed also in the course of human ontogenesis) the two centralia of the second collateral ray—the centrale radiale proximale and distale—become detached from one another during phylogenesis; only one of them remains in the place of the scaphoideum, the second, more proximal one sets in place of the intermedium and becomes the lunate. 2. The replacement of proximal elements by the centralia started much earlier in the radiale region and is finished already in primitive Reptiles. Therefore, the signs of this process during ontogenesis are less striking in the radiale region than the recapitulation of the ulnare in the form of the large styloid process of the ulna. The process younger in phylogenesis—i. e. the ulnare rearrangement—thus recapitulates more perfectly in course of ontogenesis. The traces after the detachment of the two radial centralia (joined in Reptiles—Fig. 14) which became the lunate and the scaphoid, can be seen in the dehiscence interposed during ontogenesis between the two of them and filled in by their secondary expansion.

The triquetrum must be homologised with one of the centralia if accepting Holmgren's (1933, 1952) and Kindahl's (1941a, b, 1942a, b, 1944a, b, 1949) aspect of the ulnare as an element reduced and contained in the ulnar styloid process. We have already demonstrated that our observations support their view and that during human ontogenesis a strikingly large styloid process (articulated with the triquetrum) appears temporarily and then becomes reduced—a process which may be considered a developmental recapitulation of the origin and reduction of the ulnare.

The triquetrum is, therefore, a centrale; its ulnar position can be explained in two ways. According to Holmgren and Kindahl it takes up the original position of the centrale 4 in their scheme. On the contrary, Steiner and Schmidt-Ehrenberg are unable to incorporate the triquetrum as a centrale into their scheme and they therefore hold it to be the original ulnare. In the carpus scheme, however, Steiner (1942) places the proximal centrale of the third collateral ray—the centrale ulnare proximale—as an element in extinction. We assume, therefore, that the triquetrum can be applied to Steiner's scheme as corresponding to the centrale ulnare proximale shifted in an ulnar direction by the carpale distale III (the capitate) which has in the meantime occupied the functional centre of the mammalian carpus.

In this way it is also possible to unify the views of Holmgren and Kindahl with the standpoints of Steiner and Schmidt-Ehrenberg with relation to the centralia, and to attempt the mutual identification of the centralia in both concepts (Figs. 2, 27). Accordingly centrale 1 of Holmgren's and Kindahl's scheme corresponds to the centrale radiale proximale of Steiner and Schmidt-Ehrenberg, centrale 2 corresponds to the centrale radiale distale, centrale 3 is homologous with the centrale ulnare distale. (According to Kindahl the fusion of centrale 2 and 3 occurs in Mammals; in our specimens this fusion of the centrale radiale distale and the centrale ulnare distale is visible resulting, however, in the scaphoideum.) Centrale 4 then corresponds to the centrale ulnare proximale shifted in an ulnar direction. This last homology can also be considered as convenient, because in Steiner's original scheme the centrale ulnare proximale links up with the ulnare, and the triquetrum (the centrale ulnare proximale) is also linked up closely and for a long time with the ulnar styloid process, i.e. with the original ulnare during human ontogenesis.

The pisiform is the last of the carpal elements to chondrify. During early ontogenesis it develops rather detached from the triquetrum, the close contact and the articulation between the two originates first after 25 mm C-R length. This indicates that the pisiform is really a secondary component which became the carpale during phylogenesis. It is difficult to judge from the course of ontogenesis whether the pisiforme was originally a sesamoid or not. In the course of ontogenesis all sesamoids of the hand and the foot develop later, in 50 mm long embryos. The pisiform, however, develops sooner, with only a slight retardation as against the other carpalia. This could be explained by assuming that the transformation of the pisiform from the original sesamoid into a real carpale occurred in the long phylogenetic past and its ontogenetic development in the meantime shifted to a younger ontogenetic stage. By comparing phylogenesis and its traces in the course of ontogenetic development more examples of such shifts can be found (Slabý, 1968 b).

The distal carpal row undergoes no important form changes during phylogenesis or in human ontogenesis either. The only problematic point is represented by the region of the os hamatum, the problem being as to whether the hamate contains the carpale distale IV et V or whether carpale V became extinct. According to our observations of the temporary appearance of the carpale distale V anlage in early human ontogenesis the hamate represents only the carpale distale IV. The hamulus cannot be considered a rudimentary carpale as done by Bardeleben (1885 c). The gradually developing and increasing hamulus, into which the chondrification process slowly expands, most resembles a traction apophysis entering the developing retinaculum flexorum. This view is supported by the fact that although there is no sign of independent chondrification in the hamulus (which is hence an integral hamate component) it can ossify independently, as reported by Pfitzner (1900). The carpale V anlage, situated between the base of the 5th metacarpal the hamate and the triquetrum, becomes extinct, as seen in our material. Because immediately after the disappearance of the carpale V anlage the base of the 5th metacarpal considerably increases proximally, it may be assumed that its material is partially taken into the proximal edge of the 5th metacarpal base. Although the disappearing carpale lies close to the triquetrum, we never observed its joining to the triquetrum as described by Slabý (1967 b) in Artiodactyls. The proximal position of the base of the 5th metacarpal is probably connected with the reduction of the ulnar carpal margin, where not only carpale V became extinct but also the originally larger ulnare (ulnar styloid process) was reduced a long way in the proximal direction. The carpale distale V persisting as a Vesalian bone corresponds with the conception of Thilenius (1896 a, 1897).

A summary of carpal homologies, as derived from the course of human ontogenesis, is schematically presented in Figs. 14 and 27, together with Steiner's

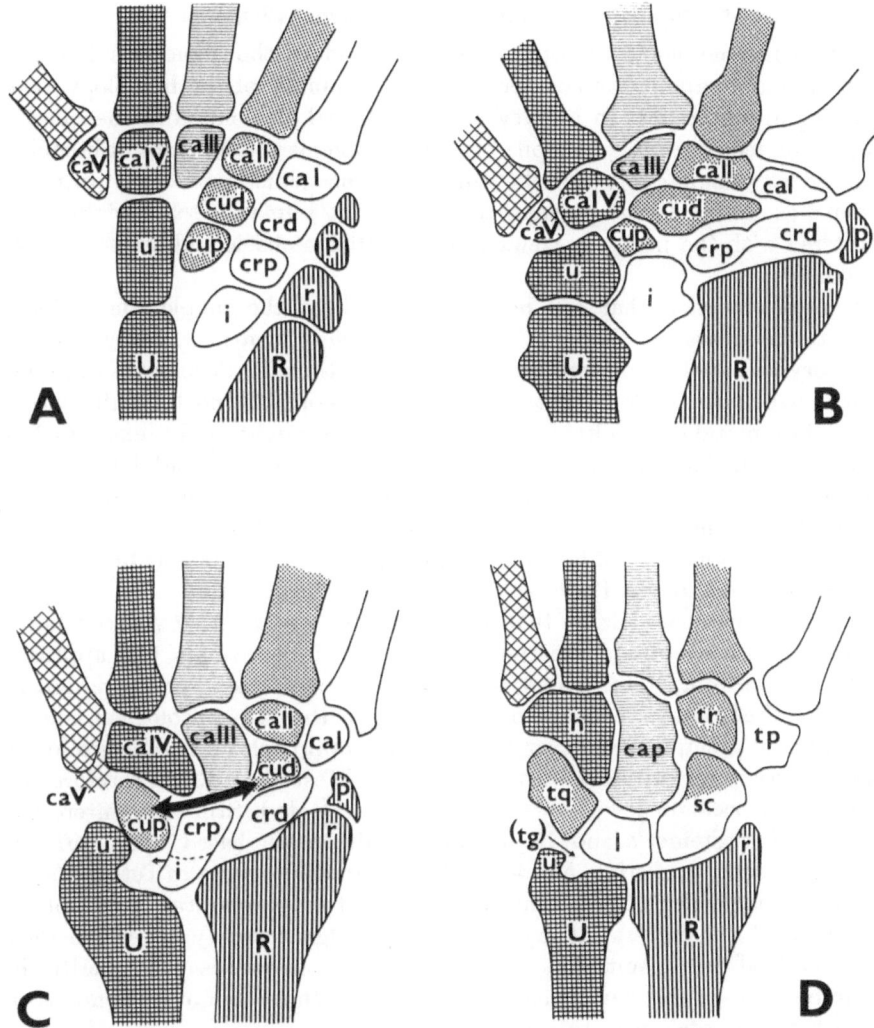

Fig. 14. A) The situation of carpal elements in single collateral rays in Steiner's scheme (according to Steiner, 1942, modified). B) Homologies of carpal elements drawn into the scheme of the carpus of Hatteria, where contrary to the literature a further bone was found at the distal radius end corresponding to the prepollex rudiment or to the radiale. In connection to it the radial part of the carpus appears as rearranged and similar to the situation in Mammals. C) The scheme of homologies obtained by comparison of Steiner's and Holmgren's schemes with results of our observations of ontogenesis, drawn into the scheme of the human embryonic hand. (Central elements of the third collateral ray are separated by the enlarged carpale distale III in Mammals.) D) The scheme of carpal homologies drawn into the carpus of the adult.
Abbreviations same as in Figs. 1–3

and Kindahl's concepts and with the correspondence of the centralia in these concepts, compared by means of their arrangement into collateral rays of the archipterygium scheme.

5. Objections to Homologies of Carpal Elements

As stated above some objections can be raised to the homologisation. One of them is doubts about the competence and possibility of the homology at all, considering all differences in literary views of carpal elements and the question of homologon recognizibility. Despite of many problems this attempt at homologisation and at bringing together the until now antagonistic concepts cannot be considered as useless. Developmental changes during human ontogenesis critically encountered with the previous views yield a sufficient basis and support to this to be done.

The next objection that can be raised is against the simple conception of four centralia, if known that e.g. Thilenius (1896a) mentions a large number of accessory carpal elements and explains most of them as developmental relics. Here it is necessary to state that some accessory bones found by Thilenius are real and interpretable in phylogenesis. The others ought to be exactified by plastic reconstructions. All these accessory elements were found by Thilenius independent in human embryos and in Thilenius's drawings it is not possible to determine whether it was only an apparent independence which, moreover, is even incomplete in some of his drawings. In spite of this Thilenius first denoted these elements and sought for their phylogenetic interpretation.

The third objection could be that our homologies are deduced without taking palaeontological conceptions of carpus development into account. Our approach, of course, starts from Steiner's and Holmgren's schools based upon comparative embryology. But Steiner's theory originated from the palaeontological concept of the uniserial archipterygium, and Holmgren's approach and palaeontological interpretations were mutually respected (comp. Westoll, 1943). Therefore neither of these aspects of development have been neglected. Still more interesting is the fact that Steiner's and Holmgren's results, both based upon different phylogenetic concepts of origin and form of the primitive carpus of Tetrapods, are agreed in the incidence of four centralia evidenced in comparative embryology. On the basis of our material it is impossible to judge the way by which these authors obtained their results, but it is possible to introduce these results critically into our findings on the developing human carpus. Our attempt at comparison has also been undertaken in this spirit.

It is also possible to object that in our homologies the situation during human ontogenesis is compared with definitive phylogenetic stages, e.g. in Sphenodon. It is, of course, a weak point of all onto-phylogenetic considerations. The literature, however, and the available material offer no other possibility.

6. Recapitulation of Observations on the Carpus in Human Ontogenesis, of Comparisons and Homologies

From subsequent changes of form and mutual relations of carpal elements during human ontogenesis and from their comparison to corresponding patterns in comparative anatomy, the following conclusions concerning the homologies of carpal elements have been drawn:

1. The radiale is contained in the distal radius end; a praepollicial rudimentary anlage visible during ontogenesis lies close to it. Steiner's view is corroborated. In the course of ontogenesis in the human temporary form changes of the distal radius end are visible suggesting its rearrangement.

2. The ulnare is homologous with the ulnar styloid process; this corresponds with Holmgren's and Kindahl's concept. During ontogenesis this is manifested by a temporary large styloid process, formed and sized similarly to other carpalia, which then becomes reduced.

3. The scaphoideum originates by fusion of two centralia. The larger of the two, situated closer to the radius, belongs to the intermedial archipterygium ray and corresponds most probably with the centrale radiale distale of Steiner's scheme (centrale 2 of Holmgren's and Kindahl's concept). The centrale normale joins it, being homologous with the centrale ulnare distale of Steiner's scheme (i.e. centrale 3 of Holmgren and Kindahl). The development of both and their fusion are visible in the course of ontogenesis.

4. The lunate corresponds to an adjacent centrale. It is obviously the centrale radiale proximale according to Steiner's classification, and centrale 1 according to Holmgren and Kindahl.

5. The fourth centrale changes into the triquetrum and probably corresponds to the ulnar shifted centrale ulnare proximale of Steiner's scheme or to centrale 4 situated in its original position according to Holmgren's and Kindahl's concept.

6. The hamatum corresponds only to the carpale distale IV.

7. Carpale distale V originates in embryos of C-R length 13–15 mm, develops only to the beginning of chondrification and disappears before reaching 17 mm C-R length. Its part is then obviously contained in the base of the 5th metacarpal and corresponds to the os Vesalianum (var.).

8. The intermedium transiently persists as a constant primordium of the os triangulare (var.) and disappears after reaching 60 mm C-R length. It is characterized by its early detachment from the blastema originally common to the lunate (the lunate is homologous with the centrale radiale proximale—centrale 1). A similar chondrification inside the ulnar articular disc belongs to the enlarged ulnare primordium and can occur together with the intermedium remnants.

9. It may be deduced from comparison of the developing human carpus with the carpus pattern in recent and fossil Reptiles that the radiale is taken into the radius in the most primitive recent Reptiles and probably in fossil Theromorphs. The recapitulation of this phylogenetically long past process in the course of human ontogenesis is therefore less evident than the recapitulation of the similar process of ulnare rearrangement which is typical only for Mammals.

7. Ontogenesis and Homologies of Human Tarsal Components

In the question of the development and homology the carpus and tarsus were usually considered together in the past. A common scheme of the basic pattern in the upper and lower limb was sought with the self-evident idea of a serial homology in both of them. Although strict homologisation between the upper and lower limb is hardly possible, the elementary similarity of the skeleton in both is evident; the pattern of the carpus and tarsus can be compared to a high degree.

In the interpretation of both the proximal and distal extremity various standpoints were taken relating to homologies. It has been supposed since Gegenbaur's (1864) time that the canonic elements, established by him, appear in the distal as well as in the proximal extremity being only differently modified. As in the carpus studies, a number of authors aimed at finding a convenient explanation of the rebuilding of canonic elements into definitive tarsalia, i.e. to find homologues with the components of the elementary scheme (Gegenbaur, 1864, 1870b, c, 1880, 1888; Albrecht, 1884, 1886; Baur, 1885a, b, c, 1886; Born, 1876b, 1880; Bardeleben, 1883, 1885a, b, c, 1894a, b; Emery, 1890, 1897a, c, 1901; Leboucq, 1886; Stieda, 1889; Wiedersheim, 1876, 1877, 1880, 1892, 1906). In these entirely comparative works attempts were made both to deduce the primi-

Table 2. *Various views concerning the*

Canonic elements of the tarsus in Tetrapods	Gegenbaur (1864)	Baur (1885 c)	Albrecht (1884)	Bardeleben (1883)	Bardeleben (1885 c)
Tibiale	talus	tibial sesamoid element	naviculare	distal part of the talus	tarsale proximale prae-hallucis = tuberositas ossis navicularis + naviculare mediale
					tibiale = caput tali
Intermedium		trigonum	inter-medium 1 = talus	proximal part of the talus, tri-gonum	intermedium 1 = corpus tali
			inter-medium 2 = trigonum		intermedium 2 = tri-gonum
Fibulare	calcaneus	calcaneus	calcaneus	calcaneus	fibulare = distal part of the calcaneus
					tarsale prox. 5 = proxi-mal part of the calcaneus
Pisiforme				tuber calca-nei	the "epiphysis" of the calcaneus
Centrale	naviculare	distal part of the talus		naviculare	c 1 = lateral part of the naviculare
					c 2 = triangulare tarsi (proximal part of the cuneiforme III)
					c 3 = proximal part of the cuboideum
Tarsale distale I	cunei-forme I	tarsale of the rudi-mentary digit		cunei-forme I	tarsale distale prae-hallucis = medial part of the cuneiforme I
					tarsale distale I = lateral part of the cuneiforme I
Tarsale distale II	cunei-forme II	cunei-forme I		cunei-forme II	cuneiforme II
Tarsale distale III	cunei-forme III	cunei-forme II		cunei-forme III	cuneiforme III
Tarsale distale IV	cubo-ideum	cunei-forme III		cuboideum	distal part of the cuboideum
Tarsale distale V		cubo-ideum			

homologies of canonic tarsal element

Bardeleben (1894a)	Emery (1897)	Weber (1927)	Broom (1930)	Holmgren (1952) Kindahl (1941–1949)	Steiner (1942)
tuberositas ossis navicularis	tuberositas ossis navicularis	os tibiale tarsi	naviculare	reduced and taken into the tibia or the talus	reduced and incorporated in the tibia
talus	talus	talus	talus	proximal part of the talus	proximal part of the talus
trigonum	corpus calcanei	calcaneus	calcaneus	proximal part of the calcaneus	distal part of the calcaneus
calcaneus	tuber calcanei				proximal part of the calcaneus
tibiale: c 1 = naviculare fibulare: c 2 = triangulare tarsi	naviculare	naviculare		c 1 = distal part of the talus .... c 2 c 3 } = naviculare .... c 4 = distal part of the calcaneus	prox. = distal part of the talus tib. .... dist. dist. } = naviculare fib. .... prox. = region of the distal part of the talus
cunei- plant. forme I dors.	cuneiforme I	cuneiforme I		cuneiforme I	cuneiforme I
cuneiforme II	cuneiforme II	cuneiforme II		cuneiforme II	cuneiforme II
cuneiforme III	cuneiforme III	cuneiforme III		cuneiforme III	cuneiforme III
cuboideum	cuboideum	cuboideum		cuboideum	cuboideum
					extinct

tive tarsus type and to homologise tarsal components in various Mammals with canonic elements (Table 2).

The quoted papers are characterized by the variability of homology deductions. This in itself demonstrates the difficulty of the problem and the impossibility of solving it only on the basis of comparative anatomy. On the other hand, these works are important for the way they included the centralia into the carpus and tarsus schemes. Except for Bardeleben (1885c) who assumed three centralia in the tarsus (and later reduced this number again to two), no other early work reckoned with more than one, maximally two centralia for the tarsus, evidently influenced by Gegenbaur. In this point all these early papers differ from the modern works where, similar to the carpus, a number of central components are assumed for the tarsus. This has again been influenced mainly by the work of Steiner (1921, 1922a, 1934, 1935, 1942) and of Holmgren (1933, 1939, 1949, 1952). Although based upon different concepts of extremity development in Tetrapods both schools employing a similar method of comparative embryology come to the conclusion that in the tarsus of Tetrapods there are four centralia that may also be identified in the mammalian foot. In the carpus as well as in the tarsus Steiner assumed four centralia oriented together with other elements inside the collateral archipterygium rays so that there are two pairs of centralia. In conformity with his concept of the carpus, Holmgren recognized a branching tarsus pattern, with the centralia accordingly dislocated and numbered (Figs. 1C, 2). Both quoted schools agreed in considering both the participation of the centralia in the origin of definitive mammalian tarsal elements and the rebuilding of some canonic tarsal elements (Kindahl, 1941a, b, 1942a, b, 1944a, b, 1949; Schmidt-Ehrenberg, 1942). Some of their views were adopted later by other authors (Slabý, 1968a; Rajtová, 1968).

As in the carpus we shall try to revise the development and homologies of the components of the tarsus. This attempt is based on previous experience that the extremities recapitulate the primitive pattern in the course of ontogenesis and that this is a way of tracing the primitive situation.

The human tarsus was studied during ontogenesis by Henke and Reyher (1874) who found the majority of the main tarsal elements to be formed already from the 5th to 6th embryonic week. Schulin (1879) found well formed tarsal primordia in the embryo of 27 mm. Leboucq established initial differentiation of tarsal elements in the 12 mm embryo. He also noted the double anlage of the calcaneus; moreover, based upon the development he homologised the triangular bone (var.) of the hand with the os trigonum of the foot (Leboucq, 1884, 1886). The chondrification process in the tarsal primordia was noted by Hagen (1900), Senior (1929), O'Rahilly, Gray, and Gardner (1957). Lazarus (1896) tried to express form changes of tarsal primordia as a process imitating forms of lower Primate tarsalia and collected evidence for the "Affenähnlichkeit" of the foetal tarsus. Tornier (1888, 1890) tended to describe phylogenetic form changes of tarsal bones. Wood-Jones (1949) mentioned the embryonic changes of the relation between the fibula and the calcaneus. Extensive observations in the mammalian tarsus during ontogenesis were made by Holmgren (1933, 1952) and Kindahl (1941a, b, 1942a, b, 1944a, b, 1949) with the aim of fixing the centralia. The ontogenesis of the human tarsus from the standpoint of joint development has been observed by Gardner, Gray, and O'Rahilly (1959).

We will, therefore, try to supplement the previous observations of tarsal ontogenesis in the human, similar to our previous observations of carpus development. In addition to form changes we will attempt to consider the development of the mutual position of embryonic tarsal elements and their participation in the definitive tarsal components.

8. Material for Observations of Tarsus Ontogenesis

For the study of tarsal elements 56 histological series of feet of human embryos and foetuses from 15 to 40 mm in C-R length were employed. One part of this material was sectioned parallel to the sole; other feet were sectioned transversally. The crown-rump lengths of embryos and foetuses employed were: 16 mm (3 feet); 17 (5), 18 (4), 19 (3), 20 (3), 21 (2), 22 (2), 23 (3), 24 (3), 25 (4), 26 (2), 27 (3), 28 (2), 29, 30 (3), 32, 33 (2), 34 (2), 35 (2), 36, 37 (2), 39, 40 mm (2 feet).

The series were stained in the same manner as in our other series, i.e. by Ehrlich's hematoxylin, Weigert's hematoxylin and eosin, and by the modified Held's hematoxylin (comp. p. 11).

The developing tarsal components were considered by applying the same viewpoints as in carpus studies (see p. 21).

9. Observations of Development of Tarsal Elements

The time sequence of developmental changes in the human tarsus corresponds in its main features with the course of development of the human carpus. On comparing them we observe a slight delay in the lower extremity, the developmental stage of the carpalia found in embryos 13—14 mm of C-R length not being attained until embryos of approximately 16—17 mm. Later on this difference diminishes. The time of origin and following chondrification sequence is in agreement with the data presented by Senior (1929) and O'Rahilly, Gray, and Gardner (1957).

The Distal End of the Fibula. We found no evidence of participation of the fibulare inside the distal fibula end in a way similar to the ulnare manifestation in form of the large ulnar styloid process. The chondrification of the fibula proceeds into its distal end very quickly, from 16 mm C-R length onward, and in embryos of 20 mm the usual fibula form is already seen. The fibula, however, differs from later developmental stages in its positional relations to the tarsalia due to the plantar-flexion of the embryonic foot.

In small embryos *the developing calcaneus* consists distinctly of two portions; they are visible especially in sections parallel with the planta pedis. In its distal part the calcaneus chondrifies sooner and from the very beginning of chondrification the cartilage is here better differentiated than in the proximal part. The cells of the distal part are arranged in an enclosed ellipsoid formation. This distal calcaneus part is oriented in the direction of the longitudinal autopodial axis. The other portion of the calcaneus differentiates proximal to this part, situated slightly lateral and towards the plantar (Figs. 15, 16). The chondrification of this more proximal primordium is delayed from the very beginning. It is completely separated from the distal part of the calcaneus only in young embryos (Fig. 16) and joins the distal part already from 18 mm C-R length onward. The

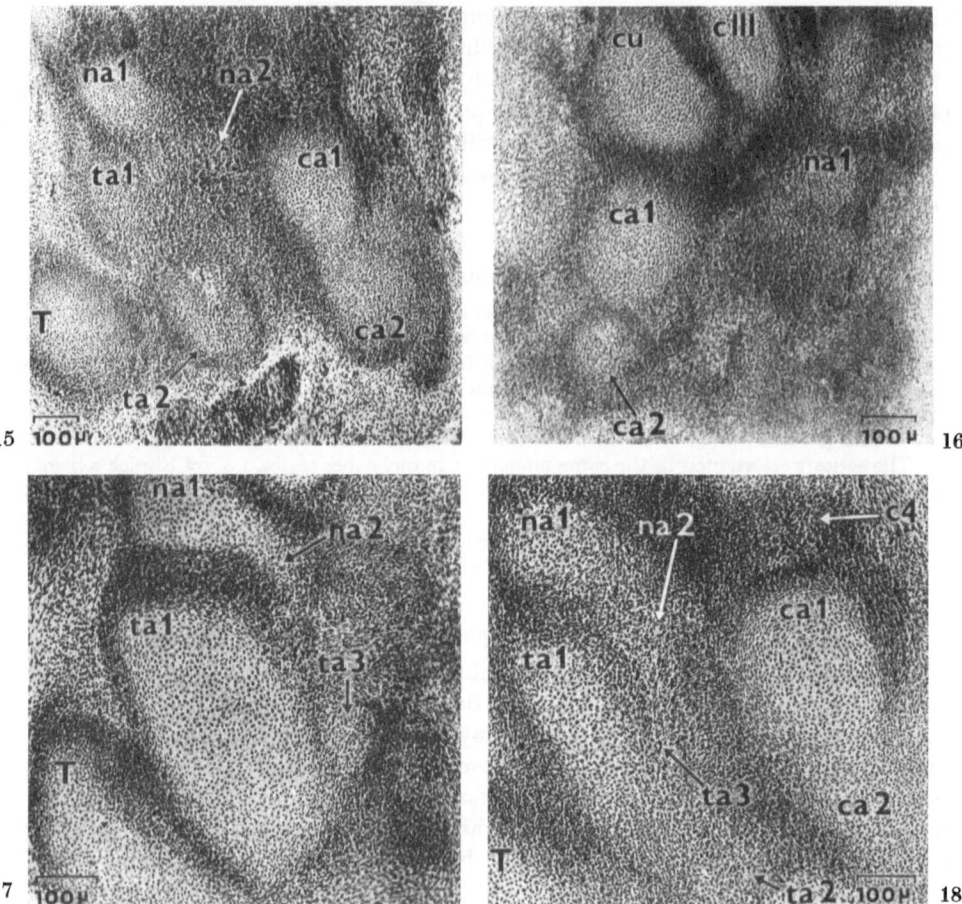

Fig. 15. Tarsal primordia of the embryo 21 mm in C–R length in the section parallel to the sole; right foot seen from dorsal. Two portions of the calcaneus are visible, the distal one is better chondrified; two chondrifications in the talus region are visible as well as two chondrification areas of the naviculare. Legend to all microphotographs in Figs. 15–26: *T* tibia; *F* fibula; *ta 1* the main chondrification in the caput and corpus tali (probably corresponding to the tibiale); *ta 2* chondrification in the region of the processus posterior tali (corresponding to the intermedium); *ta 3* chondrification in the region of the processus lateralis tali (corresponding probably to the centrale tibiale proximale); *ca 1* main calcaneus chondrification in its distal part (corresponding to the fibulare); *ca 2* chondrification in the proximal calcaneus part (corresponding to the pisiform of the hand); *na 1* main chondrification of the naviculare (corresponds to the centrale tibiale distale); *na 2* proximal chondrification of the naviculare (corresponding to the centrale fibulare distale); *cu* cuboideum; *cf I–III* cuneiforme I–III; *I–V* the metatarsals

Fig. 16. Tarsal primordia of the embryo 18 mm in C–R length, sectioned parallel to the sole (left foot seen from dorsal). Two typical calcaneus primordia are seen, the proximal is less chondrified. Some of tarsal elements are not sectioned; *c III* cuneiforme III

Fig. 17. Tarsal primordia of the embryo 20 mm in C–R length, right foot sectioned parallel to the sole and viewed from dorsal. Close to the main chondrification of the talus (*ta 1*) a chondrification in the region of the processus lateralis tali (*ta 3*) is visible. In the naviculare its two chondrifications (*na 1, na 2*) are fused already

double structure of the calcaneus is visible still later both in the orientation of cartilage cells and in the fibular shift with even a slight enlargement of the proximal part. Later on the chondrification of the distal calcaneus part extends distalwards into the loosened prochondral tissue between the calcaneus and the cuboideum.

The talus in young embryos (16—28 mm C-R length) is found to be composed of three areas of chondrifying tissue. The distal bulky area chondrifies sooner and represents the future caput and corpus tali. The second component, differently structured in young embryos, incompletely separated and delayed in chondrification, appears in the region of the future lateral process of the talus (Fig. 17). During subsequent development this element is reduced and replaced by the chondrification process expanding from the larger distal area and then forming the definitive lateral talus process. The third area, again contiguous with the main talus part and also delayed in chondrification, stands in place of the future processus posterior (Fig. 18). The chondrification at the site of the future lateral process continues in an elongated naviculare primordium, its proximal prolonged arched tip touching (Fig. 19). All the three areas fuse together by subsequent chondrification completing the typical talus form.

The naviculare primordium is found in young embryos to originate in two chondrification areas. The more distal and tibially situated one is chondrified sooner, while the chondrification of the second is delayed. The arched tip of this second anlage becomes extended proximally to the site of the future processus lateralis tali or to the early chondrified rounded primordium which precedes the processus lateralis. Both naviculare areas early join forming a prolonged arched primordium which shortens in the course of subsequent development, with a concentration to the main disto-tibial anlage. The originally proximal anlage is delayed in its development and changes into a naviculare process by which the definitive bone extends to the proximolateral side of the caput tali. Both chondrification areas forming the naviculare primordium are well visible in embryos between 16 and 20 mm in C-R length. The proximally elongated primordium part may be found in the form demonstrated in Fig. 19, up to 28 mm embryos.

A particular region is found in embryos about 18 mm in C-R length at the tibial margin of the naviculare, in place of its future tuberosity. The perichondrium of the cartilaginous primordium is here discontinuous and a condensed prochondral tissue is found in which a chondrification develops separately from the naviculare proper (Fig. 20). This distinct place of the naviculare primordium corresponds in its position with a typical skeletal variation, the os tibiale externum.

The Distal Tarsal Elements. The three cuneiformia are usually homologised with the ossa tarsi distalia, I—III. The next component of the distal tarsal row is the cuboideum. In small embryos it may be observed during ontogenesis that

Fig. 18. Tarsal primordia in the embryo of 18 mmC-R length, right foot in the section parallel to the sole, seen from dorsal. Proximal part in the lower margin of the photograph. The disposition of chondrifying tarsal primordia is seen together with the transient chondrification (*c 4*) corresponding to the centrale 4. The position of primordia corresponds maximally to the scheme of Holmgren (1933, 1952)

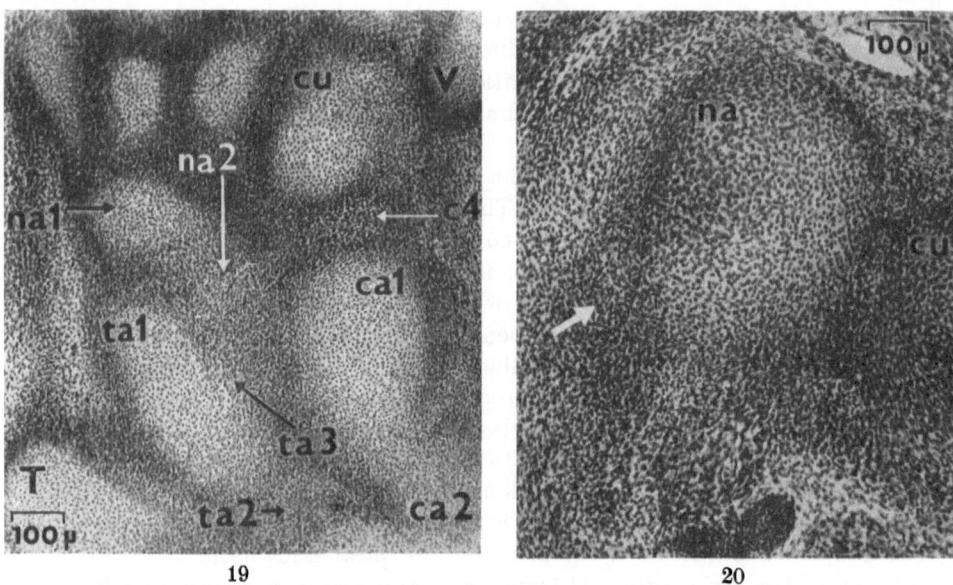

19   20

Fig. 19. Tarsal primordia of the embryo 21 mm in C-R length; right foot in the section parallel to the sole, seen from dorsal. The linked up chondrifications from the talus to the naviculare (*ta 3, na 2, na 1*) and to the other side to the transient *c 4*, are well visible

Fig. 20. The tarsus of the 19 mm embryo sectioned transversally, seen from proximal (the plantar side at the lower margin of the microphotograph). The naviculare primordium (*na*) with the joined primordium in the site of the future tuberositas ossis navicularis, with the incipient chondrification (arrow). This chondrification corresponds to the os tibiale externum

the longitudinal axes of the distal tarsal elements do not link up to the axes of developing metatarsals. The metatarsals are shifted in relation to distal tarsalia rather in a fibular direction, especially the second and third metatarsal, in addition, the metatarsal axes are at a considerable angle in relation to distal tarsalia. The longitudinal axes of distal tarsal elements are inclined in a fibular direction whilst those of the second, third and fourth metatarsals are, on the contrary, inclined tibially. The first embryonic metatarsal sets not to the distal margin of the first cuneiform but more to its tibial side, diverging strikingly from the fan of the other metatarsals. The "hooking" of the distal tarsalia towards the metatarsals is very striking and characteristic for the early embryonic period (Fig. 21). During subsequent development and growth the discrepancy of the two rows disappears, after reaching 20 mm embryo length.

We also bring an interesting observation of the 1st cuneiforme primordium which in embryos of 17—19 mm in C-R length is divided by a strip of a nonchondrified tissue into the typical cuneiforme I plantare and the cuneiforme I dorsale, both known as variations (Pfitzner, 1896). It is a constant appearance in the embryonic period (Fig. 22) and explains not only the quoted variation but also all known special types and forms of divided articular facets of the first cuneiform (Virchow, 1922).

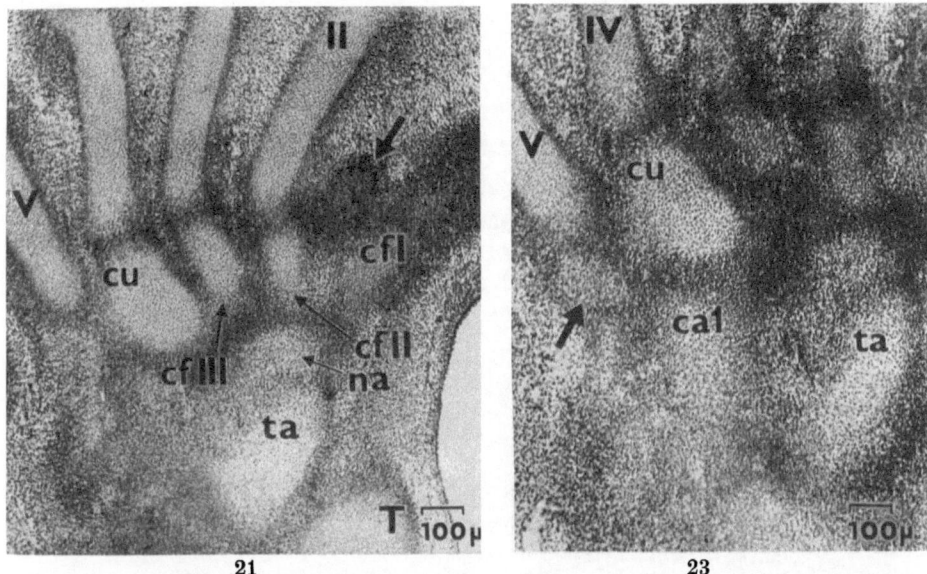

21   23

Fig. 21. Tarsal primordia of the 18 mm embryo in the section parallel to the sole. The angles between the metatarsals and the distal tarsalia are well visible. In the first intermetatarsal space the prochondral tissue of the accessory primordium of the os intermetatarscum is indicated by arrow

Fig. 23. The transiently appearing chondrification of the tarsale distale V (arrow) in the tarsus of the embryo 18 mm in C-R length. The section parallel to the sole

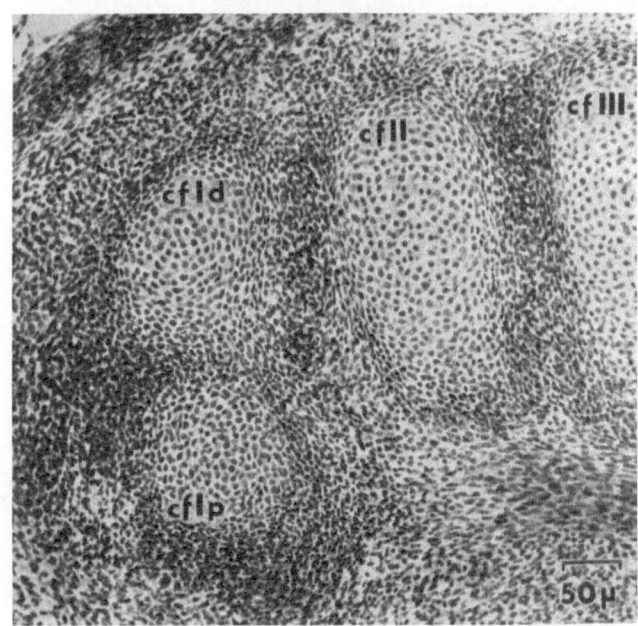

Fig. 22. Primordia of the cuneiformia in the transverse section of the foot of the 19 mm embryo (plantar side below, viewed from proximal). The cuneiforme I bipartitum contains the cuneiforme I dorsale (*cf I d*) and the cuneiforme I plantare (*cf I p*)

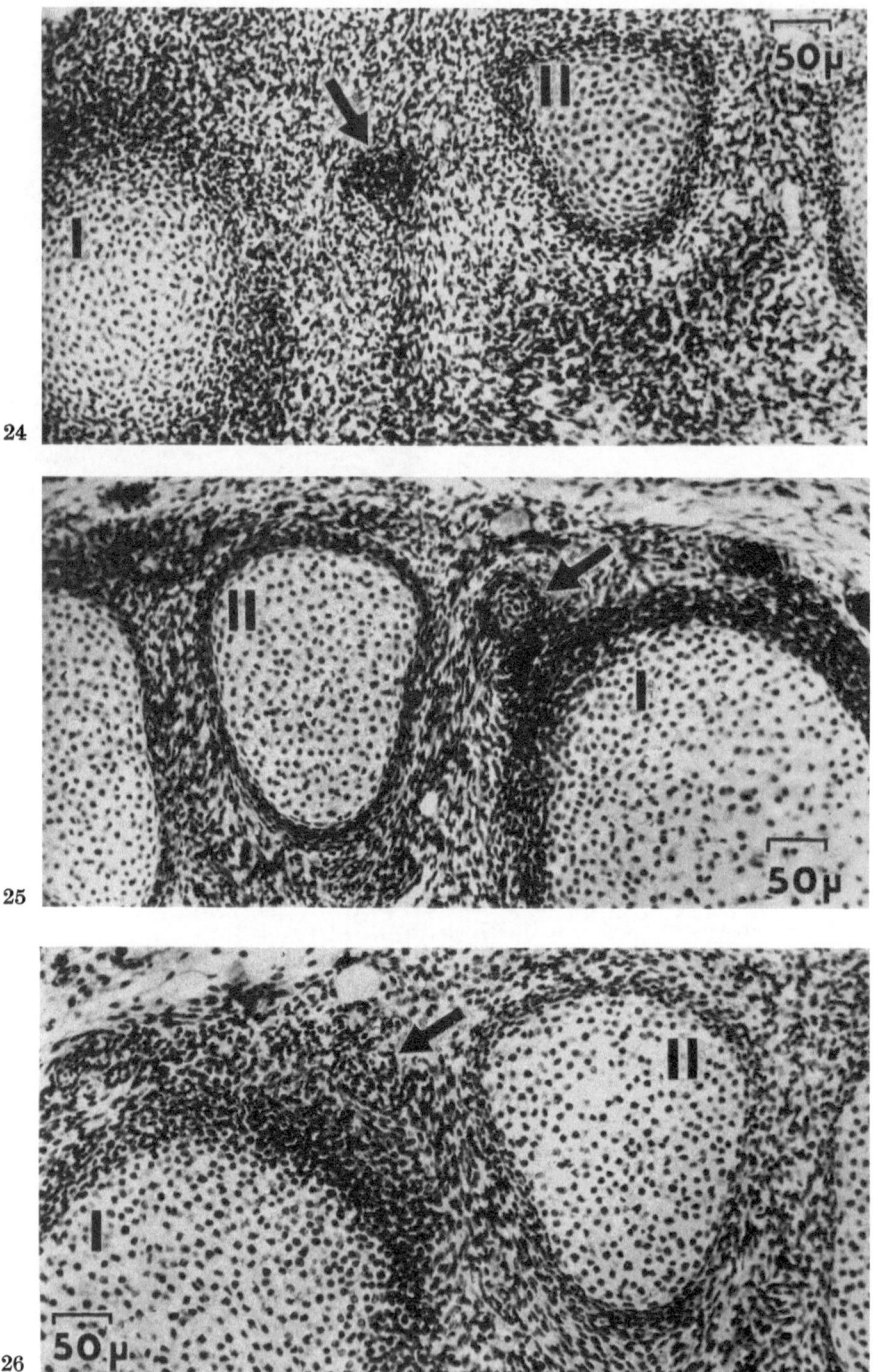

Fig. 24. Right foot of the embryo 19 mm in C-R length, transverse section viewed from proximal. Between the 1st and the 2nd metatarsals a dense primordium formed by the prochondral tissue is visible (arrow)

In the region of the cuboid primordium our observations correspond with the earlier findings on the ontogenesis of the human carpus. The cuboideum corresponds only with the carpale distale quartum. The original embryonic position of the 5th metatarsal, i.e. on the fibular side of the cuboideum primordium, is the same as that of the 5th metacarpal on the side of the hamate. In small embryos a chondrifying anlage is found proximal to the 5th metatarsal primordium in a position typical for the tarsale distale V (Fig. 23). This anlage, if accidentally independent in ossification, corresponds exactly with the Vesalian bone in form and position. The chondrifying early primordium of the tarsale distale V persists only up to 20 mm C-R length of the embryo; then it becomes extinct, being also partly taken into the base of the 5th metatarsal.

The Metatarsus. The study of developing metatarsal primordia brought a certain surprise. In embryos of 16—30 mm C-R length an accessory anlage with the character of a skeletal element is found between the primordia of the 1st and 2nd metatarsals, which in small embryos diverge at an almost double angle in comparison with other metatarsals. In small embryos of our material this anlage is formed by a dense mesenchyme, later on (between 19 and 25 mm in C-R length) it assumes the characteristics of a condensed prochondral primordium. At about 25 mm in C-R length of the embryo it may chondrify; it then quickly dedifferentiates and rapidly disappears after reaching 30 mm C-R length (Figs. 24—26, comp. Fig. 21). At the time of its full extent this primordium is ovoidly elongated and sets to the tarsus between the 1st and the 2nd metatarsals; during period of its maximum size it attains a quarter of the length of the 1st intermetatarsal space. This primordium corresponds in position and shape with a typical skeletal variation—the os intermetatarseum (Gruber, 1852); by its development to maximum size and differentiation and subsequent extinction already in the early embryonic period this primordium bears the character of a structure recapitulated in the course of ontogenesis.

10. Analysis of Observations on the Tarsus in Human Ontogenesis. Discussion and Conclusions

The homologies of tarsal elements considered by various authors differ, though not so much as the views on the homologisation of carpal elements (cf. Tables 1 and 2).

The Fibulare Problem. No signs were found indicating the participation of the fibulare inside the distal fibula end (similar to the participation of the ulnare in the ulnar styloid process). It is, therefore, necessary to look for the fibulare inside the tarsus proper, where it has also been located by the majority of authors. Steiner (1942) and Schmidt-Ehrenberg (1942) as well as Kindahl (1941a, b, 1942a, b, 1944a, b, 1949) considered the calcaneus to be a formation fused from

Fig. 25. Embryo 26 mm in C-R length, left foot, transverse section seen from proximal. The chondrified primordium of the os intermetatarseum is indicated by arrow

Fig. 26. Right foot of the 31 mm embryo in transverse section (seen from proximal). The rudiments of the primordium of the os intermetatarseum are indicated by arrow. The cells remaining in the site of the disappearing primordium differ from the surrounding mesenchyme only by their orientation

two parts; this is also supported by our observations. Steiner sees in these two portions the more distally situated fibulare and the proximal, and fibularly situated, pisiform (Fig. 27). According to Kindahl the more proximal calcaneus portion (in our specimens also the more laterally situated one) corresponds in Mammals with the fibulare, whereas the more distal (and more medially situated) portion is considered by this author as homologous with the fourth centrale, shifted fibularly like the $c4$ of the hand (Fig. 27).

The lateral position of the proximal calcaneus part as well as its delayed chondrification both support Steiner's view that the calcaneus originates by fusion of the fibulare with a homologue of the pisiform. Also a considerable distance between the distal calcaneus anlage and the developing cuboideum may be regarded as a support to the view that the distal calcaneus is no centrale. The entire pattern of this region indicates that the region of the centrale 4 can be located just into the prochondral tissue area separating the embryonic calcaneus from the cuboideum (Fig. 19).

The Intermedium. All literary data agree in localizing the intermedium in the talus, the differences concerning only the place of the talus which is considered as originating from the intermedium. It can be deduced from our series that by its position between the tibia and fibula ends the intermedium corresponds to the proximal anlage in the talus region situated in place of the future posterior process, or, if independently ossified, of the os trigonum. We also adhere to this view, since in our series of early embryonic stages (16—18 mm in C-R length) this region is observed as chondrifying differently from the main part of the future talus. In relation to the primordia of the tibia and fibula this talus portion is situated as proximal as the intermedium of the upper limb. Similarly, in both extremities the chondrification of these corresponding primordia proceeds more slowly. The agreement of the intermedia in the upper and lower limbs and of the variations originating from them was already recognized by Leboucq (1884, 1886). This view is also in agreement with other earlier authors who identified the intermedium with the os trigonum or with the proximal talus part as a whole (Albrecht, 1884; Baur, 1885c; Bardeleben, 1883, 1894a; Holmgren, 1952; Kindahl, 1941—1949; Steiner, 1942).

The Tibiale. Similarly to the fibula it was also impossible in the tibia to demonstrate any signs of the tibiale in apposition to the distal tibia end or of its recapitulation in the form of a rudimentary primordium. The tibia and its malleolus attain a shape similar to that in adult very soon (before 30 mm C-R length of the embryo). It is hence necessary to look for the tibiale (as well as for the fibulare) inside the tarsus proper. We assume therefore, unlike Steiner (1942), who considered the talus as the intermedium fused with two proximal centralia, that the original interpretation of the talus of Gegenbaur is correct. In his scheme the human talus originates by fusion of the tibiale with the intermedium. According to our observations this complex is joined by one centrale in the course of early ontogenesis. The centrale is contained in the talus, situated originally in place of the lateral process, and corresponds with the centrale tibiale proximale of Steiner's scheme or with the $c1$ of Holmgren's concept. This centrale, however, appears as an independent chondrification only for a short embryonic period, being then taken into the spreading out chondrification of the main talus portion (homologised with the tibiale).

Because the tibiale develops in the first collateral ray of Steiner's archipterygium concept, its direct continuation ought to be the prehallux. But no independent anlage was found tibial to the talus, which could be considered as an independent prehallux primordium, similar to the prepollex primordium in the hand. The existence of a prepollex and prehallux was the question extensively disputed in the older literature. Inspite of Gegenbaur's opposition, the views of Born (1876a), Emery (1890, 1897a, c, 1898, 1901), Bardeleben (1894a, b) and Wiedersheim (1892, 1906, 1907) recognizing the existence of a prepollex and prehallux gained acceptance. Rudimentary prepollex primordia were also found in Mammals by Kindahl (1941a, b, 1942a, b, 1944a, b, 1949) and Schmidt-Ehrenberg (1942). These authors, however, did not acknowledge prehallux findings or only with some doubts. Moreover, in the course of human ontogenesis we did not succeed in finding a separate rudimentary prehallux. But at the tibial tarsus margin rudimentary adjoint tarsal primordia are found developing differently from neighbouring elements. In place of the future naviculare tuberosity an unclosed perichondrium with tissue condensation appears as a less distinct primordium, in embryos of C-R length 18 mm. The next similar formation is the plantar part of the first cuneiform (this cuneiform is divided into two parts in small embryos). The constant embryonic primordia (in adults known as variations) of the tibiale externum and the cuneiforme I plantare could be considered to be the rudiments of the primitive extremity first collateral ray—i.e. the rudiments of the tarsal sector of the prehallucial anlage.

The Centralia and their Relation to the Naviculare and to the Calcaneus. Most authors agree in considering the naviculare as corresponding with central elements. Only Albrecht (1884) and Baur (1885c) assumed a different homology of the naviculare (comp. Table 2). In newer concepts, according to Steiner as well as to Kindahl, the naviculare corresponds with two central elements. In our series the naviculare is observed as specifically shaped during ontogenesis. Its main tibial primordium joins the fibular portion which is delayed in chondrification, and extends proximally to the early chondrification situated in place of the future processus lateralis tali (v.s.). The position and shape of the primordia here looks as though cut out from Holmgren's (1933, 1952) and Kindahl's (1941—1949) general scheme, where centralia 2 and 3 link up to a prolonged arch with centrale 1 (which is here seen as the early temporary chondrification in place of the processus lateralis tali—Figs. 1C, 27). Although the definitive naviculare form does not correspond to the full extent of the embryonic chondrifying primordia, in any case the naviculare can be homologised with the centrale 2 and 3 according to Holmgren and Kindahl compared with the two distal centralia (centrale tibiale distale and centrale fibulare distale) of Steiner's scheme. The primordium adjacent to the naviculare in place of the future tuberositas ossis navicularis or the variable os tibiale externum has already been mentioned as most probably corresponding with the rudiments of a prehallucial ray. Rajtová (1968) also observed the naviculare originating from two components in the guinea-pig, and the prehallux primordium situated first at the tibia end and then joining the tarsus (talus) margin. It has been demonstrated above that the centrale tibiale proximale of Steiner's scheme (centrale 1 of Holmgren and Kindahl) situated at the beginning of development in place of the future processus lateralis tali is later pushed back and replaced by the chondrification of the main talus part expanding into the lateral process of the talus. From this $c1$ two arch-formed streams of the prochondral tissue and of early chondrification proceed distally to the tibial and fibular side (exactly according Holmgren's and Kindahl's concept). The tibial part represents both areas of the naviculare primordium. The fibular part proceeds between the distal part of the developing calcaneus and the cuboideum. This V-shaped region may be regarded as the area of central elements. It is situated in the region of the future sinus tarsi; all three ends of this area may be regarded as centralia, the centrale 1 being situated at the proximal edge of this region, centrale 2 and 3 on the tibial distal end and the centrale 4 on the fibular distal end (Figs. 19, 27). The rudiments of the $c1$ and the remains of the $c3$ (which is not taken into the naviculare in full original extent) and $c4$ then evidently become the source of a number of accessory elements known in the literature (Pfitzner, 1896; Lanz and Wachsmuth, 1938; Marti, 1947; O'Rahilly, 1953, 1957; Slabý, 1968a) as variations situated directly distal to the lateral process of the talus, between the talus, calcaneus and the naviculare. The ossicle found as variation in place of $c1$ is the os sustentaculi, the calcaneus secundarius and the cuboideum secundarium may be regarded as derivatives of the extinct $c4$ and the talus secundarius as a part of the original $c3$ which was not included into the naviculare.

The Tarsalia Distalia. The division of cuneiforme I into the cuneiforme I plantare and the cuneiforme I dorsale, transient in the course of embryonic development, suggests that the prehallucial ray extends to the cuneiforme I plantare, which may be assumed as its rudiment. In the cuboideum region our findings are in agreement with those in the upper limb. The cuboideum represents only the tarsale distale IV, the tarsale distale V being a temporary independent chondrification which becomes extinct without fusing with the primordium of the cuboid.

It may be deduced from the above analysis that, contrary to the carpus, the canonic elements remain in the human tarsus. These canonic elements fuse with some of the centralia (or replace some of them) so that in the foot all rows of tarsal elements are preserved. The prehallucial ray becomes reduced by joining the other tarsus and the canonic elements come together in the tibiofibular direction and fuse with the centralia. The differences in our homologisation from that of Holmgren and Steiner are schematically demonstrated in Fig. 27. The elements of the primitive tarsus participate in the formation of human tarsal primordia in the following manner:

The talus originates by fusion of the tibiale, forming its main part, with the intermedium, representing the region of the os trigonum, and with the centrale tibiale proximale ($c1$) which first originates in place of the future lateral process, being later replaced by the chondrification expanding from the primordium of the main talus part.

The calcaneus originates by the union of the fibulare, which forms the distal part, with the homologon of the pisiform forming the proximal calcaneus part.

The naviculare develops by fusion of two centralia, which may be homologised with the centrale tibiale distale and centrale fibulare distale of Steiner's scheme or with the centralia 2 and 3 according to Holmgren. The tuberosity of the naviculare chondrifies separately at first, being a part of the rudimentary prehallux ray—i. e. the tarsale (centrale) praehallucis.

The cuneiforme I results from the fusion of the originally separate dorsal and plantar parts. The dorsal part is the tarsale distale I, whilst the plantar part corresponds most probably with the distal end of the prehallux primordium.

The cuneiforme II is homologous with the tarsale distale II, *the cuneiforme III* is the tarsale distale III.

The cuboideum is the tarsale distale IV. The tarsale distale V appears transiently as a small islet of early chondrification and soon becomes extinct. Part of it is probably taken into the 5th metatarsal base as the material of its tuberosity or of the variable os Vesalianum.

The Metatarsus. During the ontogenesis of the metatarsal region a peculiar initial position of the metatarsals has been observed in relation to distal tarsalia. The metatarsal primordia do not link up exactly to the tarsalia, and, in addition, the longitudinal axes of tarsalia and of metatarsals are mutually inclined at a considerable angle. There is no explanation of this phenomenon.

The next point of interest in the embryonic metatarsus is the constant occurrence of the transient primordium of the os intermetatarseum during early embryonic stages. With relation to this skeletal variation, which has been noted a number of times and is quoted as a typical and known one (Gruber, 1852, 1877, 1879; Pfitzner, 1896; Thilenius, 1896a, 1897; Schwalbe, 1917; Tokmakoff, 1928; Martj, 1947; O'Rahilly, 1953, 1957; Slabý, 1968a), three opinions were expressed: it was considered either an element persisting from the phylogenesis of the foot skeleton (Pfitzner, 1896) or as the sesamoid bone (Tokmakoff, 1928) or the separated process of the first cuneiform (Schwalbe, 1917). Slabý (1968a) mentions that "phylogenetic evidence can scarcely be found for the theory which considers this bone a persisting ancestral metatarsal element". The explanation of this accessory primordium which appears in human ontogenesis, is very difficult. In position and shape it corresponds to the typical os intermetatarseum. The manner of its development indicates that it is a phylogenetically ancient element manifested in the course of ontogenesis. It seems that the os intermetatarseum in adults is nothing but an accidental persistence of this constant embryonic anlage.

To answer the question of the phylogenetic origin of the intermetatarseum it is at first necessary to refute Tokmakoff's opinion that the accessory ossicle is a sesamoid, because all sesamoids of the human hand and foot develop later, in embryos of about 50 mm in C-R length, while the element concerned is formed already in 16 mm embryos. It is also necessary to refute Pfitzner's opinion considering the intermetatarseum as an ancient persisting metatarsal or tarsal element. In palaeontology there is known neither a case of six elements in the distal tarsal row nor an increased metatarsal number in Theromorphs; in theromorph Reptiles not even a prehallux has been noted and all known Theromorphs are five-toed (Broom, 1930; Romer and Price, 1940; Romer, 1956). Only Romer and Price (1940) noted that in some Theromorphs the first toe diverged at a

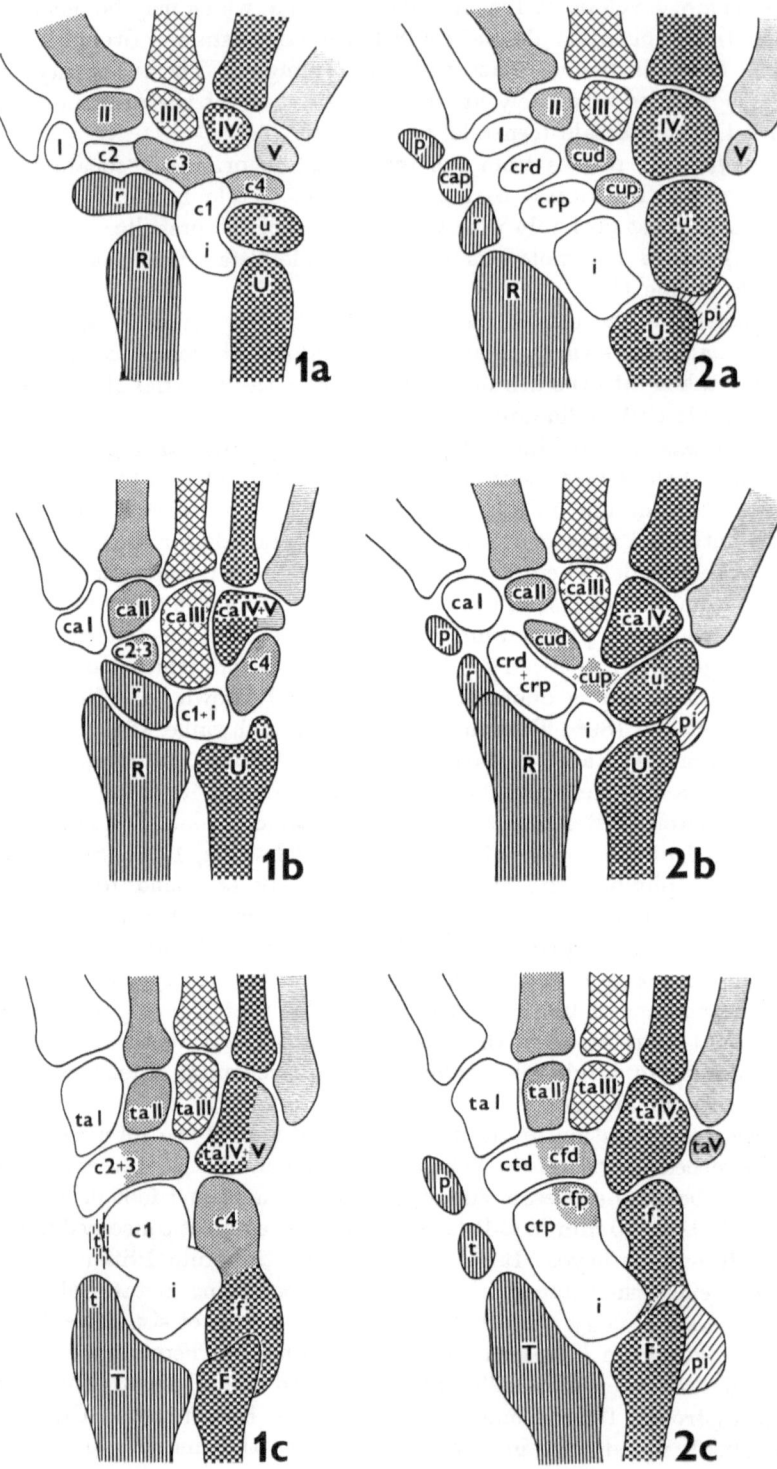

Fig. 27. Summary of homologies of carpal and tarsal primordia: *1* according to Holmgren (1933-1952) and Kindahl (1941–1949) (1 a–c); *2* according to Steiner (1942) (2 a–c); *3, 4* our conclusions demonstrated in the hand and foot of human embryo (3 b–c) and drawn into the schemes of the hand and foot skeleton in adult (4 b–c). Single collateral rays of Steiner's general scheme (*2 a*) are transferred for comparison also into Holmgren's scheme (1 a) and into our concept. Legends same as in Figs. 3–23; *pi* pisiforme, *cap* carpale praepollicis; *taph* tarsalia praehallucis; c_{1-4} centralia according to Holmgren

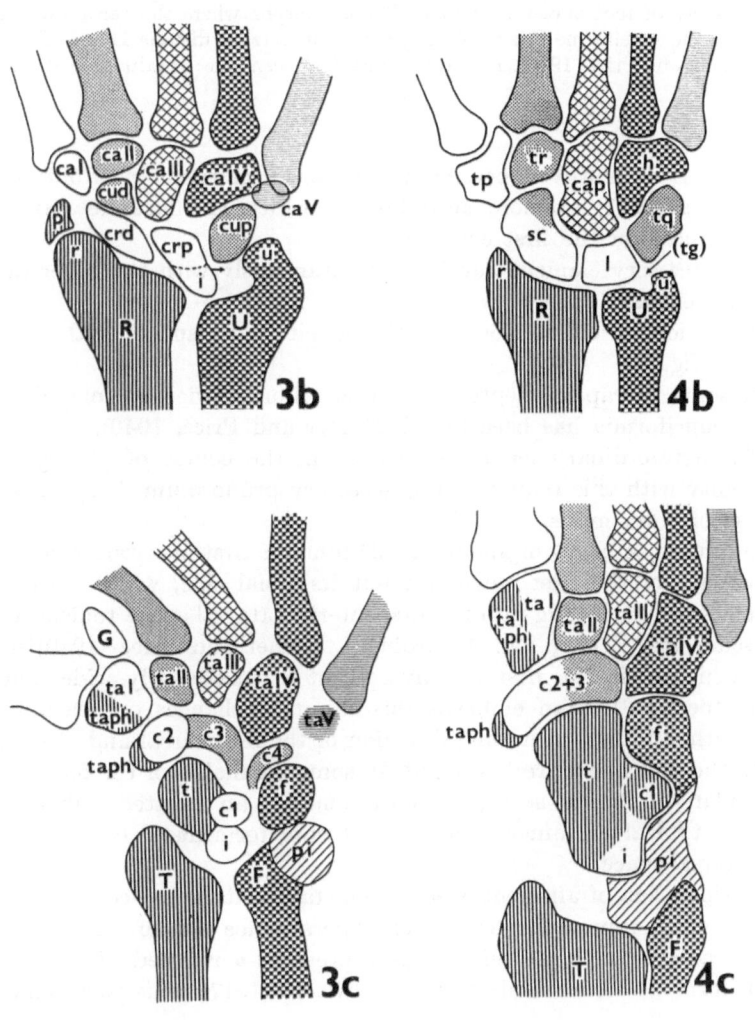

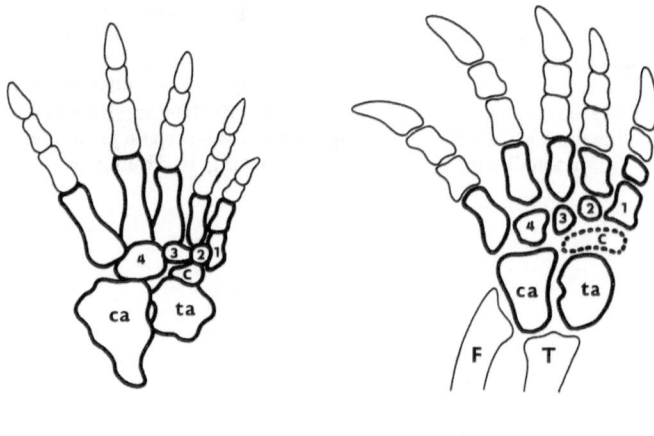

BAURIA   EMYDOPSIS

Fig. 28. Schemes of foot skeleton of fossil Thermomorphs where the tarsale distale I (corresponding to the cuneiforme I) is much longer than the tarsalia distalia II and III. (According to Romer and Price, 1940). *1–4* tarsalia distalia; *c* centrale; *ta* talus; *ca* calcaneus

wider angle. It is, however, possible to find some morphological data on behalf of Schwalbe's (1917) opinion, according to which the intermetatarseum is a separated process of the first cuneiform:

1. The accessory element develops simultaneously with the other tarsal and metatarsal elements.

2. It develops in connection with the cuneiforme I and II with a secondary separation (Fig. 21).

3. In some therapsid Reptiles a 1st cuneiform twice so long (Fig. 28) as the other cuneiformia has been found (Romer and Price, 1940).

4. This extraordinary length is reduced in the course of phylogenesis and in conformity with this reduction the accessory primordium disappears early in the course of ontogenesis.

5. In human embryos of about 22—27 mm the first metatarsal does not join the distal side of the first cuneiform but its tibial side, while the distal part of the cuneiform extending into the first intermetatarsal space touches the intermetatarseum anlage (Fig. 29). Accordingly, Romer and Price (1940) note that in some Pelicosauria the first toe diverges at a considerably wider angle than the other toes. In human embryos this situation changes on reaching 30 mm of C-R length, and later a normal direction of the metatarsal and of its articular line (with the first cuneiform) is found. In some anomalies of the foot (pes inversus) a similar situation is seen (Fig. 30) resembling an arrested embryonic situation with a typical prominence of the first cuneiform distal edge into the first intermetatarsal space.

In consideration of all mentioned circumstances it can be concluded that the intermetatarseum represents the accidental persistence of a constant and transient embryonic anlage and that this anlage represents a reduced distal part of the first cuneiform, as assumed already by Schwalbe (1917). This part is most prob-

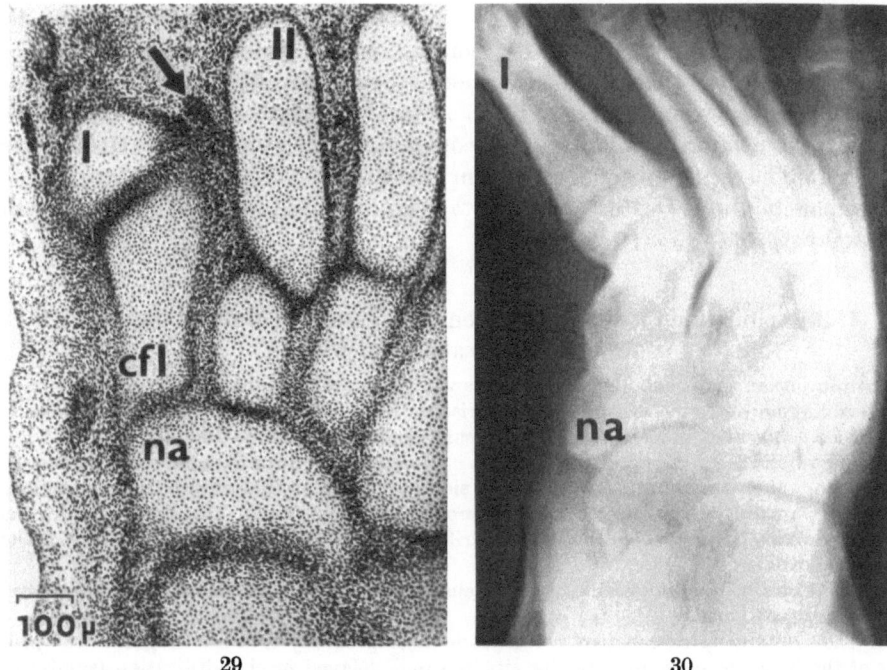

Fig. 29. Tarsal primordia of the embryo 27 mm in C-R length, right foot, sectioned parallel to the sole. The contact between the primordia of the cuneiforme I and the 1st metatarsal stands obliquely so that the 1st metatarsal diverges at a considerable angle. The rudiment of the primordium of the os intermetatarseum is indicated by arrow

Fig. 30. The relation between the cuneiforme I and the 1st metatarsal, similar to that in embryos (Fig. 29) is seen in the congenital malformation of the foot (pes inversus) in a girl 16 years old

ably the distal prolongation of the 1st distal tarsale, known in phylogenesis and seen in the course of ontogenesis as a specific form of the first cuneiform and as the intermetatarseum anlage. The reduction of this superfluous anlage occurs together with typical position changes of the first metatarsal and of its articulation with the first cuneiform. The process represents a specific reduction development of material originally more bulky in the course of phylo-ontogenetic development, with the transient independence of the superfluous material.

With regard to the collateral rays of the primitive extremity in Steiner's concept, the elements can be situated as follows (Fig. 27):

The first collateral ray contains the tibia, tibiale (inside the talus), the os tibiale externum (normally extinct in the region of the navicular tuberosity), and the cuneiforme I plantare (observed in the course of ontogenesis). All tarsal components of this first ray are fused with the tibial margin of the tarsus.

The second ray then contains the intermedium (os trigonum), the centrale tibiale proximale ($c1$) transiently originating in place of the future processus lateralis tali, the centrale tibiale distale (Holmgren's and Kindahl's $c2$) contained in the naviculare, and the cuneiforme I dorsale with the first metatarsal and toe.

The third collateral ray includes the centrale situated originally between the calcaneus and the cuboideum which according to our material either gets extinct or persists in form of the variable calcaneus secundarius or the cuboideum secundarium (Holmgren's and Kindahl's $c4$, centrale fibulare proximale of Steiner's concept), the centrale fibulare distale contained in the naviculare (Holmgren's and Kindahl's $c3$), the second cuneiform and the second metatarsal and toe.

The cuneiforme III with the 3rd metatarsal and toe correspond to the fourth collateral ray.

11. Recapitulation of Observations on the Tarsus in Human Ontogenesis of Comparisons and Homologies

On the basis of the chondrification of tarsal primordia, on their interrelations in the course of human ontogenesis and on comparison with earlier literary views, the following conclusions concerning the homologies of tarsal elements have been drawn:

1. The tibiale is contained in the talus. It is joined by the Intermedium as the processus posterior (or the os trigonum). At the lateral side of the talus the centrale tibiale proximale ($c1$) exists transiently in place of the future processus lateralis tali. The definitive processus lateralis develops by expansion of the chondrification from the corpus tali in place of the reduced centrale.

2. The fibulare is contained in the calcaneus forming its distal, during ontogenesis more medially situated part.

3. The proximal calcaneus part corresponds most probably to a homologon of the pisiform of the hand, being more laterally situated and delayed in chondrification (similar to the pisiform of the hand). The relatively independent chondrification of the two calcaneus components is striking during early ontogenesis.

4. The naviculare originates by fusion of two centralia, the centrale tibiale distale and the centrale fibulare distale of Steiner's concept, $c2$ and $c3$ according to Holmgren. The picture of the embryonic naviculare primordia with their relation to the $c1$ (in place of the processus lateralis tali) and to the distal calcaneus end strikingly resembles Holmgren's general scheme of the autopodium.

5. The $c4$ is transiently formed in young embryos between the distal end of the calcaneus and the cuboideum primordium.

6. In the course of human ontogenesis in embryos of 18 mm in C-R length an independent chondrification may be found in place of the tuberositas ossis navicularis. The cuneiforme I primordium is divided into a dorsal and plantar part. The anlage in the naviculare tuberosity corresponds to the variable os tibiale externum tarsi and together with the cuneiforme I plantare primordium probably represents the prehallucial ray.

7. The tarsalia distalia proper begin with the dorsal cuneiforme I and contain the three cuneiformia and the cuboideum; the later being only the tarsale distale IV.

8. The tarsale distale V originates as a small primordium during ontogenesis, persists for a short period and then disappears. Its part probably corresponds to the tuberosity of the 5th metatarsal and to the os Vesalianum (var.).

9. The embryonic metatarsals are typically shifted in a fibular direction and inclined by their longitudinal axes tibially in relation to the longitudinal axes of distal tarsal elements.

10. In the first intermetatarsal space a transient primordium of the os intermetatarseum is found constantly, originating already in young embryos. Its maximal extent with possible chondrification is found in embryos of 25 mm C-R length. Then it disappears rapidly. The course of its ontogenesis suggests a formation recapitulated during ontogenesis. It probably represents the extinct distal part of the originally longer first cuneiform.

11. The embryonic tarsus contains all the canonic elements, and its four centralia may be established. With the exception of $c4$ no element gets completely reduced, all of them persist either in form of accessory tarsal elements or as parts of primordia of definitive tarsal elements. The general trend of tarsus development is represented by the tibio-fibular narrowing of tarsus disposition with fusion of the centralia with canonic elements.

12. Comparison of Developmental Changes in the Hand and Foot Skeleton

Comparing the development of hand and foot and reconsidering the homologies and relations of single elements to skeletal rays established by Steiner (1942) some changes are deduced, which, however, respect and imply some of the anterior schemes of carpus and tarsus homologies. In the course of development of the hand as well as of the foot the signs of incidence of four centralia can be found and corresponding homologies can be assessed. An attempt has also been made at overcoming the differences between Holmgren's and Steiner's schools in the interpretation of the centralia.

The hand and the foot both have some specific primitive features: maintainance of the basic arrangement of collateral rays, participation of the centralia, developmental recapitulation of the first collateral ray rudiments (prepollicial and prehallucial rudiments) in the carpal and tarsal region. The basic scheme then changes for the hand and for the foot with resulting differences between them. The sequence of changes in the hand is characterised by the proximodistal shift of carpal rows, while in the foot the course of developmental changes results in the tibiofibular condensation of elements and their fusion. The most characteristic feature in development of the hand (as seen in our material as well as in literature) is the exchange of proximal row canonic elements for the centralia. The most characteristic pattern in the foot is the maintainance of canonic elements and their fusion with the centralia resulting in the tibiofibular condensation of the tarsus followed by the clasping together of the widely opened fan of metatarsal primordia. In connection with it the prehallux rudiments firmly join the tarsus.

The hand and the foot then differ considerably in their definitive form, both in elements participating in the autopodium formation and in their mutual fusion into definitive bone primordia. By the participation of all canonic elements the foot appears to be more primitive in development, but it immediately reaches high specialization. This combination of primitive and specialized features is found also in the course of development of muscles in the foot.

The human hand and foot are formations closely similar in pattern only at the beginning of their development. During their entire subsequent development they continually differ in structure. Neither the hand nor the foot maintained the original pattern of the extremity of Tetrapods and the application of this abstract general scheme is possible only to early embryonic stages of the human (or generally mammalian) hand and foot.

IV. Development and Homologies of Intrinsic Musculature of the Hand and Foot
A. Problem of Muscle Layers of the Hand and Foot

The fundamental question concerned in developmental studies of hand and foot muscles is that of the origin and homologies of the muscle layers. The attempts at classification and homologisation of palmar muscle layers appeared in the literature a long time ago. Cunningham (1878a) on the basis of studies on Marsupials (Thylacinus, Phalangista, Phascogale) divided the palmar muscles, and later (1878b) on the basis of more extensive studies, also the plantar muscles

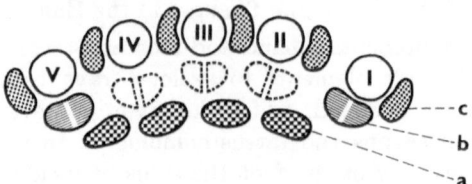

Fig. 31. Scheme of Cunningham's concept of layers of the palmar musculature: *a* the palmar layer of adductors; *b* intermediate layer of flexors; *c* dorsal layer of abductors. Elements drawn by dotted line became extinct according to Cunningham

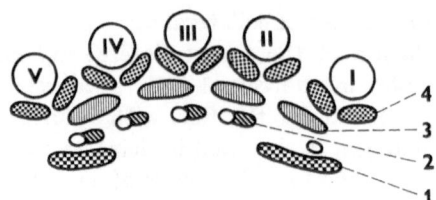

Fig. 32. Bardeleben's general scheme of layers of the palmar musculature: *1* the flexores breves superficiales; *2* the lumbricales; *3* the contrahentes or flexores breves medii; *4* the flexores breves profundi, interni (the palmar interossei) and externi (the dorsal interossei). The change of position of the flexores breves externi by their migration was supposed

into three groups (Fig. 31): the palmar (plantar) layer of adductors, the intermediate group containing the paired muscles on the palmar side of the metacarpals together with the flexor pollicis brevis and the flexor digiti minimi brevis, and the dorsal group also according to Cunningham including the abductor pollicis brevis and the abductor digiti minimi. The muscles of the dorsal group situated between the metatarsals were considered by Cunningham to be the homologues of the human dorsal interossei. For the intermediate group an extinction of most elements was assumed by Cunningham, the abductor pollicis and the abductor digiti minimi being its only rudiments in man. Cunningham's view was further elaborated by Young (1880) and Brooks (1886a, b). Cunningham, however, in the meantime (1882) revised and modified his original view in that the part of muscles of the intermediate group changed into the palmar interossei, while the remaining ones disappeared, and that in the palmar group only its first most radial muscle persisted as the adductor pollicis. This view was accepted by Thane (1892); the original classification of muscle layers (Cunningham, 1878a, b; Young, 1880; Brooks, 1886a, b), modified by Primrose (1899), was also employed by Wood-Jones (1944a) who, in agreement with other authors, considered the adductor pollicis as a part of the palmar group of deep intrinsic musculature.

Another classification of hand muscles was carried out by Bardeleben (1890). This author recognized five muscle layers generally in the mammalian hand and foot (Fig. 32): 1. The flexores breves superficiales, situated palmar or plantar to the long flexor tendons. 2. The flexores breves lumbricales, originating inside the flexor tendon layer. 3. The mm. flexores breves medii or mm. contrahentes or mm. adductores (contracteurs des doigts of French authors) characterized in

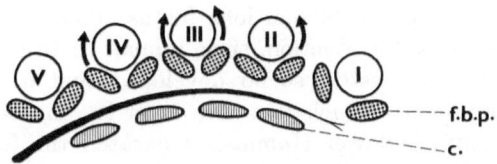

Fig. 33. Scheme of supposed changes of position by which the flexores breves profundi (*f.b.p.*) become the dorsal and palmar interossei. According to Keith (1949) modified. The layers of contrahentes muscles (*c.*) and the interossei are separated by the ulnar nerve

the hand (Forster, 1916) and in the foot (Ruge, 1878a) by their position between the flexor tendons and the deep palmar branch of the ulnar nerve (deep plantar branch of the fibular plantar nerve) and corresponding with the palmar layer of Cunningham's division; Bardeleben situated these muscles as separate from the interossei while they were considered by Cunningham as the palmar interossei. 4. and 5. The mm. flexores breves profundi—interni et externi—situated originally as a single layer, in man divided into the interossei palmares and dorsales; according to Bardeleben they should correspond with Cunningham's intermediate and dorsal layers. The homologies of layers in both systems and in the two mutually is disputable.

Comparative considerations of homologies were joined by a new standpoint, the study of ontogenesis: Ruge (1878a) described the migration of the primordia of mm. interossei in the foot from the plantar side into the intermetatarsal spaces. He stated that the dorsal and plantar interossei were originally situated at the same level, and then migrated from it. Conforming views were adopted by Windle (1883), Schomburg (1900), Bardeen and Lewis (1901), Lewis (1901/02), Gräfenberg (1905/06) and Bardeen (1907). All these embryological studies confirm the identity of the dorsal and palmar interossei with the layer primarily situated palmar to the metacarpals, i.e. with the deep short flexors. On this basis, in connection with Bardeleben's concept (1890), a scheme of origin of the interossei by migration from the flexores breves profundi layer (Fig. 33) was elaborated, according to which each member of the twins of the flexores breves profundi beneath the metacarpals became one of the palmar or of the dorsal interossei. This scheme of interossei origin (Fig. 33) was employed up to a short time ago (Campbell, 1939; Keith, 1949), modified for the hand and foot only by the position of the axis in respect to which the symmetric shifts of muscle primordia were claimed.

Some comparative studies, however, point against the concept of the origin of the interossei by the migration of deep short flexors. McMurrich (1903, 1907, 1927), Ribbing (1909, 1938), Stjernman (1932) and Howell (1936) from the phylogenetic standpoint considered the dorsal interossei as derived from some of the flexores breves profundi, but presumed that they are also joined by some more dorsal muscle elements. According to Campbell (1939) these concepts were elaborated in order "to bring the theory into agreement with the indisputable evidence of Ruge and the embryologists", since in comparative anatomy a larger number of layers of hand muscles were known in lower Tetrapods. McMurrich (1903) tried to demonstrate these dorsal components in the transverse sec-

tion of the hand of the human 60 mm long foetus. This is, however, the result
of a theoretical comparative deduction, since human foetuses, aged like the one
quoted, have their muscle system so far developed that it is quite impossible
to recognize the components which joined to form the muscle.

Ribbing (1909, 1938) in lower Mammals separated the flexores breves profundi as the palmar interossei from the so-called mm. interdigitales, situated
more dorsally and denoted also as the mm. interossei dorsales. He then noted
either the duplication, or, on the contrary, the absence of these dorsal interossei
in various Mammals; describing the flexores breves profundi he mentioned that
in the genera Cebus and Homo the seemingly extinct halves of mm. flexores
breves profundi are fused with the mm. interdigitales. His concept is analogous
to McMurrich's view, being derived from the alternative symmetric position of
the human dorsal and palmar interossei with regard to the third finger. A similar
view from the comparative standpoint was assumed by Forster (1916) who
considered a far advanced reduction of the corresponding palmar element (again
in the genera Cebus and Homo) and an inverse fusion: the fusion of the palmar
element with the dorsal one, so that the palmar element apparently disappears.

These views, however, are in contradiction to the observations of Ruge
(1878a) and of other embryologists who claim the unilaminar origin of the interossei followed by their migration. Our previous observations demonstrated two
possibilities of origin of the dorsal interossei: we followed the origin of the first
dorsal interosseus in the course of human ontogenesis by fusion of two neighbouring primordia of the flexores breves profundi layer entering symmetrically
into the first intermetacarpal space in human embryos (Čihák, 1960b, 1963b, c).
We also assessed that the mm. interossei dorsales II, III and IV each originated
by the joining of one primordial element from the flexores breves profundi layer
with one more dorsally situated intermetacarpal anlage (Čihák, 1963b, c). Similar
results in the comparative anatomy of Primates were achieved by Lewis (1965)
who observed the origin of all dorsal interossei by the fusion of the palmar and
dorsal elements.

A quite different manner of solving these questions was attempted by Kadanoff (1958). On the basis of findings of muscular variations of the extensores
digitorum breves muscles and of the occurrence of branches of the radial nerve
reaching to the dorsal surface of dorsal interossei, this author assumed that the
extensores digitorum manus breves are progressively reduced elements, the
rudiments of which then join the dorsal interossei from the dorsal side, either
in the form of a muscle rudiment or as material where the nerve supply by the
radial nerve solely documents its origin from an extensor. The significance of
branches of the radial nerve as a proof of his view is, however, doubtful, as
shown by Sunderland's (1946) observation of the low incidence of such branches
and of the impossibility of distinguishing whether these are motor or sensory.

It is evident from the quotations of earlier observations that most authors
agree that the interossei originate solely from the layers corresponding to the
flexores breves profundi of Bardeleben's scheme or also from some more dorsally
situated primordia. Because according to these observations the contrahentes
take no part in the development of deep layers of hand musculature, their situation in relation to hand musculature ought be recognized. Gräfenberg (1905/06)

thought that three contrahentes muscles form the adductor pollicis and that the fourth becomes extinct. According to Ribbing (1938) only the most radial contrahens muscle forms the adductor, whilst the others disappear; according to Forster (1916) the contrahentes change into the ligamentum metacarpeum transversum profundum. The transient existence of contrahentes primordia during human ontogenesis and their extinction has already been described (Čihák, 1963 b, c, 1967 a, 1969 c). Later on these observations were completed by studies of the special manner of their extinction (Čihák, 1967 b, 1968 a, b, 1969 c). These observations are summarized in the present publication. An unknown point was the manner of development of the adductor hallucis and its relation to the contrahentes layer of the foot (Čihák, 1969 a). For recognizing the development and homologies of the interossei the following questions raised on the basis of literary contradictions must be clarified and answered: a) How the paired flexores breves profundi situated beneath the metacarpals change into the interossei in the hand and the foot. b) If the third (dorsal) layer of Cunningham's division really exists as an independent layer, or if it is identical with the mm. flexores breves profundi externi, since it is known that in Mammals both the flexores breves profundi, externi et interni, are one layer beneath the metacarpals. c) Whether Campbell (1939) was right in considering that the Marsupials have one additional dorsal layer calling it the mm. flexores digitorum minimi, or McMurrich (1903, 1907, 1927) was right when supposing a similar layer for Man as well, denoting it the mm. intermetacarpales.

The solution obtained by studies of the interossei manus in human onto-genesis (Čihák, 1963 b, c, 1967 a, 1968 b, 1969 c) appears to be plausible for the development of the interossei, especially for the question of layers of the flexores breves profundi and the intermetacarpales, and is summarized in the present publication. The development of these muscles and muscle layers will be compared with the ontogenesis of the interossei in the human foot, since certain changes may be anticipated due to foot specialisation. Because in all interossei the question of their insertion, i.e. of ontogenetic changes in their insertion—as supposed by Baumann (1951)—is not sufficiently clear, its solution from the standpoint of development of the dorsal aponeurosis of fingers will also be attempted. The participation of accessory muscle elements, described previously (Čihák, 1963 b, c, 1968 b, 1969 c) will be reconsidered as well. In all these questions the development of the hand and foot will be compared, concerning the course of development and the structures involved. The supplying nerve branches in embryonic and adult hands were taken into account as the most exact sign in following the muscles and layers of muscle primordia.

These complex studies have demonstrated that comparative anatomy in itself may be insufficient for the solution of a developmental problem and so may the mere study of ontogenesis. An attempt was therefore made to link up both these viewpoints. The present observations start by the study of ontogenesis, comparative anatomy is employed for the correction and for the developmental explanation of the results. Unclear points in observed facts and employed nomen-clature between embryology and normal and comparative anatomy were removed by employing the nomenclature of comparative anatomy for the embryonic human hand. Therefore Bardeleben's nomenclature of autopodial muscle layers has been accepted as the basis of the following considerations; the further dorsal layer is denoted by McMurrich's term, the mm. intermetacarpales (intermeta-tarsales).

B. The Mm. Contrahentes

1. Mm. Contrahentes in the Course of Development of the Human Hand

To answer questions of the developmental relations of the contrahentes muscles in Man, given in the previous chapter, attention has been drawn to the ontogenetic development of those primordia in the human hand where they are situated in the palm as a layer between the flexor tendons and the ulnar nerve. The course of the nerve in the palm and in the sole (nervus ulnaris, n. plantaris lateralis) was previously assessed by Ruge (1878a) and by Forster (1916) as the demarcation line between the contrahentes and the interossei layers. The study of the contrahentes layer is naturally connected with the study of the onto-genesis of the human adductor pollicis and adductor hallucis, which originate inside this layer.

2. Material for Studies of the Development of the Mm. Contrahentes in the Human Hand

The development and transformations of the contrahentes layer were followed in three steps. In the first step 70 hands of human embryos and foetuses from 10 to 75 mm in C-R length were employed (Čihák, 1963c). This first study demonstrated the temporary existence of a complete contrahentes layer and the subsequent gradual extinction of its ulnar half during human ontogenesis. The second study (Čihák, 1967b) followed up the process of devel-opment and the time of extinction of the contrahentes layer. In the third study (Čihák, 1968a, b, 1969c) and in the present publication the differentiation process and the manner of the contrahentes layer extinction are demonstrated in 82 hands of human embryos and foetuses from 10 to 75 mm in C-R length.

C-R lengths of embryos and foetuses employed: 10 mm, 12, 13.6, 14, 15 (2 hands), 15.5 (3), 16 (2), 16.5 (4), 17, 17.5 (4), 18 (4), 19 (6), 19.5 (3), 20 (4), 20.5 (3), 21 (6), 22 (2), 22.5 (2), 23 (4), 25 (5), 25.5, 26 (3), 27 (2), 28 (2), 29 (3), 30 (2), 32 (2), 35 (2), 40, 45, 50, 56, 65, 75 mm.

The hand musculature of embryos of 15.5 mm and of 21 mm in C-R length was recon-structed. The staining of histological series and the technic of reconstructions are described on p. 10–11.

3. Observations of Development and Extinction of the Contrahentes Layer in Human Ontogenesis

In the embryo of 10 mm in C-R length only suggestions of future meta-carpals and an unclear primordium of the future carpal skeleton can be found. The dense mesenchyme offers no possibility of even approximately determining the sites of future muscular blastemas. Similarly, in the 12 mm embryo the mesenchyme of the future palmar musculature can hardly be recognized. The common blastema of deep intrinsic muscles already appears in the 13.6 mm long embryo of our material. This blastema can be clearly distinguished from the skeletal primordium on the one side and from the denser blastema of the flexor digitorum profundus tendons on the other. The contrahentes layer is as yet neither differentiated nor detached from deeper structures. The ramus pro-fundus nervi ulnaris passes through the blastema common for all the intrinsic hand muscles, which is situated palmar to the carpal and metacarpal primordia;

the main part of the blastema is situated on the palmar side of the nerve. At this stage the more bulky part of the blastema is that for the future contrahentes layer. In the embryo of 14 mm in length the whole situation already appears to be more explicit. Accordingly to the course of the deep palmar branch of the ulnar nerve, the common blastema of deep intrinsic muscles becomes clearly differentiated into a superficial and a deeper layer, the former being still more bulky (Fig. 34).

The two layers of primordia of the deep palmar musculature are closely adherent to the ulnar nerve in the region of its transverse course across the palm (Figs. 35, 39). Both layers—in some embryos between 15 and 17 mm in C-R length not yet quite exactly contoured—are well differentiated in all embryos from 18—28 mm of C-R length (Figs. 35, 36). The above mentioned division of the blastema of the palmar musculature at the level of the crossing ulnar nerve gives rise on one side to a constant deep primordia layer corresponding to the layer of flexores breves profundi in Bardeleben's scheme (i.e. to the interossei), and on the other side to a constant more superficial layer corresponding to the contrahentes muscles. The homology of this more superficial layer with the contrahentes muscles of lower Mammals and lower Primates is also supported by the subsequent fate of this primordial layer. Therefore the term *"contrahentes layer"* will be employed for it in subsequent descriptions.

The contrahentes layer is anchored on the ulnar side in the blastema of hypothenar muscles, at the level of the future flexor digiti minimi brevis. On the ulnar side it extends more proximally. It then continues to the radial side in the form of a thin plate. This plate becomes thinner in the middle of the palm and gets more bulky again towards the thenar eminence (Fig. 36). The contrahentes layer becomes detached from the hypothenar blastema directly palmar to the stem of the ramus profundus nervi ulnaris, before the nerve turns to cross the palm. On the sagittal section through the hand (Fig. 37) the contrahentes layer is seen extending far proximally. The reconstructions of the general form of this layer demonstrate that in younger embryos the layer is not yet fully developed. Its full extent is not achieved until 19 mm embryos (Čihák, 1967 b).

The contrahentes layer is distinctly separated from the more dorsally situated layer of the flexores breves profundi as well as from the more palmar layered tendons of the flexor digitorum profundus by loose mesenchyme (Fig. 38). On the contrary, at the level of the crossing nerve both layers are attached so closely to the ulnar nerve that the impression arises that the nerve even pierces a single blastema (Fig. 39). The difference, however, is demonstrated by cell orientation. The cells in the proximal part of the contrahentes layer are oriented transversely to the palm, whilst those in the flexores breves profundi layer are mostly longitudinally directed. Distal to the nerve arch both layers are again separated by the mesenchyme and the contrahentes layer gradually disappears in the distal direction.

The differentiation of the layer is different in its ulnar and radal ihalves. In the ulnar half the cells remain in the form of less differentiated elements with nuclei larger than those of surrounding fibroblasts. The contrahentes layer cells distinctly differ from those of the loose mesenchyme. However, they do

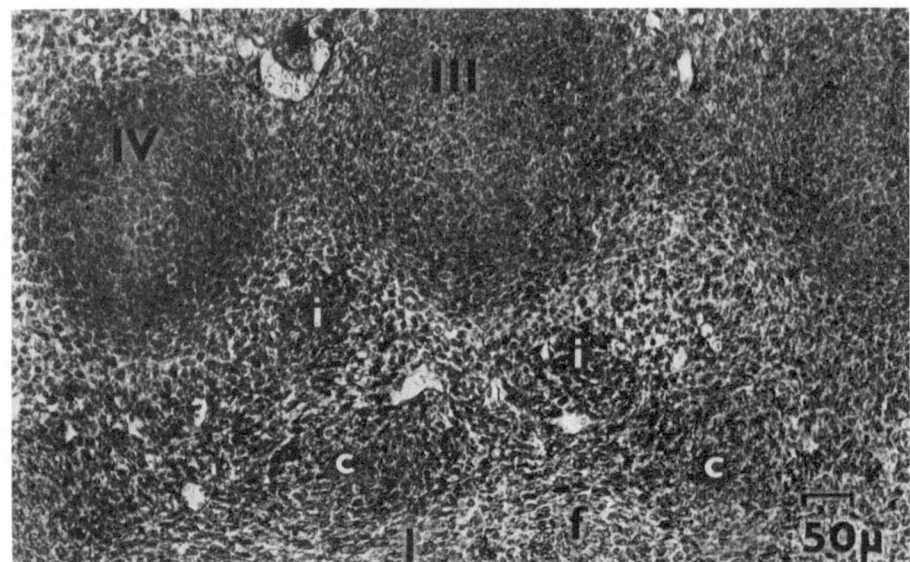

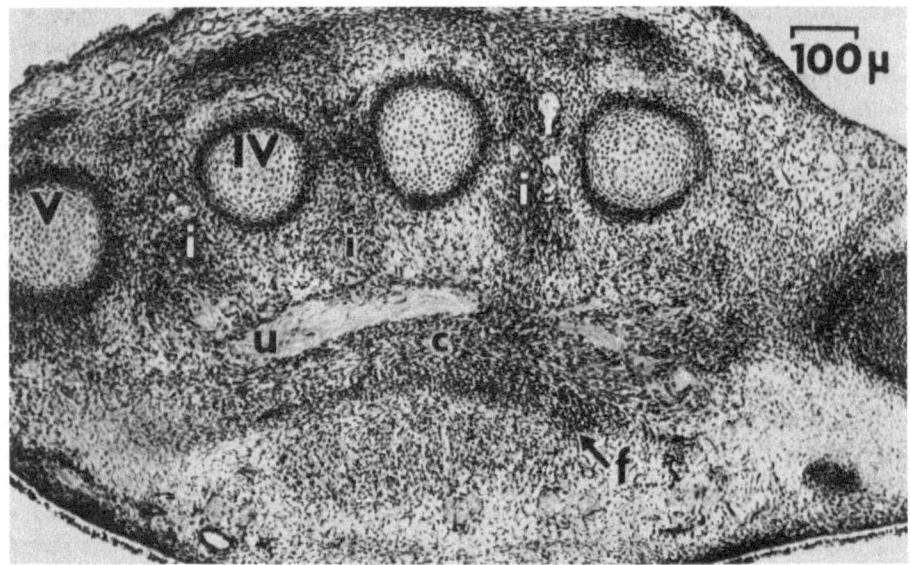

Fig. 34. Left hand of the embryo 14 mm C-R length, transverse section seen from proximal, the dorsal side of the hand above in the microphotograph. (In this manner all microphotographs of transverse sections of hands and feet are oriented.) Palmar to the interossei primordia (*i*) relatively bulky primordia of the contrahentes layer (*c*) are visible; *IV, III* the metacarpal primordia; *l* primordium of the lumbricalis; *f* primordium of the tendon of flexor digitorum profundus (Čihák, 1968a)

Fig. 35. Transverse section of the left hand of the 19 mm embryo. The course of the ulnar nerve (*u*) in the palm separates the interossei primordia (*i*) from the contrahentes layer (*c*); both layers are closely adjacent to the nerve; (*f*) a dense primordium of flexor digitorum profundus tendons

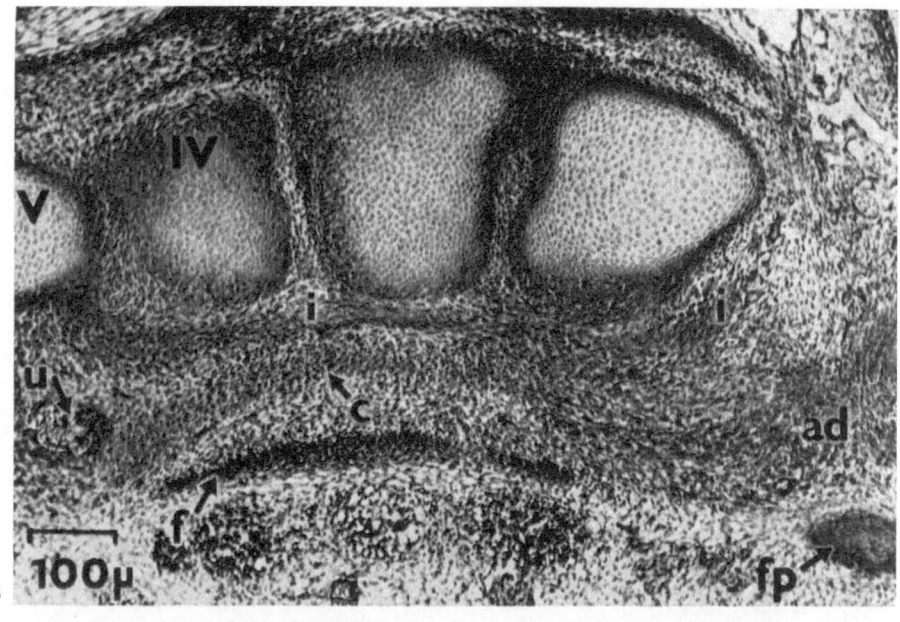

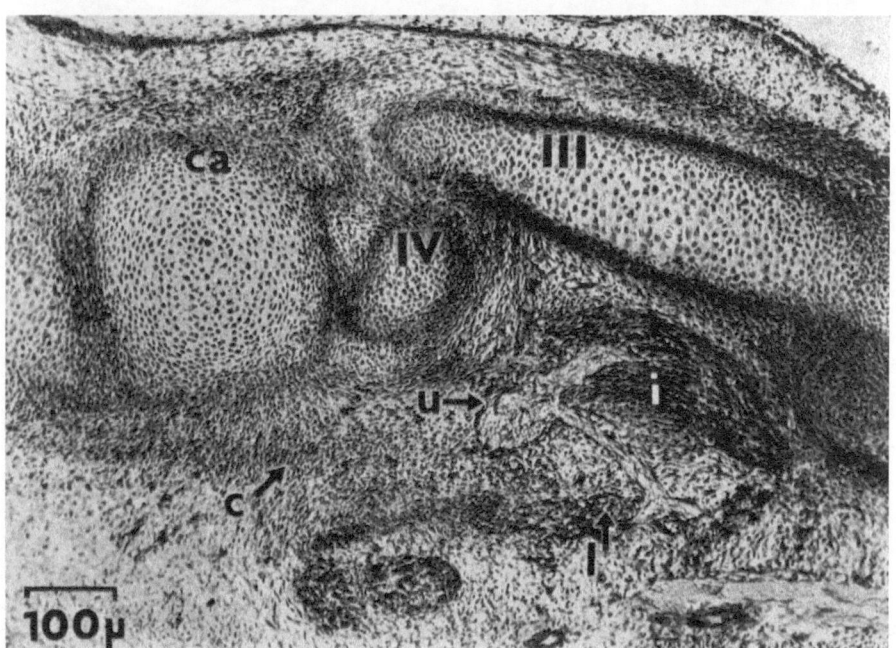

Fig. 36. Transverse section of the left hand of the embryo 20.5 mm in C-R length. The contrahentes layer (c) is visible in its full extent; it adjoins the hypothenar primordia on the ulnar side (u ulnar nerve) and on the radial side it differentiates to form the adductor pollicis (ad); f tendon primordia of the flexor digitorum profundus; fp flexor pollicis longus (Čihák, 1967b)

Fig. 37. Embryo 19 mm in C-R length, right hand, sagittal section (in the microphotograph the dorsal side is above, proximal side on the left). The contrahentes layer (c) is visible from the level of the proximal row of carpal primordia; l the lumbricalis and the branch of the ulnar nerve (u) entering it; i primordium of the interosseus with the entering branch from the ulnar nerve; ca the capitatum; III, IV metacarpals (Čihák, 1967b)

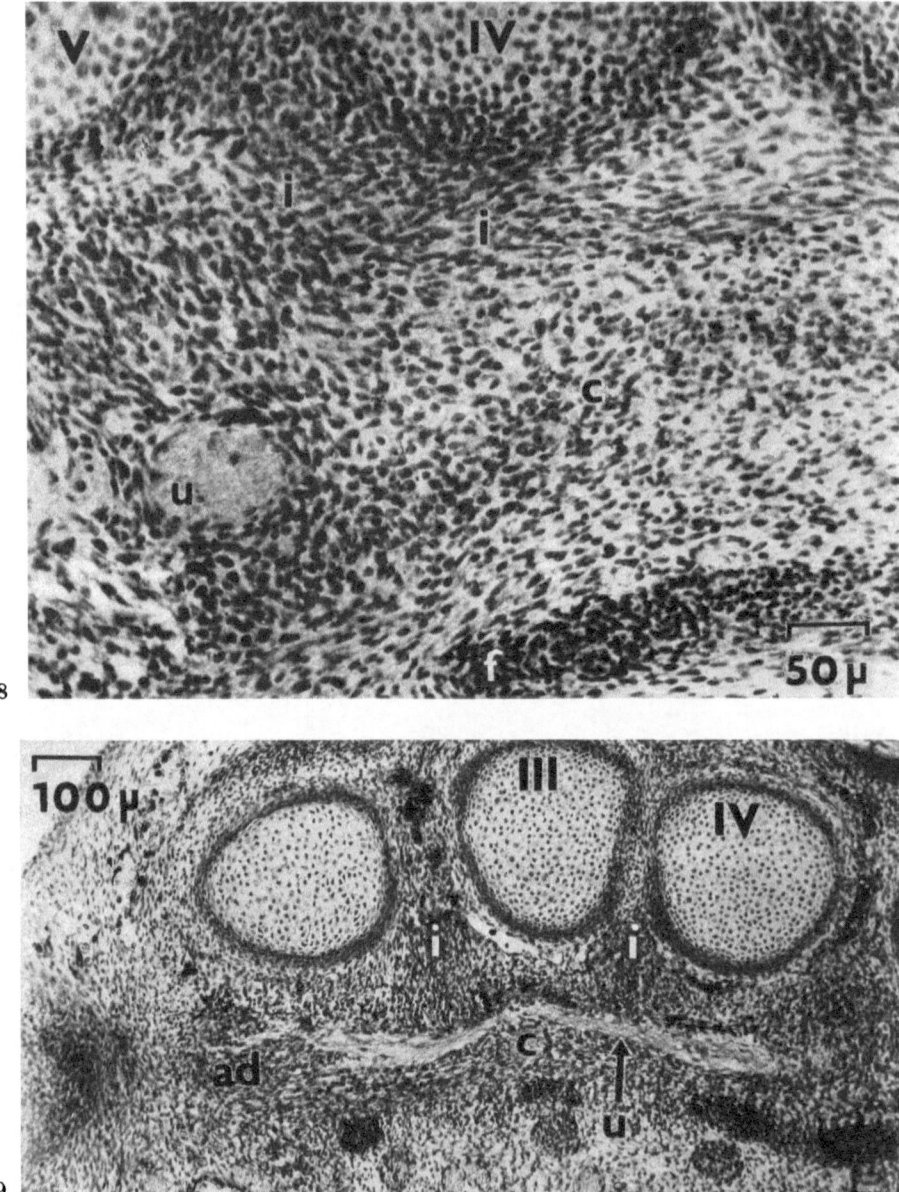

Fig. 38. Embryo 17 mm in C-R length, left hand, transverse section; the contrahentes layer (c) is distinctly different from the surrounding loose mesenchyme being separated by it from the deeper layer of interossei primordia (i) as well as from the more superficial layer of tendons of the flexor digitorum profundus (f); u ulnar nerve (Čihák, 1967b)

Fig. 39. Right hand of the embryo 22.5 mm ,transverse section. To the ulnar nerve (u) the layer of the interossei (flexores breves profundi) is closely joined from the dorsal side (i), the contrahentes layer adheres to it from the palmar side (c); the contrahentes layer forms the adductor pollicis (ad) on its radial side. III, IV the metacarpals

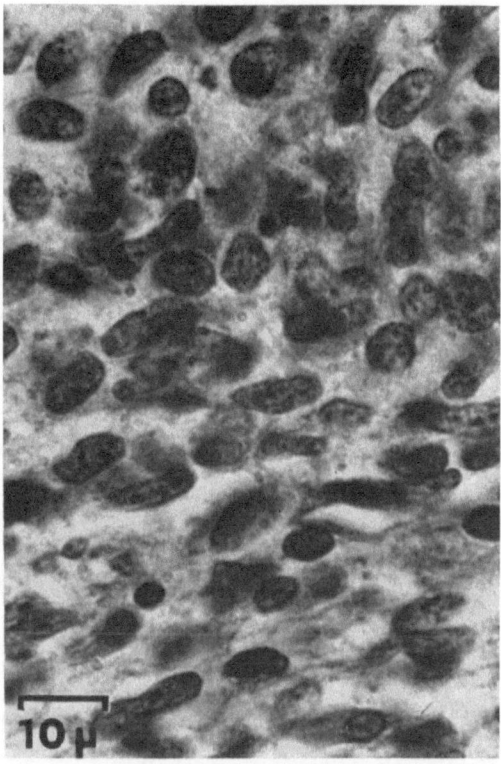

Fig. 40. The nuclei of the cells in the contrahentes layer (above) are distinctly different from the cells in the surrounding mesenchyme (below). Embryo 17 mm in C-R length, right hand, transverse section

not proceed in further differentiation (Fig. 40). No myofibrils were found in these elements by light microscopy.

In the radial half of the layer larger elements develop, differentiating already in embryos of about 20 mm into typical myoblasts of the adductor pollicis anlage and proceeding in further differentiation in the manner typical for muscle. This difference is also seen in the nerve supply. No innervation of the layer was found in the ulnar half.

Three parts of the contrahentes layer can be distinguished according to the cell pattern and to subsequent fate (i.e. according to the mode of development or of gradual changes and extinction):

The radial part of the layer, relatively bulky in the transverse section, represents the anlage of the future m. adductor pollicis (Figs. 36, 41, 55).

The ulnar part of the layer, situated medially to the previous one, extends in an ulnar and distal direction from the coursing ramus profundus nervi ulnaris; it projects distally in three, later only into two distinct slips (Fig. 55).

The proximal part of the layer, documented in previous communications (Čihák, 1963c, 1967a, b), extends from the proximal margin of the primordium

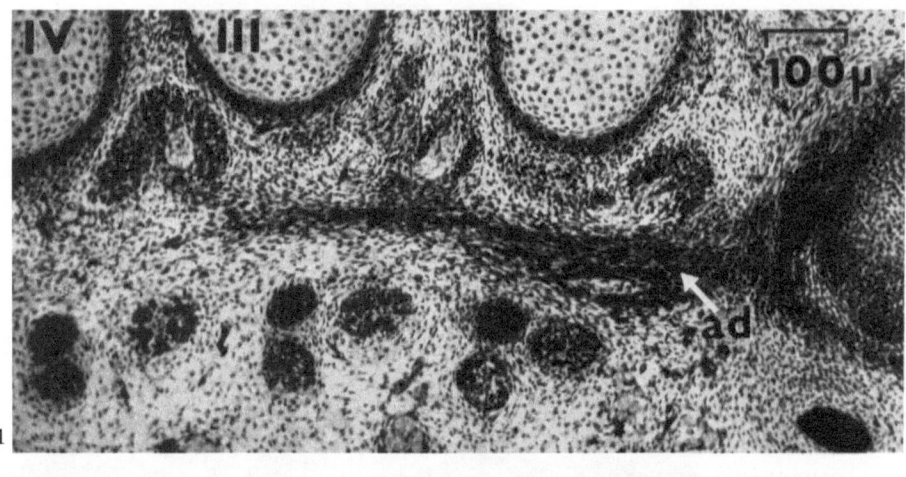

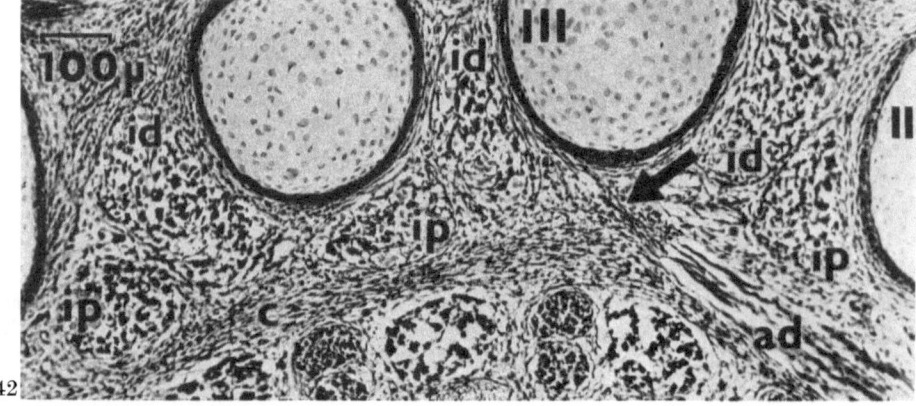

Fig. 41. Embryo 19 mm C-R length, left hand, tranverse section. The adductor pollicis (*ad*), differentiated in the radial part of the contrahentes layer, remains in this stage without contact of its origin with the metacarpals. Its insertion to the capsule of the metacarpophalangeal joint of the thumb is already formed (Čihák, 1967 b)

Fig. 42. Left hand of the embryo 32 mm C-R length, transverse section. The transiently denser contrahentes-plate (*c*) joins the adductor pollicis primordium (*ad*). The adductor (*ad*) is in this stage for the first time fixed to the 3rd metacarpal (*III*) — indicated by arrow; *id*, *ip* primordia of the dorsal and palmar interossei (Čihák, 1968 a)

up to the transverse course of the r. profundus nervi ulnaris through the palm and joins the radial part of the layer with the ulnar one (Fig. 55).

Each part of this layer develops further in its own manner:

The radial part of the layer gradually differentiates into the primordium of both heads of the adductor pollicis. It then undergoes all typical changes of the muscular primordium, from myoblasts to myotubes and toward muscle fibres. Two branches of the ulnar nerve end inside of this bulky muscle primordium, and accordingly, this primordium is divided into a superficial and deeper

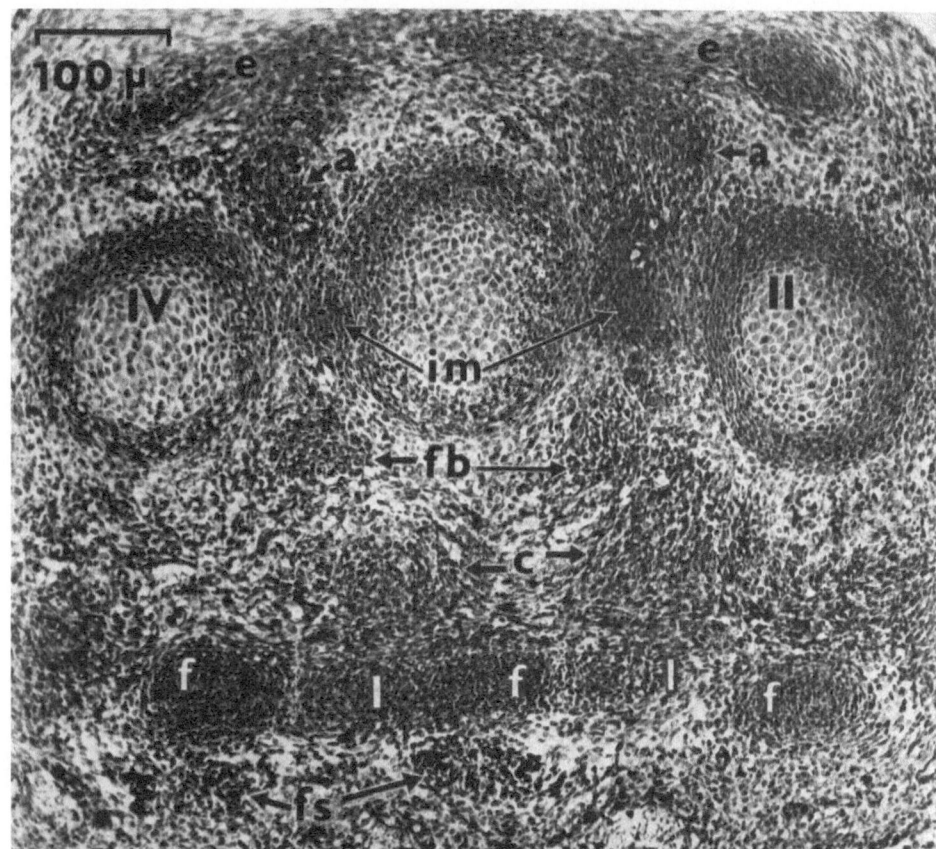

Fig. 43. Embryo 15.5 mm in C-R length, left hand, transverse section. In this stage all layers of primordia of the hand muscles are already differentiated; *fs* slips of the flexor digitorum superficialis to the fingers, *f* layer of tendons of the flexor digitorum profundus with lumbrical muscles (*l*), *c* the contrahentes layer; *fb* flexores breves profundi layer (the basal layer for the interossei); *im* layer of intermetacarpal primordia; *a* primordia of the interossei dorsales accessorii; *e* the layer of extensor tendons (Čihák, 1968a)

sector which then differentiate into the transverse and the oblique heads of the adductor pollicis. In earlier embryonic stages the two muscle components are still not joined by their origins to the metacarpal primordia (Fig. 41), being even far distant from the metacarpals. Their joining up with the skeleton occurs secondarily after reaching 32 mm of C-R length (Fig. 42). On the other hand, the insertion of the adductor pollicis is fixed to the perichondrium of the first metacarpal end and to the developing capsule of the thumb metacarpophalangeal joint already from 19 mm embryos (Fig. 41).

The ulnar part of the layer in younger embryos is still compact and to a variable extent distal to the ulnar nerve (Fig. 55). The future distal slips lie on the layer in the form of distally projecting tubercles (Fig. 46). These are quite thick in embryos between 14 and 17 mm in C-R length (Figs. 34, 43, 44, 45).

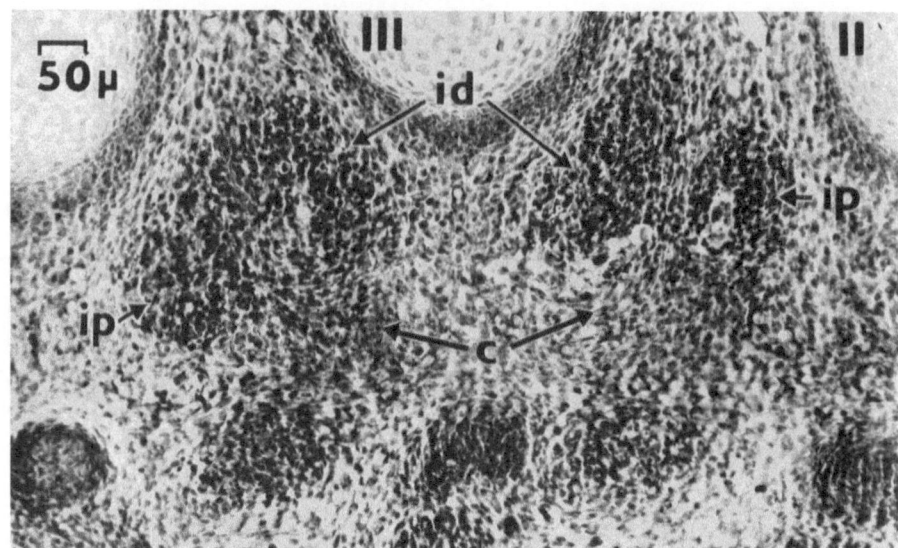

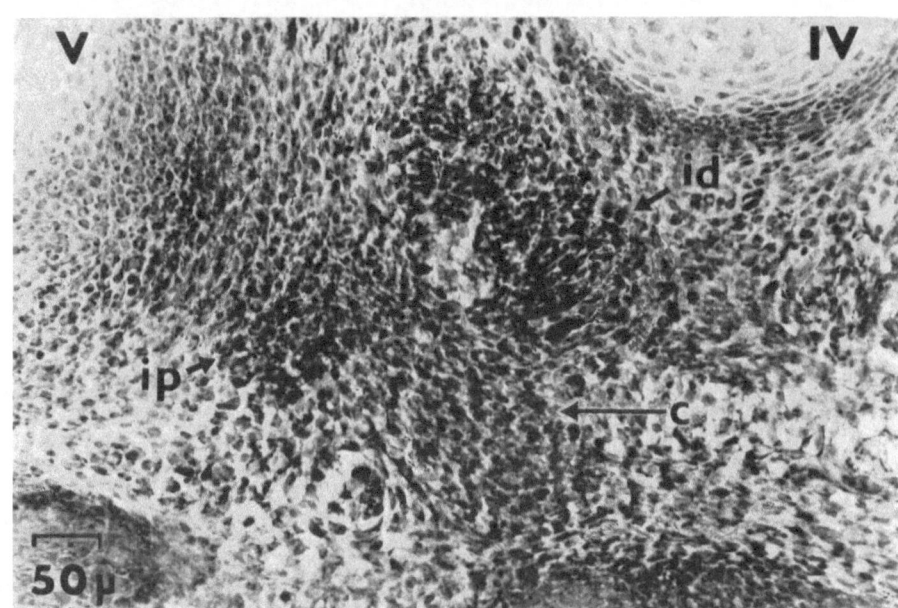

Fig. 44. Left hand of the 16.5 mm embryo, transverse section. The interossei primordia in the 2nd and 3rd intermetacarpal spaces start to differentiate into the palmar and dorsal interossei (*ip*, *id*); between the palmar and dorsal interosseus of the space the strip-like residua of the contrahentes layer (*c*) attach (Čihák, 1968a)

Fig. 45. The detail from another section of the same series as in Fig. 44. The relatively bulky strip-like residuum of the ulnar part of the contrahentes layer (*c*) is attached between the primordia of the dorsal (*id*) and palmar interosseus (*ip*) in the 4th intermetacarpal space (Čihák, 1968a)

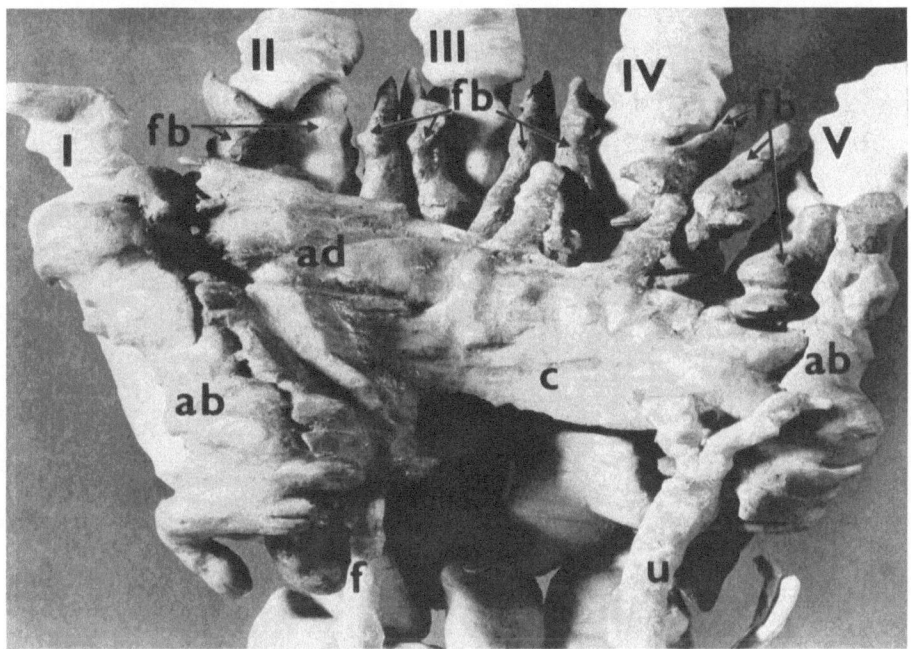

Fig. 46. Reconstruction of the contrahentes layer (c) of the embryo 21 mm C-R length. The radial part of the layer represents the future adductor pollicis (ad) the ulnar part projects into strips to beneath the intermetacarpal spaces (3rd and 4th); fb couples of twins of flexores breves profundi primordia in the intermetacarpal spaces; I–V skeleton of fingers; ab abductor pollicis brevis and abductor digiti minimi; f tendon of the flexor pollicis longus; u ulnar nerve

In agreement with these indicated tubercles the ulnar part of the layer disintegrates in the meantime into longitudinal slips, which in smaller embryos fade out gradually in the distal direction. In distal parts of intermetacarpal spaces these slips are interposed between the primordia of lumbrical muscles and of the interossei so closely that a dense nonseparated material appears in the intermetacarpal spaces (in the 4th, 3rd and distal to the adductor anlage also often in the 2nd space). This material is composed of the primordium of the lumbricalis, the slip of the contrahentes layer and of both interossei primordia and of the dorsal material of the dorsal interosseus (Fig. 47). The condensation of the material from all these layers into the distal sector of the intermetacarpal space furnishes evidence of the unfinished differentiation of layers proceeding in a proximodistal direction. In older embryos the slips, into which the ulnar part of the layer disintegrates, are more clearly contoured. The entire ulnar layer part, coherent (Figs. 44, 46, 48, 55) or already disintegrated into slips (seen in transverse section as condensations of cells — Figs. 45, 55), obtains a slender junction with the interossei primordia (Fig. 49). The fragments of the contrahentes layer are seen in transverse sections attached by a stalk (Fig. 49) between the primordia of the two interossei of the relevant intermetacarpal space. The whole complex (together with the interossei primordia) has the form of a leaf

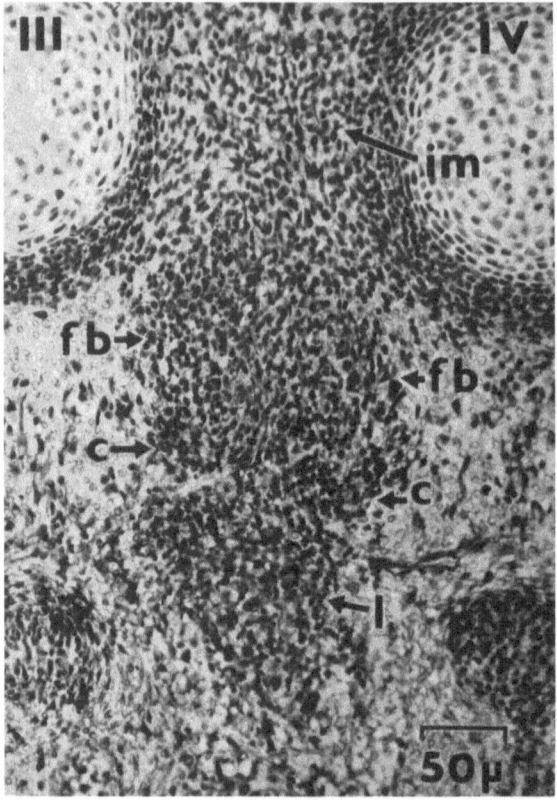

Fig. 47. Right hand of the 19.5 mm embryo, transverse section. The material from various
layers of primordia is condensed beneath distal sectors of intermetacarpal spaces. The material
from the lumbricalis primordium (*l*) from the contrahentes layer (*c*) from the layer of flexores
breves profundi (*fb*) and from the layer of intermetacarpal primordia (*im*) is contained
(Čihák, 1968a)

with branch and a stalk in transverse section, or it may be compared to the form
of the spade in playing cards (Figs. 48, 49, 54). The parts of the material remaining at the sides of the stalk join the palmar surface of the interossei, the stalk
itself is attached to the mesenchyme between the two primordia of the interossei
(Figs. 49, 50).

This described situation is well visible in embryos between 18 and 25 mm
in C-R length. The level of differentiation of the ulnar part of the layer attains
at first the stage of premyoblasts which, however, differ from the cells of surrounding mesenchyme by the form of nuclei (Fig. 40) but do not continue in
further development (Čihák, 1967b). Later, from about 25 mm C-R length
onward, the cell nuclei lose their specific form, more resembling fibroblasts both
in the strip-like residua of the ulnar layer part (Figs. 50, 51) and in the residual,
transversely oriented proximal part. After this stage (from about 27 mm in C-R
length) the strips fuse definitively with and between the interossei primordia.

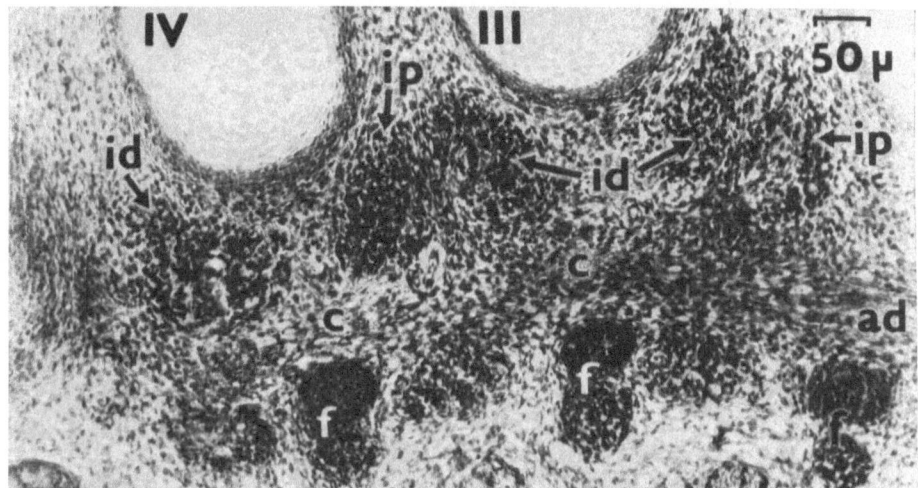

Fig. 48. Left hand of the embryo 16 mm in C-R length, transverse section. The contrahentes layer (c) is continuous but is already fixed between the primordia of the interossei of the 2nd to 4th intermetacarpal spaces; *id* dorsal interossei primordia; *ip* primordia of palmar interossei; *f* tendons of the flexor digitorum superficialis and profundus. The contrahentes layer continues radiad into the adductor pollicis (*ad*). (Čihák, 1968a)

From 27 mm C-R length onward the residua of the ulnar part of the layer—i. e. the strips coursing distal from the ulnar nerve—adjoin the interossei primordia more closely. The contact of the interosseus anlage with the rudiment of the contrahentes layer is best seen in a sagittal section: the rudiment of the contrahentes layer is impressed into the interosseus anlage, the stream of its cells is at first directed distally; it then suddenly turns toward the palm and fades out (Fig. 52). This pattern of the ulnar part of the contrahentes layer is the last one seen, in embryos between 28 and 32 mm. From this stage onward this layer can no longer be followed.

The described splitting of the ulnar layer part into strips extends transiently also into *the proximal part of the layer* which disintegrates and loosens. This situation is maintained up to 27 mm of C-R embryo length. Later on the proximal part of the layer again appears more strikingly. It appears anew as a mesenchymal plate in its typical position, but more compact, than it was before attaining 28 mm of C-R length. No premyoblasts are found, only the early connective tissue is present. The plate has the form and position of a "contrahent-plate" joined to the adductor pollicis, known in comparative anatomy as constant in anthropoid apes. It appears after the C-R length of 28 mm and disappears after reaching 32—35 mm (Fig. 42). In embryos from 35 mm onward only a loose mesenchyme is found in place of the contrahentes plate, without any trace or even rudiments of the contrahentes layer. The loose mesenchyme remaining in place of the contrahentes layer indicates the site of the future deep palmar fascia which has yet to be differentiated in embryos about 50 mm in C-R length.

Besides the observed process of extinction of the contrahentes layer other formations and their changes may be followed in the neighbourhood of contra-

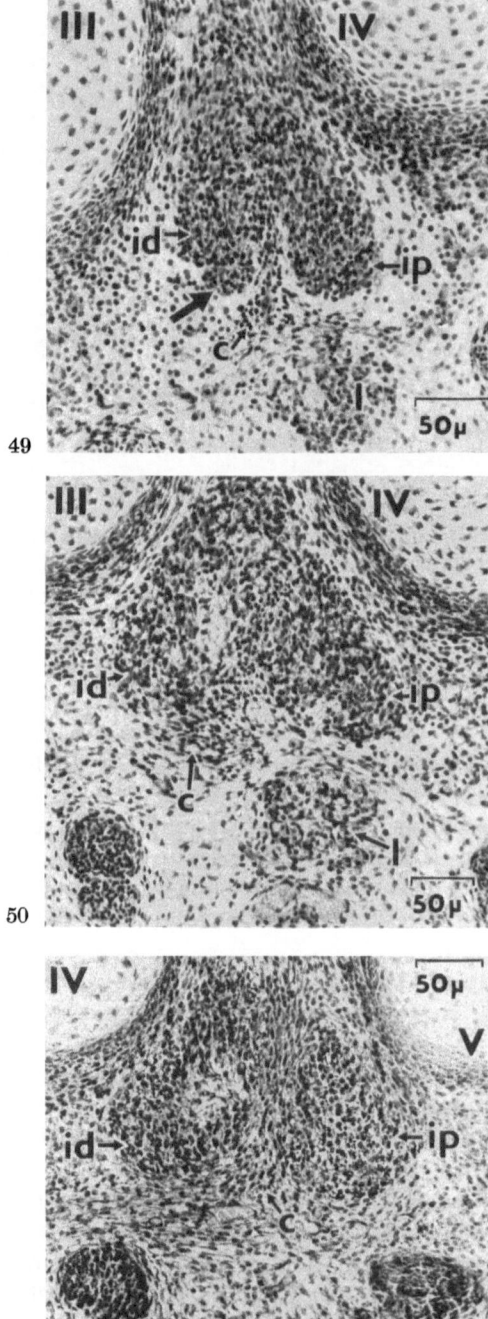

49

50

51

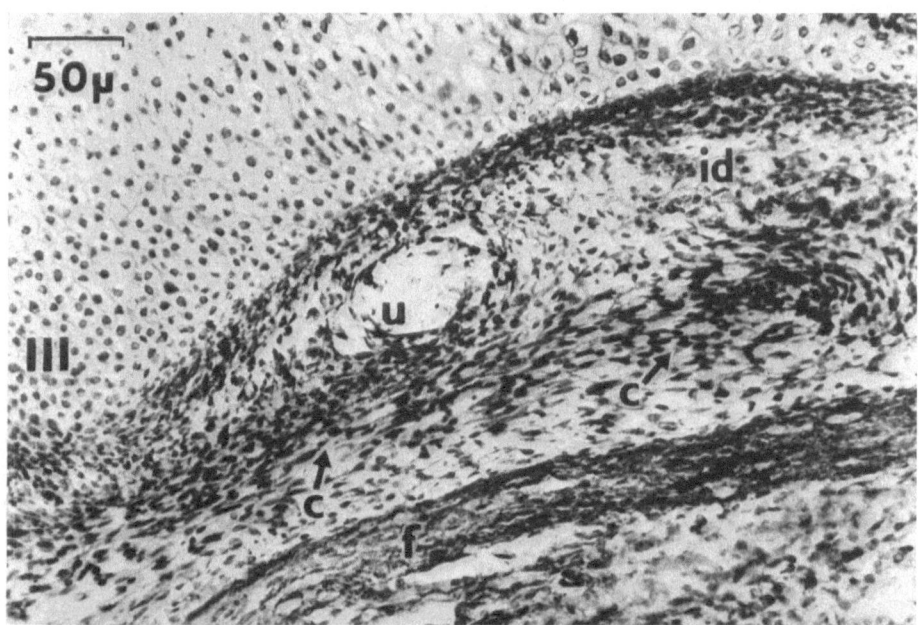

Fig. 52. Right hand of the embryo 28 mm C-R length, sagittal section (dorsal side above, distal direction to the right). The residuum of the contrahentes strip is fixed to the interosseus anlage; *III* third metacarpal; *id* dorsal interosseus of the third intermetacarpal space; *u* ulnar nerve; *c* contrahens; *f* anlage of the flexor digitorum profundus tendon for the 3rd finger. (Čihák, 1968a)

hentes rudiments. In embryos from 17 mm C-R length onward the residua of the ulnar part of the layer are pressed in between the corresponding lumbrical muscle and the mesenchyme by which the primordia of the palmar and dorsal interosseus of one intermetacarpal space are separated. It is in the region where the lumbricalis elongates in a palmo-dorsal direction and courses between the two interossei. The residuum of the contrahentes slip hence represents a sagittal junction between the lumbricalis and the mesenchyme interposed between the

Fig. 49. Embryo 18 mm C-R length, right hand, third intermetacarpal space in transverse section. The residuum of the contrahentes layer (*c*) is fixed between the primordia of the dorsal and palmar interosseus (*id, ip*) in form of a slender stalk. The arrow indicates the material of the contrahentes layer joining the interosseus primordium; *l* lumbricalis muscle. (Čihák, 1968a)

Fig. 50. Right hand of the embryo 23 mm in C-R length, transverse section, 3rd intermetacarpal space. The residuum of the contrahentes layer (*c*) joins partly the interosseus dorsalis primordium, partly passes into the mesenchyme between the two interossei primordia; *l* the lumbricalis. (Čihák, 1968a)

Fig. 51. Right hand of the 27 mm embryo, transverse section. The contrahentes residuum (*c*) fixed between the interossei primordia is formed now only by cells of the primitive connective tissue. (Čihák, 1968a)

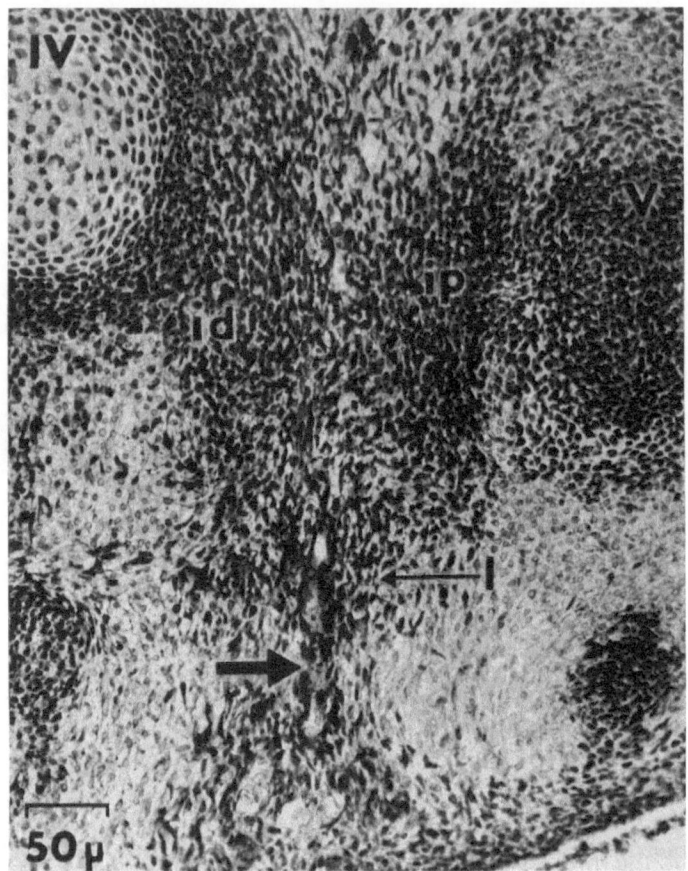

Fig. 53. Right hand of the 19.5 mm embryo, transverse section. The arrow indicates a mesen-chymal strip containing the blood vessel, passing from the subcutaneous region (from the digital vessels and nerves) to the lumbricalis primordium (*l*) which joined the contrahens rudiment and together with it the interossei primordia. 4th intermetacarpal space. (Čihák, 1968a)

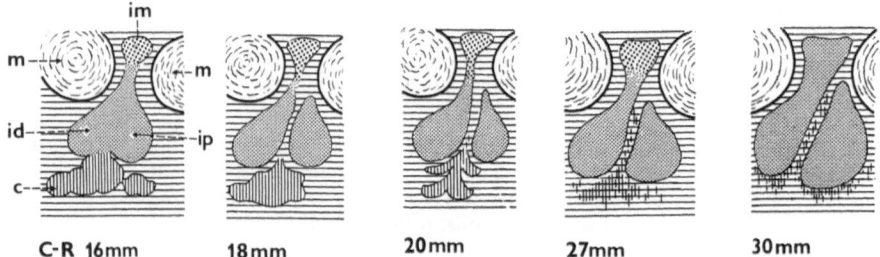

Fig. 54. Scheme of gradual extinction of the strip-like residuum of the contrahentes layer and of its fusion with the primordia of the interossei. Abbreviations same as in the micro-photographs; *m* metacarpals

two primordia of the interossei. This mesenchyme and later the connective tissue obliquely inserted between the two interossei is known as the "cloison oblique" of French authors. (Testut and Latarjet, 1948.) Concurrently, at the level of metacarpal heads a similar sagittally situated strip differentiates in the superficial mesenchyme and contains a perforating blood vessel and a nerve branch passing into the depth (Fig. 53). This strip has no relation to the palmar aponeurosis since this is not yet developed. The superficial strips of mesenchyme together with the distal ends of the rudimentary contrahentes slips—both joined to the lumbricalis anlage and between the two interossei primordia of the corresponding space—are in fact the first indications of sagittal septa developing inside the palm. They still end between the interossei, inside the "cloisons obliques". Later, between 40 and 60 mm of C-R length the "cloisons obliques" diminish and lose their importance. In the meantime new septa are formed by connective tissue coursing through intermetacarpal spaces in a dorso-palmar direction, between the lateral surfaces of the metacarpals and the interossei—the so-called "fibres perforantes" (Legueu and Juvara, 1892; Testut and Latarjet, 1948), or the "cloisons sagittales" (Paturet, 1951). These bundles do not link up in their development with the formations observed before which were connected with the disappearing ulnar part of the contrahentes layer. The "cloisons sagittales" ("fibres perforantes") appear as late as in embryos of 50 mm and are not seen well developed before 75 mm of C-R length.

4. Discussion and Conclusions from Observations of Ontogenesis of the Contrahentes Layer in the Human Hand

The contrahentes layer of the human embryonic hand may be considered to be a formation which appears transiently in the course of human ontogenesis according to the recapitulation rule. The development of this primordial layer culminates in human embryos between 19 and 28 mm in C-R length.

The mode of extinction of the layer and the complexity of this process cannot be fully reviewed from the phylogenetic standpoint, since there is no comparative material in which the process of extinction of this layer can be followed. In Primates up to the Cercopithecoids the contrahentes are well developed (Jouffroy and Lessertisseur, 1959; Jouffroy, 1962). In Anthropoid apes a well developed adductor pollicis occurs, the ulnar layer part being transformed into a contrahentes-plate ("Contrahentesplatte" — Forster, 1916). This situation is still found in older embryos (28—35 mm in length), and the temporary occurrence of this plate in the human embryo may be considered a recapitulation of a phylogenetically more ancient structure.

According to their form and course in embryos the strip-like contrahentes layer residua in the third and fourth intermetacarpal spaces may be taken to be the homology of the contrahentes III and IV of Marsupials, Insectivores and lower Primates. The less developed residuum appearing in the distal sector of the second space (distal to the adductor pollicis anlage) probably corresponds with the distal remnants of the contrahens II, the main part of which is taken into the adductor pollicis primordium. The adductor probably corresponds to

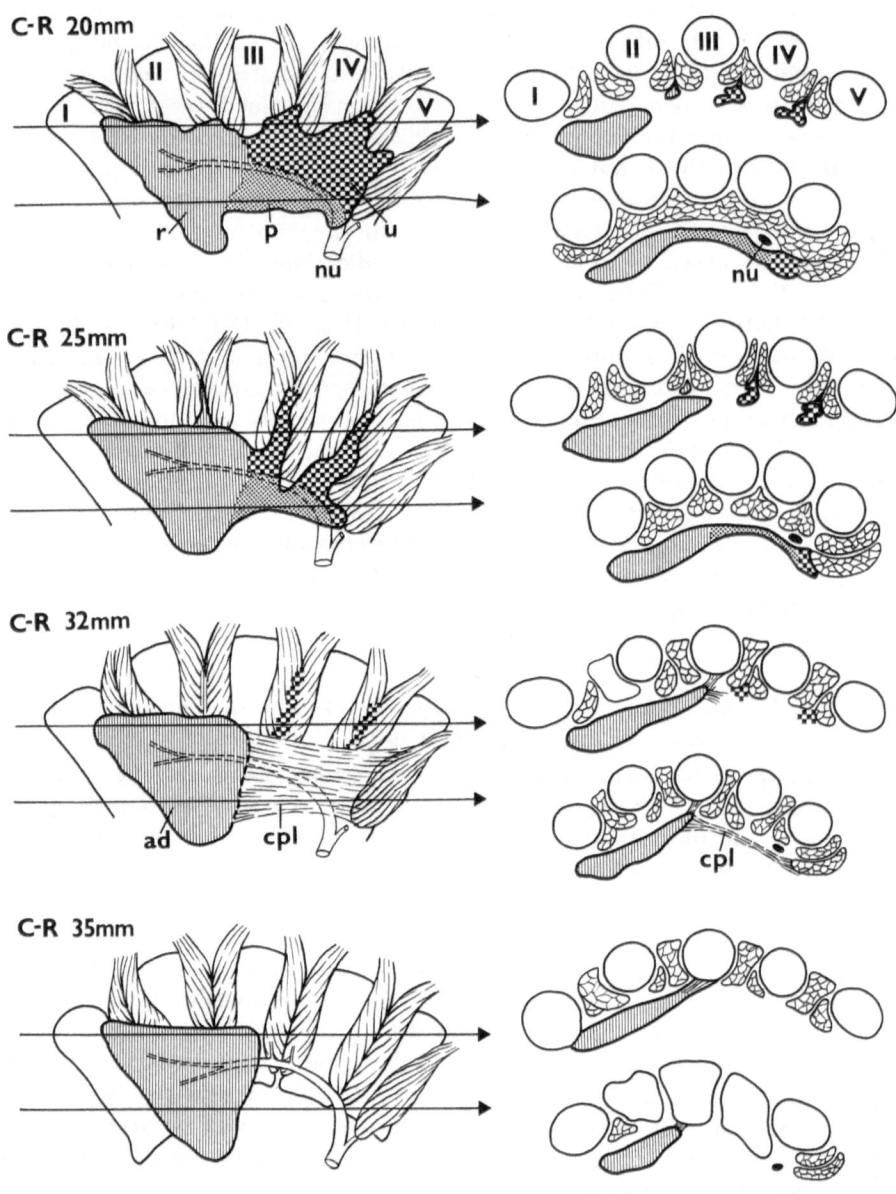

Fig. 55. Scheme of maximal extent of the contrahentes layer and of its subsequent changes up to the extinction. Schemes of transverse sections indicate the differences in shape of this layer seen in histological series of various stages and the differences seen at various levels of the same hand; *I–V* the metacarpals; *r* radial part of the contrahentes layer; *u* ulnar part of the contrahentes layer; *p* proximal part of the contrahentes layer; *nu* ulnar nerve; *ad* the differentiated adductor pollicis primordium; *cpl* the contrahentes plate; between the metacarpals the twins of the interossei primordia (flexores breves profundi layer) are visible

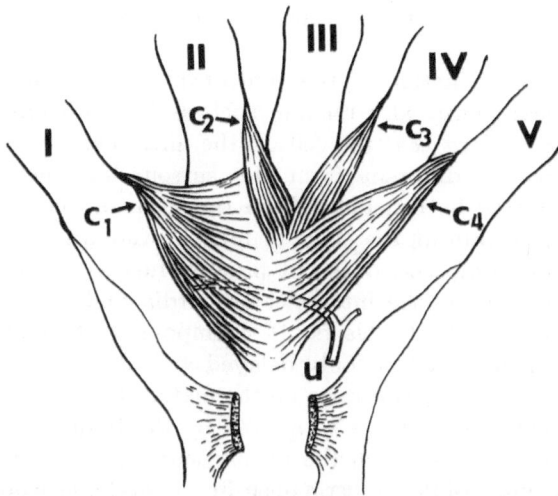

Fig. 56. Scheme of typical pattern of the contrahentes layer in the mammalian hand; left hand, palmar aspect; I, V first and fifth finger; u ulnar nerve; c_{1-4} the contrahentes muscles I–IV (for the 1st, 2nd, 4th and 5th finger). (According to Čihák, 1968a)

the first contrahens and to a greater part of the second (not to one or to three contrahentes, as claimed in the literature — Gräfenberg, 1905/06; Ribbing, 1938).

In lower Mammals the contrahentes are mostly well developed in Marsupials (Fig. 56). According to Forster (1916) they are not found in the hand of Mono-tremes. Kajava (1911), who minutely observed the intrinsic muscles of the Monotreme hand, also did not mention these muscles. In the Insectivores this layer is found well developed but contains only three muscles in the Centetidae, Solenodontidae and Potamogalidae (Dobson, 1882; Leche, 1900). A similar situation is found in the transitional group to the Primates, in the Tupaiidae (Carlsson, 1922; Clark, 1924, 1926). In other Insectivores this layer is either reduced or absent altogether, e.g. in the Erinaceidae, Talpidae (Dobson, 1882; Leche, 1900; Forster, 1916). Because these muscles are well developed in Marsu-pials and also in most other mammalian orders, their absence in some Insecti-vores remains an unclear point. According to Cunningham (1882) the trend of the contrahentes layer is to recede towards marginal fingers or to be reduced into an aponeurosis. However, the fact that in Erinaceus the contrahentes are absent but the deeper flexores breves profundi are found perforated by the coursing deep palmar branch of the ulnar nerve (Čihák, 1960b, 1963b) suggests that there may be some traces of the extinct layer. This phylogenetically interest-ing point deserves further attention. It is also of interest that Trnková and Dylevský (1969), when revising the arrangement of hand musculature of the rat in connection with the above question, demonstrated the existence of three contrahentes muscles in opposition to the literature. In the hand of the rat in the course of ontogenesis a contrahentes layer of complete extent is formed, being much thinner in place of one absent muscle, and during subsequent development single contrahentes muscles separate; the layer in place of the absent muscle fades out.

In the course of extinction of the contrahentes layer during human onto-genesis some unclear points also remain, such as the differentiation of cells in the blastema. It is evident that the cells of the ulnar part of the well developed contrahentes layer are different from the surrounding mesenchyme (Čihák, 1967b, 1969c). As may be concluded from the form of nuclei, the cells of the contrahentes layer remain at the stage of initial differentiation into myoblasts. Their differentiation, however, does not proceed further. In the meantime the material of the layer joins the interossei primordia and later a plate appears, composed only of typical fibroblasts. It is impossible to distinguish whether the development of myoblasts is only delayed and then continued after fusion with the interossei, or on the contrary, all the material is replaced by fibroblasts. The former possibility seems to be supported by the frequent finding of muscle strips covering the ulnar nerve on the palmar surface of the interossei in adult hands. It was also impossible to distinguish in our material whether the residua of the contrahentes layer after fusion with the interossei primordia became parts of the perimysium or of the contractile tissue. No striking signs of the cell death were found by light microscopy in the contrahentes layer.

The residua of the contrahentes layer may be manifested in man in form of muscle variations. Flower and Murie (1867) described a muscle shaped as an adductor of the 5th finger in the hand of a Bushwoman; it was evidently the persisting m. contrahens IV. Le Double (1897) also knew this muscle and denoted it the "tenseur d'articulation métacarpo-phalangienne du petit doigt".

It may be concluded from the observation of the extinction of the contra-hentes layer during ontogenesis that the ligamentum metacarpeum transversum profundum does not develop from this layer, as supposed by Forster (1916). Raven (1936) also admitted that the distal margin of the transverse head of the adductor hallucis corresponds in its position to these ligaments. Jouffroy and Lessertisseur (1959) accepted Forster's view and drew attention to the reci-procal relation of the fading out contrahentes layer on one side and the appear-ing transverse ligamentous strip on the other. Against this concept stands the fact that in Prosimians the full set of contrahentes muscles normally exists together with the ligaments between metacarpal heads. It may be stated that neither the components of tendon sheaths nor the ligamentum metacarpeum trans-versum profundum develop from the rudiments of the contrahentes layer, nor do these rudiments join the lumbrical muscles of the hand, as could be supposed from the spatial relation of these primordia in younger embryos. The observa-tions also reveal that the development of the so-called "cloisons sagittales" of French authors bears no relation to the extinction of the contrahentes layer and that the "cloisons" contain none of the extinct structures of the layer, no contra-hentes rudiment.

The development and early extinction of the mm. contrahentes of the human hand as a transiently differentiating layer of embryonic muscle primordia provi-des evidence of the conservative manner of hand development and a perfect example of an ontogenetic recapitulation of a pattern extinct in course of the phylogenetic past.

5. Recapitulation of Observations on the Ontogenesis of the Contrahentes Layer in the Human Hand

The contrahentes layer in Mammals is situated between the flexor tendons and the deep palmar branch of the ulnar nerve. The complete layer is absent in adults; in the course of ontogenesis it develops to an extent similar to that in lower Mammals. The layer originates before reaching 14 mm of C-R length of the embryo. Observations revealed the following:

1. A radial, ulnar and proximal part can be distinguished in the developing layer of the contrahentes blastema. Each of them proceeds in an own manner during ontogenesis.

2. The radial part gradually differentiates into the adductor pollicis.

3. The ulnar part, extending distal and ulnar to the course of the ulnar nerve through the palm, disintegrates between 20 and 25 mm of embryo length into longitudinal strips gradually joining the interossei primordia and the mesenchyme situated between them (in the corresponding intermetacarpal space).

4. The reduction and fusion of strips of the ulnar part proceeds in the form changes over a stalk-shaped residuum (in transverse section) fixed between and to the interossei primordia. The contrahentes residua fade out definitively after reaching 28 mm of C-R length.

5. The proximal part of the layer, which joins the radial and ulnar parts proximally to the coursing ulnar nerve, fragments at first similar to the ulnar part; before extinction it still transiently strengthens into a plate similar to the so-called "contrahent-plate" of anthropoid apes. It then fades out concurrently with the ulnar part.

6. The adductor pollicis is homologous with the first contrahens muscle and with the major part of the second one. The residuum in the 2nd intermetacarpal space corresponds to the remnants of the m. contrahens II. The residua of the ulnar part of the layer are homologous with the mm. contrahentes III and IV.

7. The transient occurrence of the complete contrahentes layer during ontogenesis of the human hand manifests a developmental recapitulation of a form developed and extinct in the course of the phylogenetic past.

6. The Layer of Mm. Contrahentes during the Ontogenesis of the Human Foot

It was in the planta pedis where Halford (1863) for the first time employed the term mm. contrahentes for the muscular layer situated in some Primates between the tendons of the long toe flexors and the course of the ramus profundus nervi plantaris lateralis. Comparative studies all showed that this muscle layer was a constant component of the musculature of the sole as well as of the palm (Ruge, 1878a, b; Cunningham, 1878a, b, 1882; Young, 1880; Brooks, 1886; Primrose, 1889; Bardeleben, 1890; Thane, 1892; Leche, 1900; Ribbing, 1909, 1938; Forster, 1916; Stjernman, 1932; Keith, 1949; Howell, 1936; Campbell, 1939; Jouffroy, 1962). Bardeleben's general classification of muscle layers in the mammalian autopodium (1890), which we accept in general features, was held as universally applicable to the hand and foot. The views of previous authors concerning homologies of muscles and muscle layers were also projected generally for the autopodium of the upper and lower extremities.

Therefore all previous findings in the ontogenesis of hand muscles are correlated with the course of development of the human foot; the justification of the generally accepted serial homology of upper and lower extremities will be reconsidered on the basis of this comparison. From the morphological standpoint it is interesting to compare the development of the contrahentes layer in the human hand and foot, especially because the human foot is very specialised in its morphology and function.

The question, therefore, arises, as to whether and in what manner the contrahentes layer develops as a primitive structure within such a specialised organ as the human foot. An attempt to find the embryonic layer from which the human adductor hallucis differentiates and to compare it with the ontogenesis of the contrahentes layer of the hand will hence be made. The different pattern of the adductor pollicis and adductor hallucis intensifies interest in a comparison of the development of both.

7. Material for Studies of Development of the Mm. Contrahentes of the Human Foot

The development and the transformations of muscle primordia in the layer between the tendons of long finger flexors and the course of the ramus profundus nervi plantaris lateralis were studied in histological series of 70 feet of human embryos and foetuses from 12 to 60 mm in crown-rump length. Most series were cut transversely, since transverse sections offer the best possibility of following muscle layers; five series were cut sagittally for control. The C-R lengths of the employed embryos were: 12 mm, 13, 14, 15, 15.5 (2 feet), 16 (3), 16.5 (3), 17 (5), 17.5 (2), 18 (3), 19 (2), 20 (3), 21 (4), 22 (2), 23 (2), 24 (2), 25 (2), 26 (2), 27 (2), 28 (2), 29 (2), 30 (3), 31 (2), 32 (2), 33 (2), 34 (2), 35 (2), 36, 37, 38, 40 (2), 46 (2), 54 (2), 60 mm.

The staining of histological series is described on pp. 10 and 11. The observations of the contrahentes layer of the foot are compared with corresponding developmental stages in the embryonic human hand. The comparative data of the contrahentes layer in Mammals are quoted from the literature.

8. Observations of the Development and Changes in the Contrahentes Layer during the Ontogenesis of the Human Foot

It has been possible to find and to specify in the human foot all layers of essential and accessory blastemas of the intrinsic muscles described in the embryonic human hand (cf. Čihák, 1963 b, c, 1967 a, b, 1968 a, b, 1969 a, c). Accordingly between the layer of flexor tendons and the deep branch of the lateral plantar nerve a layer of mesenchymal and later muscular blastemas is found, in the same situation as the contrahentes layer in the hand. This layer is, therefore, termed *the contrahentes layer* in accordance with that of the hand. The layer conforms to that of the hand only in its general position; it differs from the contrahentes layer both in its general form, its development and its differentiating components.

In embryos up to 17 mm in C-R length intrinsic muscles of the foot are very poorly differentiated. Although the primordia of the tarsal skeleton are already in the prochondral stage and the metatarsals are undergoing chondrification, the intrinsic muscular layers are quite indistinct. Only the layer of long flexor tendons is visible in transverse section as a darkly stained dense cellular strip which is a point of orientation for the position of other muscle layers. Only after reaching 17 mm C-R length of the embryo do the blastemas of future muscle layers and of some typical ligaments start to be visible. Thus there is a certain delay as compared with the hand, visible in all the further development, up to the stages when muscle primordia become attached to the skeleton. (A similar delay of the foot in comparison with the hand has also been ascertained in the course of development of the skeleton.)

In the 17 mm long embryo the primordium of the ligamentum plantare longum can be distinguished beneath the calcaneus. Just distal to crossing the primordium of the peroneus longus tendon, the primordium of the ligament passes into a broader layer which comes into contact with the tibially turning deep branch of the lateral plantar nerve. This is the contrahentes layer. At the level of the metacarpal bases this layer is quite thick, more bulky than that of the hand (Fig. 57). On the fibular side, the layer starts from the m. abductor digiti minimi primordium and extends in a tibial direction; on transverse section the layer is slightly vaulted in its proximal part suggesting the future transverse arching of the foot. The ramus profundus nervi plantaris lateralis runs in the thickest part of the contrahentes layer between it and deeper blastemas. In the 17 mm embryos the contrahentes layer adheres very closely to the nerve (Fig. 58). This site also has a shape most similar to that of the embryonic human hand. The contrahentes layer extends in a tibial direction to come into contact with the elongated anlage of the m. flexor hallucis brevis.

From 18 mm C-R length onward there is a difference in the level of differentiation between the anlage of the flexor hallucis brevis and the contrahentes layer, the contrahentes layer being less differentiated. In 18 mm long embryos the material of the layer is concentrated rather to its tibial side, it can be well distinguished from the developing primordium of the long plantar ligament and acquires the shape of the oblique head of the adductor hallucis (Fig. 59). Further distal sections show only some distal residua of the layer on the plantar side of the deeper primordia of the 4th, 3rd and sometimes also of the 2nd intermetatarsal space; after a very short course the primordia of mm. lumbricales join these residua of the contrahentes layer from the plantar side (Fig. 61). The contrahentes layer is a long way from the intermetatarsal spaces due to the relatively plantar position of the primordia of the interossei (Fig. 59). In embryos of 17 and 18 mm C-R length no traces of the contrahentes layer are found in sections proceeding in a distal direction toward the metatarsal heads. At this stage also the primordium of the caput transversum of the adductor hallucis is not differentiated and at its site there is no evidence of denser mesenchyme nor any other suggestion of a future muscle anlage. The strip-like rudiments of the layer beneath the third and fourth intermetatarsal spaces are also quite short and not conspicuously formed. This is a significant difference from their conspicuous shape in the embryonic hand (Figs. 66, 67). Thus, the stage of 17 and 18 mm C-R length is characterized only by a basic differentiation of the contrahentes layer which is better differentiated in its external form and cytology at the site of the caput obliquum of the adductor hallucis and which in the fibular half extends distally beyond the course of the lateral plantar nerve only in the form of two rudimentary strips (Fig. 66).

In the stages between 20 and 24 mm of C-R length the contrahentes layer in the foot is already better differentiated. The cytologically well distinguished primordium of the oblique head of the adductor hallucis is joined to the less differentiated fibularly extending contrahentes layer (Fig. 59). As in the hand, it is thus possible to distinguish the tibial part of the layer developing typically into the oblique head of the adductor hallucis and the fibular part of the layer, less differentiated, extending distally and tibially to the course of the lateral plantar nerve (Figs. 59, 66). Between 20 and 24 mm of C-R length strip-like primordia appear in this fibular part beneath the primordia of muscles of the 4th and 3rd intermetatarsal spaces (Figs. 60–62). They are not so long and distinct as those of the embryonic hand but the basic resemblance in shape is striking

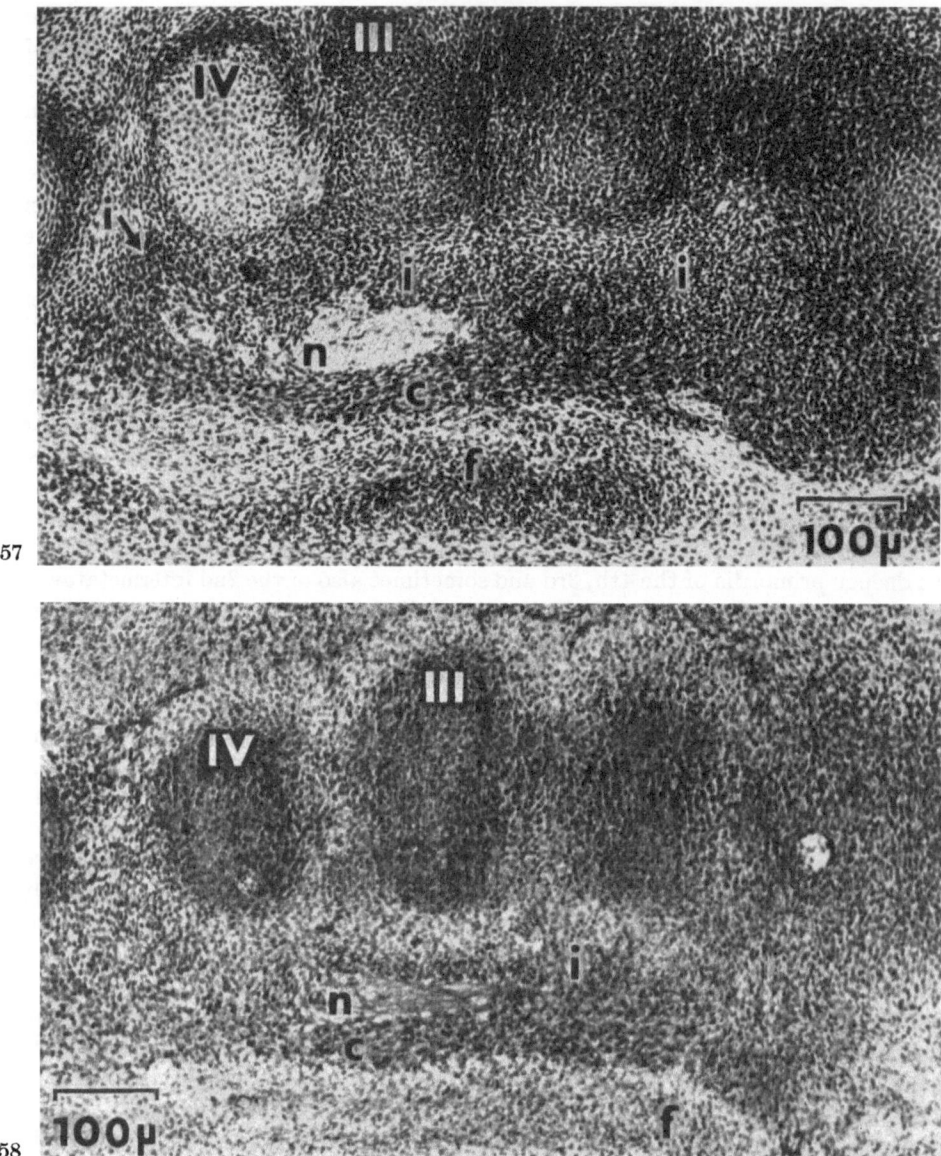

Fig. 57. Left foot of the embryo 17 mm in C-R length, transverse section. The contrahentes layer (c) is situated between the primordia of flexor digitorum longus tendons (f) and the course of the lateral plantar nerve (n); i material for the future interossei; III, IV the metatarsals. (Čihák, 1969 a)

Fig. 58. Left foot of another embryo of 17 mm, transverse section. The contrahentes layer (c) and the flexores breves profundi layer (for the future interossei) (i) closely adjoin the coursing lateral plantar nerve (n); III, IV metatarsals; f flexor tendons (primordia). (Čihák, 1969 a)

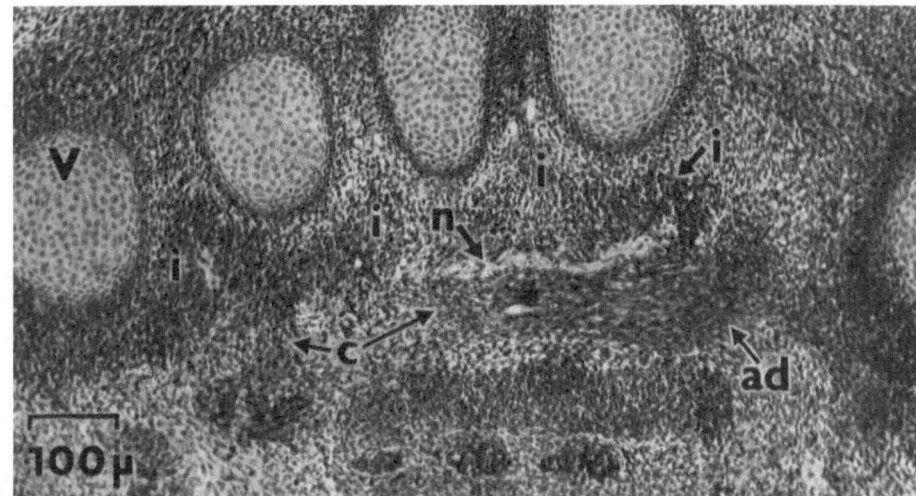

59

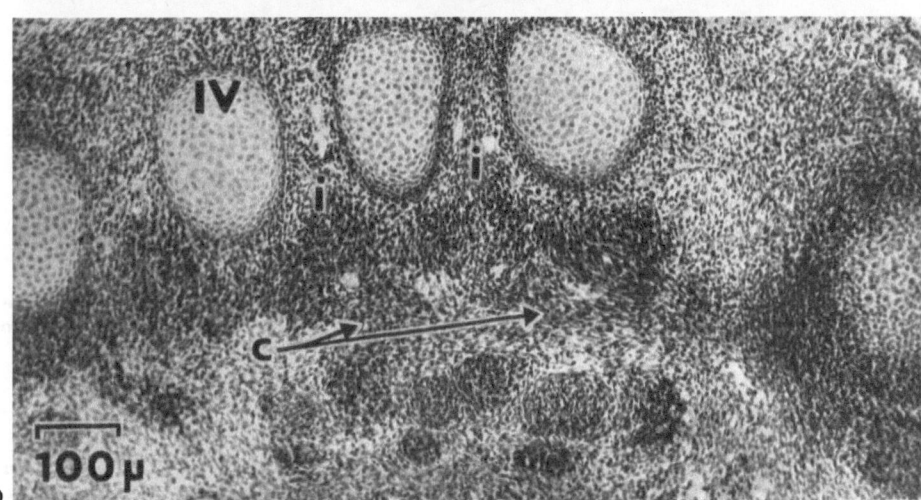

60

Fig. 59. Left foot of the embryo 20 mm in C-R length, transverse section. The tibial part of the contrahentes layer (c) develops into the adductor hallucis (ad), the fibular part remains in form of a non-differentiated mesenchyme. Beneath the interossei primordia (i) in the 4th intermetatarsal space a strip-like residuum of the layer is formed; n nervus plantaris lateralis. (Čihák, 1969a)

Fig. 60. Left foot of the embryo 20 mm in C-R length, same as in Fig. 59, sectioned more distally, transverse section. The contrahentes layer (c) is divided into strips beneath the intermetatarsal spaces; this pattern corresponds to the position of the contrahentes muscles in the foot of lower Mammals; i material for the future interossei. (Čihák, 1969a)

(Fig. 67). These strips become extinct during further development of the embryonic foot and fade out in the continuous mesenchymal sheet (Figs. 62, 66). During this period the strip-like residua also join between the interossei primordia,

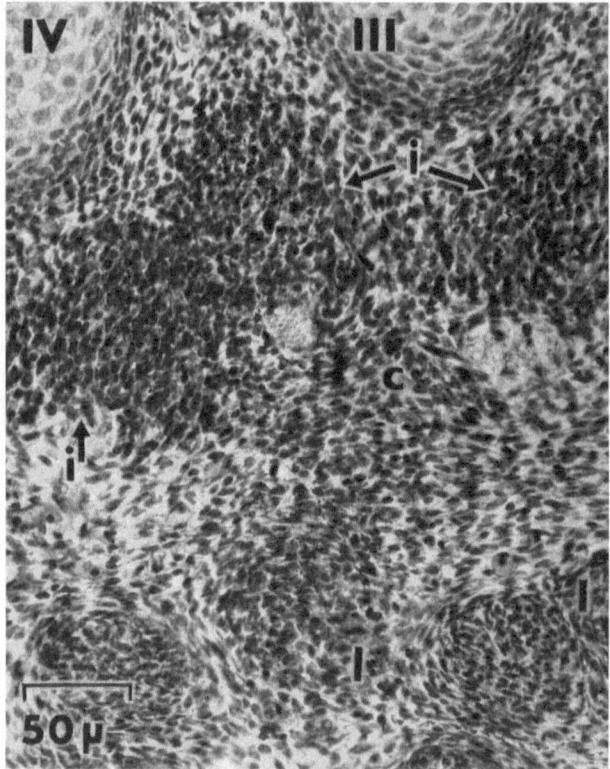

Fig. 61. The same section as in Fig. 60, detailed view of the primordia in the 3rd intermetatarsal space; *i* interossei primordia; *c* the strip of the contrahentes layer (corresponding to
the contrahens III—of the 4th digit); *l* lumbricalis primordia. (Čihák, 1969a)

as in the hand (Figs. 61, 62, 66). However, they do not fuse with the interossei
during subsequent development, remaining inside the mesenchymal sheet proper.

After extinction of the strip-like primordia in embryos ranging from 25 to
30 mm in C-R length the fibular part of the contrahentes layer is composed of
an equally distributed mesenchyme. It is distinguishable from the loose mesenchyme on its plantar side as well as from the more dense primordia of the interossei. Even at this stage the transverse head of the adductor hallucis is not yet
formed (Fig. 63).

Only after reaching 30 mm C-R length does the fibular part of the contrahentes layer start to differentiate (at the level of insertion of the oblique head of
the adductor to the thumb metatarsal) into the transversally situated bundles
of the future transverse head of the adductor hallucis (Fig. 64). During further
development this muscle component becomes still more distinct; the supplying
branch from the arch of the lateral plantar nerve entering distally into the
primordium is also visible (Fig. 64). Both the oblique and the transverse heads
of the adductor continue to be connected by mesenchyme which is a rudiment

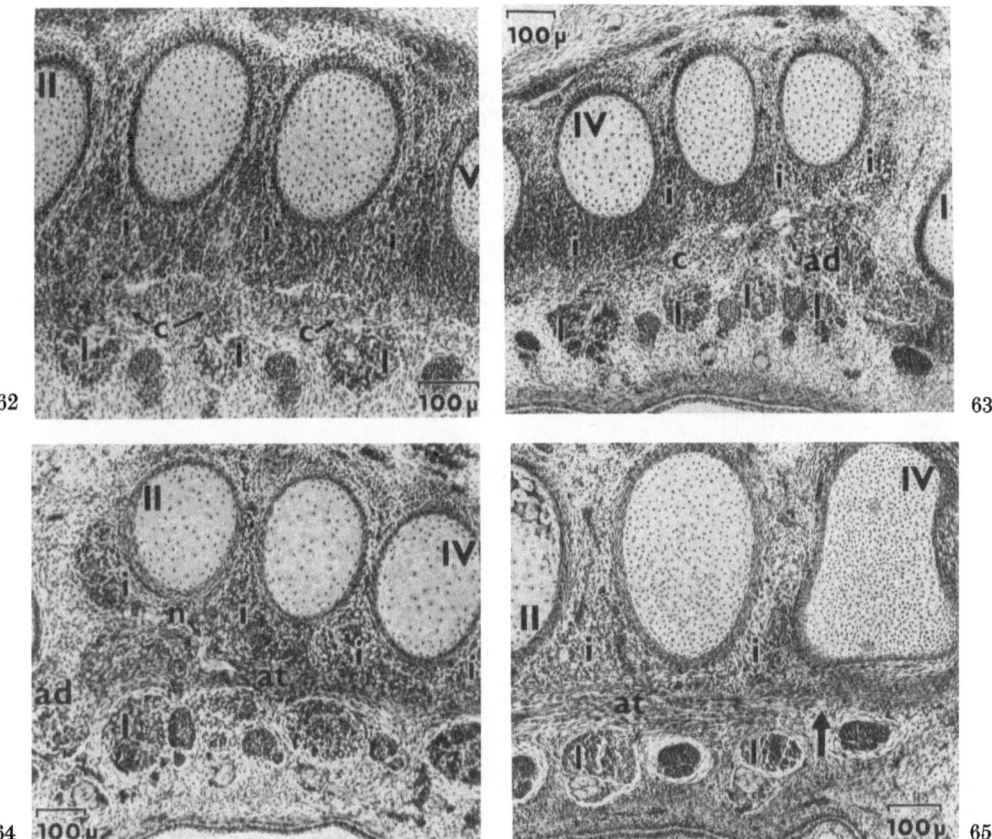

Fig. 62. Embryo of C-R length 24 mm, right foot, transverse section. The strip-like residua of the contrahentes layer (c) join transiently to and between the interossei primordia, similar to the hand. In this stage the contrahentes strips are connected by a continuous mesenchymal layer; in the fibular part of the contrahentes layer the strips soon disappear and the layer remains in form of the continuous mesenchymal sheet. (Čihák, 1969a)

Fig. 63. Left foot of the 28 mm embryo, transverse section. The tibial part of the contrahentes layer is formed as the caput obliquum of the adductor hallucis (ad), the fibular part (c) remains in form of a non-differentiated mesenchyme; the transverse head of the adductor is not yet formed; i the interossei primordia; I, IV the metatarsals. (Čihák, 1969a)

Fig. 64. Right foot of the embryo 30 mm in C-R length, transverse section. The caput transversum musculi adductoris hallucis is for the first time in this stage well formed in distal sectors of the contrahentes layer; II, IV metatarsals; ad oblique head of the adductor hallucis; at transverse head of the adductor hallucis; i interossei primordia; n supplying branch for the transverse adductor head coming from the lateral plantar nerve in a distal direction; l primordium of the first lumbricalis. (Čihák, 1969a)

Fig. 65. Right foot of the 54 mm embryo, transverse section. The arrow indicates the first joining of the adductor hallucis (transverse head) to the primordium of capsule of the metatarsophalangeal joint of the 4th finger; in this stage the primordium of this transverse adductor head is not yet fixed to the perichondrium of the metatarsals; II, IV metatarsals; i interossei primordia; at transverse head of the adductor. (Čihák, 1969a)

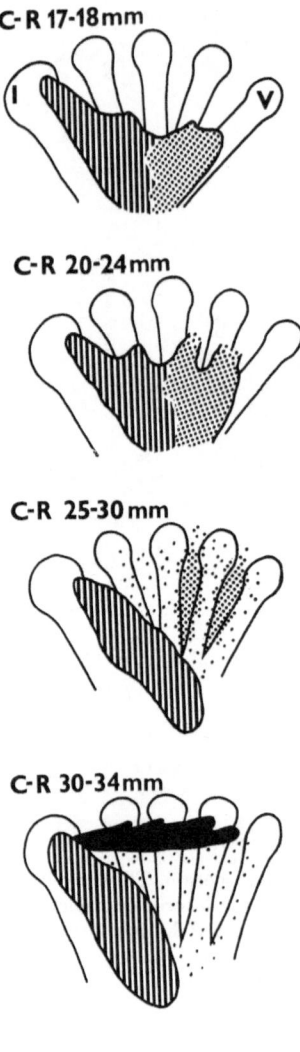

C-R 17-18mm

I   V

C-R 20-24mm

C-R 25-30mm

C-R 30-34mm

Fig. 66. Scheme of subsequent changes of shape of the contrahentes layer in the course of ontogenesis of the human foot. The differentiation of strips of the layer suggesting the four contrahentes muscles (the phylogenetically ancient pattern) is characteristic for younger stages. The extinction of strips, the change of the fibular part of the layer into the mesenchymal sheet and the secondary differentiation of the transverse head of the adductor is seen in later stages. The stages are outlined in approximately equal size, the tibial part of the contrahentes layer is shaded with vertical lines, the fibular part is dotted, transverse head of the adductor drawn in black. (According to Čihák, 1969a)

from the former wider contrahentes layer. The supplying nerve branches from the lateral plantar nerve enter the primordia of both heads of the adductor hallucis from the dorsal side; the supplying branch of the oblique head represents a terminal part of the nerve stem of the lateral plantar nerve, while a special twig branches off in the distal direction into the transverse head (Figs. 64, 108).

Even after 35 mm in C-R length the anlage of the transverse head was not yet attached to the skeleton; it remains a long way from the metatarsals, separated from them by the bulky primordia of the interossei. The attachment to the metatarsals occurs secondarily in embryos of 50 mm C-R. Even there the transverse head is not attached to the skeleton but only to the primordia of the capsules of the metatarsophalangeal joints (Fig. 65). The origin of the caput obliquum of the adductor hallucis on the skeleton is also secondary and develops at the same time. The only primary origin of the oblique head is on the anlage of the long plantar ligament.

In contrast to the development of the ulnar part of the contrahentes layer in the hand no steady development of strips of the fibular part of the contrahentes layer with their characteristic mode of extinction (which is so typical for the ontogenesis of hand muscles—Čihák, 1967b, 1968a, b, 1969c) can be found during the ontogenesis of the human foot. The two strips in the fibular part of the contrahentes layer also develop during the ontogenesis of the foot; they are not nearly as distinct as they are in the hand and they do not become extinct by joining the interossei. Although in slight contact with the interossei primordia (Fig. 62), these strips in the foot disappear gradually in the homogeneous fibular part of the contrahentes layer (Figs. 62, 63). In the distal part of this layer the caput transversum m. adductoris hallucis differentiates secondarily in another direction.

9. Discussion and Conclusions from Observations of the Ontogenesis of the Contrahentes Layer in the Human Foot

In comparative anatomy, the mm. contrahentes digitorum pedis are particularly well developed in Monotremes, Marsupials, Insectivores, Proimians, Platyrrhines and in some catarrhine monkeys (Dobson, 1882; Leche, 1900; Clark, 1924, 1926; Jouffroy and Lessertisseur, 1959; Jouffroy, 1962). In anthropoid apes the contrahentes muscles of the 2nd, 4th, and 5th toe (i.e. the m. contrahens II, III et IV) are greatly reduced. In Prosimians contrahens II is always the most reduced, being even absent in several species. There is a difference in size between the bulky first contrahens (contrahens hallucis) and the slender contrahentes of other digits in all Primates (Champneys, 1871/72; Langer, 1879; Hepburn, 1891/92; Kohlbrugge, 1897; Primrose, 1899; Leche, 1900; Straus jr., 1930; Jouffroy and Lessertisseur, 1959; Jouffroy, 1962).

It may be concluded from this comparison that the temporary appearance of the complete contrahentes layer during the ontogensis of the human foot can be considered a developmental recapitulation of a pattern typical in the phylogenetic past. This recapitulation of the layer during ontogenesis of the human foot proceeds in exact conformity with the pattern of these muscles in lower Primates and in lower Mammals in general. During ontogenesis there is a definite predominance of the tibial part (i.e. of the contrahens I—the future oblique head of the adductor hallucis). The part of the layer projecting to the 2nd toe is almost undeveloped; it fuses with the oblique head of the adductor. Only sometimes is its small rudiment visible. This pattern again resembles that in the Prosimians, where the thinnest or even absent muscle is that for the 2nd toe. The two rudimentary strip-like primordia in the fibular part of the layer are evidently homologous with the contrahens IV (adductor digiti minimi) and with the contrahens III (adductor digiti IV). These primordia, however, are transient and quite rudimentary, and soon disappear. The transverse head of the adductor hallucis first develops after these normal components of the layer corresponding to the normal set of contrahentes muscles of lower mammals have disappeared. A comparison with the foot of Prosimians demonstrates that the transverse head of the adductor is a secondary pattern which in Prosimians develops in addition to their full set of four normal contrahentes. It is, therefore, impossible to homologise this transverse head of the adductor hallucis with any of the four normal contrahentes. This difference between the caput transversum of the adductor and the mm. contrahentes of the foot was already noted by Brooks (1888) as distinguishing the adductor transversus from the "adductor opponens".

The development of this layer from the pattern in lower Primates to that in Man thus occurs by disappearance of the contrahens II, III et IV together with the secondary development of the transverse head of the adductor. Successive stages of this developmental process are maintained in Anthropoid apes. The ontogenesis of this layer in the human planta thus proceeds in agreement with phylogenesis. The ontogenesis of the contrahentes layer in the human foot proceeds from the very beginning as a combination of a phylogenetically old pattern recapitulating during ontogenesis and a specializing process. The specialized development of the oblique head of the adductor is accentuated from the beginning, the unimportance of the fibular part of the contrahentes layer is manifested. The secondary development of the head of the transverse adductor is also the result of the specialized development.

As in the human hand, also in the foot of the adult, the contrahentes layer can be manifested by the occurrence of further rudimentary adductors. The adductor of the 2nd toe was observed by Cunningham (1882). Le Double (1897) quoted similar observations of Danseux and denoted the accessory muscle the "adducteur du second orteil".

The oblique head of the adductor hallucis is homologous with the contrahens I and evidently includes the contrahens II which remains as a separate muscular component during ontogenesis only in the distal part beneath the intermetacarpal space, in the form of a thin rudimentary anlage. The caput transversum of the adductor is not homologous with the normal contrahentes and corresponds to the transverse head of the adductor hallucis of lower Primates, where this head is also present, together with all other contrahentes and transverse to their direction. The nerve supply of the transverse head by an independent twig branching off from the stem of the lateral plantar nerve in a distal direction also indicates that this head is a separate component, not only a part of a spread out oblique adductor.

It may be deduced from the course of ontogenesis of the contrahentes layer that although the human foot is morphologically highly specialized and functionally adapted, primitive structures appear during ontogenesis, differentiating transiently to the same or similar extent as in lower Mammals. This pattern, however, quickly disappears and the development is concurrently stigmatized by the specialization of the foot. Accordingly, from the beginning of development the oblique head of the adductor develops conspicuously more swiftly in its form and cytology than other parts of the layer. Developmentally original structures— the contrahentes of the 4th and 5th toes—disappear very early. The caput transversum is characteristic only for Primates, appearing late in the phylogenesis. In the course of human ontogenesis this component develops conformably as a last one.

10. Recapitulation of Observations on the Ontogenesis of the Contrahentes Layer in the Human Foot

The contrahentes layer originates in the course of ontogenesis of the human foot as in the ontogenesis of the hand, being absent in adults and known only in comparative anatomy. The observations of its development and extinction revealed the following:

1. The layer originates to an extent analogous to that in lower Primates, before the embryo reaches the C-R length of 17 mm, when this layer is already well discernible.

2. During ontogenesis of the foot inside this layer a tibial and fibular part may be distinguished, according to the form and the manner of development.

3. The tibial part of the layer early obtains the form of the caput obliquum of the adductor hallucis. The fibular part projects in strips of mesenchyme which pass distally on the palmar sides of the interossei primordia of the 4th, 3rd and sometimes of the 2nd intermetatarsal spaces.

4. From 20 to 24 mm C-R length the caput obliquum of the adductor hallucis is well differentiated in its form and cytology, while the strips in the fibular part of the layer remain in the stage of poorly differentiated mesenchyme.

5. Between 25 and 30 mm C-R length of embryos, the fibular part of the layer changes into a continuous layer of mesenchyme, where the strips disappear.

6. After reaching 30 mm C-R length the caput transversum of the adductor hallucis differentiates at the level of distal metatarsal ends in the fibular mesenchymal part of the layer, transverse to original strips of the layer.

7. Comparison with lower Primates reveals that the caput obliquum of the adductor hallucis is homologous with the contrahens I and with a major part of the contrahens II, the embryonic strips beneath the 3rd and 4th intermetatarsal spaces correspond to the mammalian contrahens III et IV. The caput transversum is not homologous with any of the typical contrahentes of the mammalian foot.

8. The occurrence and subsequent changes of the entire contrahentes layer in the human embryonic foot bears the character of a developmental recapitulation, which soon disappears being overlapped by the process of foot specialization.

11. Comparison of Dominant Ontogenetic Features of the Contrahentes Layer in the Human Hand and Foot

During ontogenesis the contrahentes layer of the human hand fully recapitulates the primitive phylogenetic pattern with a full set of four contrahentes muscles (Čihák, 1967b, 1968a, b). The developing blastema of this layer in the human hand is apparently well distinguishable by its form and cytology from the surrounding mesenchyme and from other layers of muscle primordia. The recapitulating primitive pattern remains for a relatively long time. Phylogenetically extinct structures of the hand are fully developed as blastemas and primordia during human ontogenesis; they disappear gradually by their rearrangement and fusion with another layers of primordia. The parts of the contrahentes layer, which disappear in the third and fourth intermetacarpal spaces, first join the interossei primordia of their intermetacarpal spaces and then (relatively reduced in size) fuse with the interossei (Čihák, 1968a, b).

In the human foot the contrahentes layer also recapitulates the primitive pattern of four muscles, but only as indications of muscle forms. The contrahentes blastema of the human foot, however, is well discernible, but from the beginning the centre of its differentiation is the bulky primordium of the oblique head of the adductor hallucis. The recapitulating primitive pattern remains only for a very short time. Unlike the ontogenesis of the hand, the structures disappearing in course of phylogenetic development of the human foot are only slightly

PALMA　　PLANTA

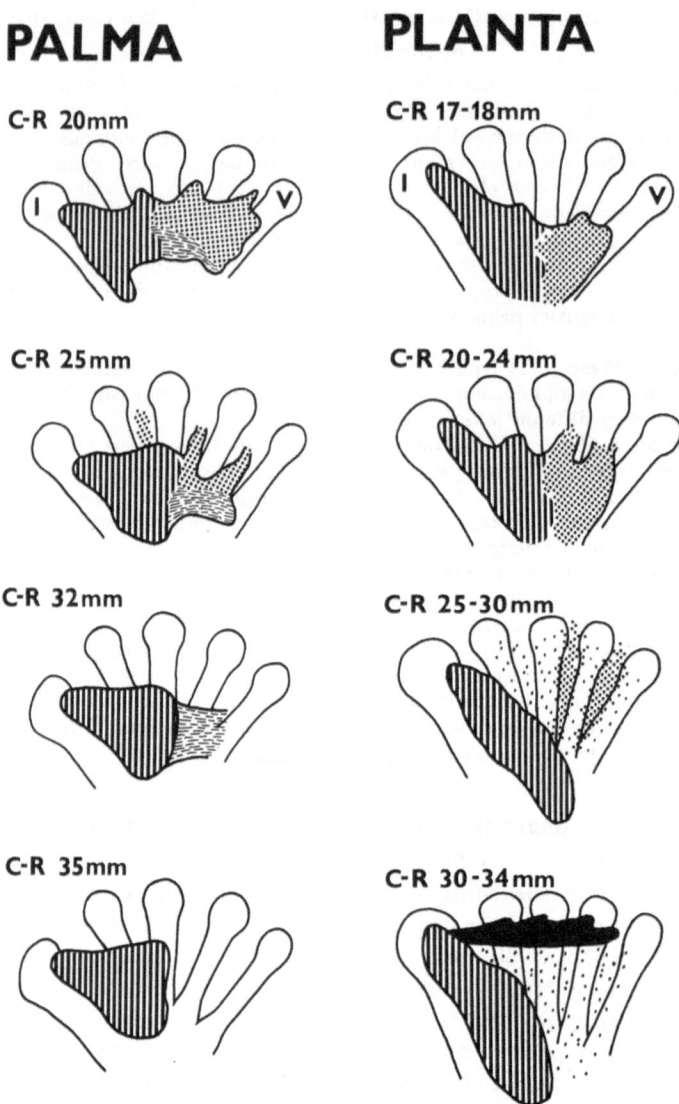

C-R 20mm　　　　C-R 17-18mm

C-R 25mm　　　　C-R 20-24mm

C-R 32mm　　　　C-R 25-30mm

C-R 35mm　　　　C-R 30-34mm

Fig. 67. Comparison of developmental changes of the contrahentes layer in the human hand and foot; proximal part of the layer in the hand shaded with transverse lines, transverse head of the adductor hallucis is black. (According to Čihák, 1969a)

developed during ontogenesis. They disappear quickly, they do not maintain their form and they change into an indefinite layer of mesenchyme. The fusion with the primordia of the interossei is also indicated but there is no real fusion which can be seen in the hand. It is also possible that some of the tissue of the contrahentes rudiments joins the primordia of the lumbrical muscles which are in close contact. Contrary to the hand, during development of the foot there appears a secondary structure inside the contrahentes layer—the transverse head of the adductor hallucis. The concordance and differences of the contrahentes layer development in the hand and foot are summarized in Fig. 67.

The comparison demonstrates that in the human hand the complete development of the primitive structure and its gradual extinction is recapitulated during ontogenesis while in the human foot this recapitulation is only suggested, combined during the entire course of development with the display of the developmental specialization of the contrahentes layer, in accordance with the morphological specialization of the foot in general. (By this developmental specialization in the contrahentes layer the development of the caput obliquum m. adductoris hallucis is accentuated. In comparison with its rapid development in form and cytology the fibular part of the layer remains at the level of poorly differentiated blastema.) The transverse head of the adductor hallucis has no homologue in the human hand.

The joining up of the developed adductor to the skeleton during ontogenesis is late in the hand as well as in the foot; in the hand it appears sooner (from 32 mm C-R length), while in the foot this joining up does not appear before 50 mm C-R length.

C. The Mm. Interossei and the Layers of their Embryonic Primordia
1. Mm. Interossei in the Course of Development of the Human Hand

Since the deep palmar branch of the ulnar nerve represents the division of the layers of intrinsic muscle primordia, it is necessary to look for the primordia of the interossei only on the dorsal side of the nerve. Therefore, the development of blastemas and primordia originating dorsally to the ulnar nerve were studied partly on the palmar side of metacarpal primordia, partly between the metacarpals. The origin of blastemas and the main features of development of the primordia of the interossei has already been described (Čihák, 1963 b, c, 1967 a, 1968 b). Many of these previous observations now appear in new light and with new interrelations in connection with the development of other layers of muscle primordia (cf. pp. 59–63, 105). This especially concerns the participation of accessory primordia on the dorsal side of the dorsal interossei. Their occurrence not only influences the morphogenesis of the interossei but also originates the development of the dorsal aponeurosis of fingers.

The development of the mm. interossei pedis will be described further and the interossei development in the hand and foot will be compared.

2. Material for Studies of the Development of the Mm. Interossei of the Human Hand

The development of the interossei manus was followed in three consecutive studies. In the first study (Čihák, 1960 b) the origin of the first dorsal interosseus from two neighbouring components was established by means of comparative anatomy and a comparison with the fundamental stages of human embryonic development. In the next study (Čihák, 1963 b, c) on 70 hands of embryos from 10 to 75 mm C-R length, the difference in development between the first dorsal interosseus and the other dorsal interossei was assessed. The third step of this study is represented by a summary of observations of proper primordia of the interossei and of the accessory primordia. This study, summarized in the present publication, is based upon observations in 86 hands of human embryos and foetuses from 10 to 75 mm in C-R length.

The C-R lengths of employed embryos were: 10 mm, 12, 13.6, 14, 15 (2 hands), 15.5 (3), 16 (2), 16.5 (4), 17, 17.5 (4), 18 (4), 19 (6), 19.5 (3), 20 (4), 20.5 (3), 21 (6), 22 (2), 22.5 (2), 23 (4), 25 (5), 25.5, 26 (3), 27 (2), 28 (2), 29 (3), 30 (2), 32 (2), 33, 35 (2), 36, 38, 40, 45, 50, 56, 60, 65, 75 mm.

Muscle primordia of the hand of embryos 15.5 and 21 mm in C-R length were reconstructed. The staining of histological series and the technic of reconstructions are described in pp. 10–11.

3. Observations on the Development of the Interossei Manus

In embryos between 19 and 25 mm in C-R length the complete division of the deep palmar blastema into two layers of primordia is always visible (Figs. 35, 36, 39). The more superficial of these layers corresponds to the mm. contrahentes of comparative anatomy; its further differentiation and fate have been described above. The deeper layer represents the primordia of the future interossei (Figs. 35, 36, 68). In the first study of this layer we supposed (in conformity with the literature) that its material migrates into the intermetacarpal spaces, pulling along its nerves. Now the study of a larger number of embryos reveals that muscle primordia are formed and differentiated in situ so that the migration into intermetacarpal spaces does not proceed in a proper sense of this term, and that the shift and expansion of primordia inside of these spaces results from the differential growth of involved formations.

In comparison with Bardeleben's scheme (1890) of hand musculature this deep layer of palmar muscle primordia, situated dorsal to the ulnar nerve and partly extending into intermetacarpal spaces, can be identified with the layer of the so-called mm. flexores breves profundi of comparative anatomy. While studying its development it was soon evident that dorsal to this layer and separate from it there develop further primordia, each in the 2nd, 3rd and 4th intermetacarpal spaces (Fig. 68). It was, therefore, necessary to add one more dorsally situated layer to Bardeleben's scheme, the so-called mm. intermetacarpales (according to McMurrich, 1903, 1907). In description of the primordia therefore the terms primordia of the flexores breves profundi layer and intermetacarpal primordia or primordia of intermetacarpal muscles are employed, according to their relevance to a certain layer. (The general situation of the primordia is demonstrated in Fig. 68.)

The large layer of flexores breves profundi primordia, extending from the first to the fourth intermetacarpal spaces and going beyond to the ulnar margin of the fifth metacarpal and to the radial margin of the first one, is already distinctly formed in embryos from 13.5 mm in C-R length of the studied material. At this stage the layer is poorly differentiated. In embryos of 14 and 15 mm C-R length the differentiation of the layer is better and the layer divides into parts for the future primordia of the flexores breves profundi in intermetacarpal spaces (Figs. 34, 43). From 16 mm C-R length onward these primordia are already quite distinct (Figs. 44, 48). There is a general rule that in Mammals the flexores breves profundi are arranged in twins (Fig. 32), each couple of muscle twins being beneath one metacarpal bone. In man, however, these twins stand apart, originating coupled in new pairs, each of them on the palmar margin of the correspond-

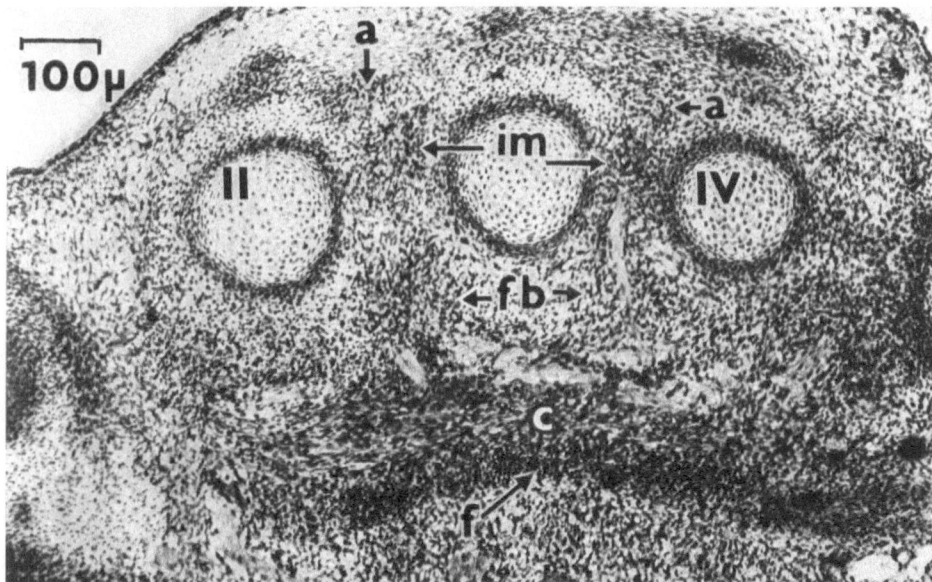

Fig. 68. Right hand of the embryo 19.5 mm in C-R length, transverse section. Distribution of primordia layers in the hand and their mutual relations. *II, IV* metacarpals; *f* primordia of tendons of the flexor digitorum profundus; *c* the contrahentes layer, separated by the course of the ulnar nerve from the layer of flexores breves profundi (*fb*); *im* intermetacarpal primordia; *a* primordia of the interossei dorsales accessorii. The interossei dorsales II–IV originate by fusion of the primordium from the flexores breves profundi layer with the intermetacarpal primordium

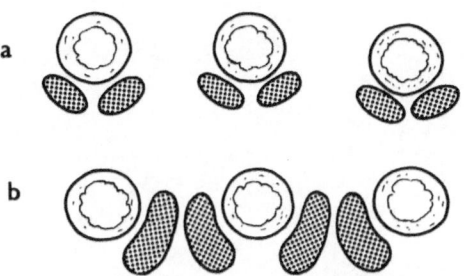

Fig. 69. Arrangement of the couples of twins of flexores breves profundi muscles (or corresponding primordia) *a* in lower Mammals, in relation to single metacarpals; *b* in Primates, in relation to intermetacarpal spaces

ing intermetacarpal space (Fig. 69). Both elements of the twins are independently innervated. The original scheme of development of the interossei solely from the flexores breves profundi, as quoted e.g. by Keith (1949), supposes a simple migration of single elements of these couples symmetrically according to the axis of the third finger. The primordia situated toward the axis are thought to migrate further dorsally and to become the dorsal interossei, the remaining primordia, averted from the axis, become the palmar interossei (Fig. 33). Our previous

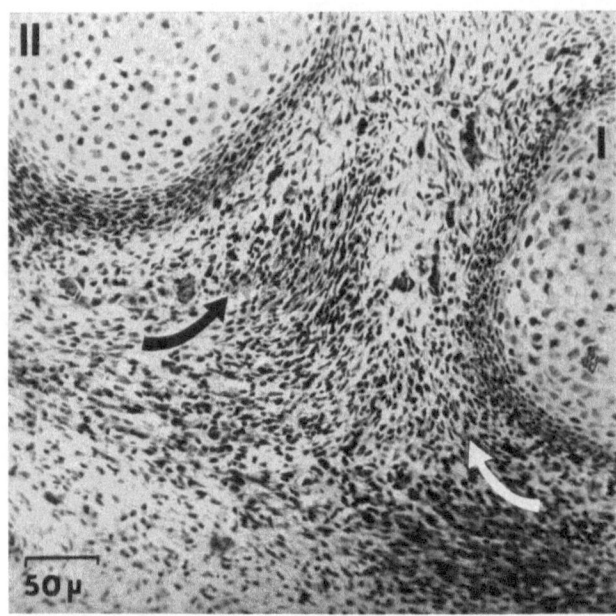

Fig. 70. Left hand of the embryo 19 mm in C-R length, transverse section. Two primordia are entering the first intermetacarpal space (arrows) and join to form the primordium of the first dorsal interosseus. *I, II* metacarpals. Both primordia belong to the flexores breves profundi layer

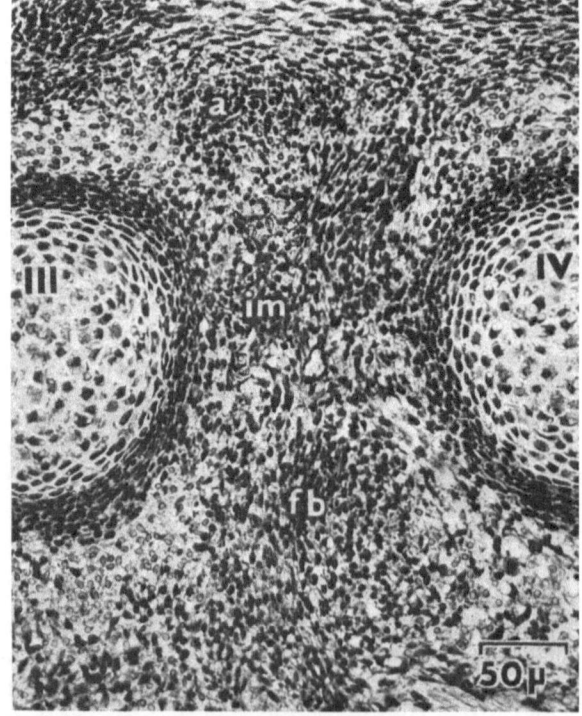

Fig. 71. Right hand of the embryo 19.5 mm in C-R length, transverse section, 3rd intermetacarpal space. Three layers of primordia for the interossei: *fb* primordia of the flexores breves profundi layer; *im* intermetacarpal primordium; *a* anlage of the interosseus dorsalis accessorius; *III, IV* metacarpals

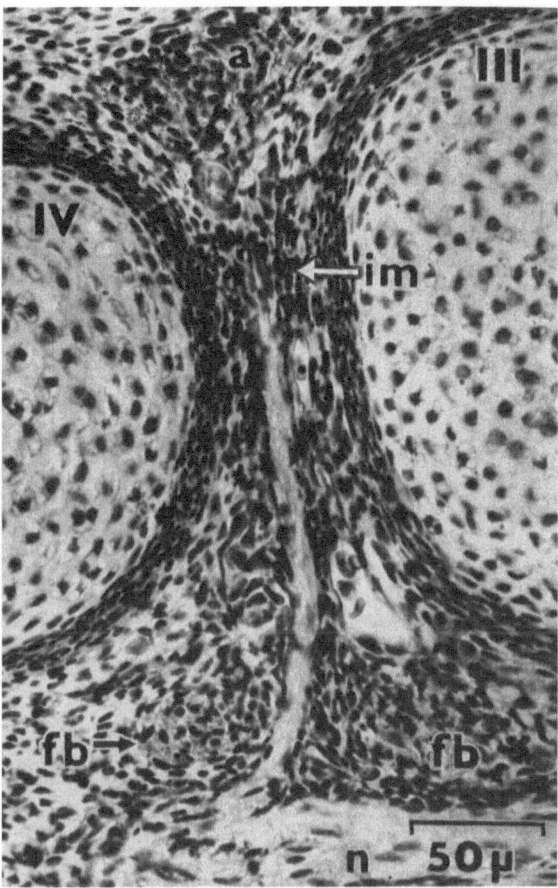

Fig. 72. Left hand of the embryo 19 mm in C-R length, transverse section, 3rd intermetacarpal space. The branch of the ulnar nerve perforates the intermetacarpal space and supplies
the intermetacarpal and dorsal accessory primordium; *n* deep palmar branch of the ulnar
nerve; *fb* primordia of the flexores breves profundi layer; *im* intermetacarpal primordium;
a anlage of the interosseus dorsalis accessorius; *III, IV* metacarpals. (Čihák, 1963b)

publications demonstrated that this scheme is invalid and that the dorsal interossei develop in a different way in the first intermetacarpal space and in other
intermetacarpal spaces.

In the first intermetacarpal space the pattern of the interosseus dorsalis I
differs from the other dorsal interossei in that from the beginning of development
the material is found entering the intermetacarpal space from the two sides, i.e.
from the radial and the ulnar side. This material hence represents the primordia
of the two neighbouring flexores breves profundi joining to form the m. interosseus
dorsalis I (Figs. 70, 101). The intermetacarpal primordium is absent in man in
the first intermetacarpal space, contrary to the situation in Mammals in general,
where this element is still normal even in Prosimians (Lewis, 1965). In
conformity with this double anlage there are also two supplying branches of the

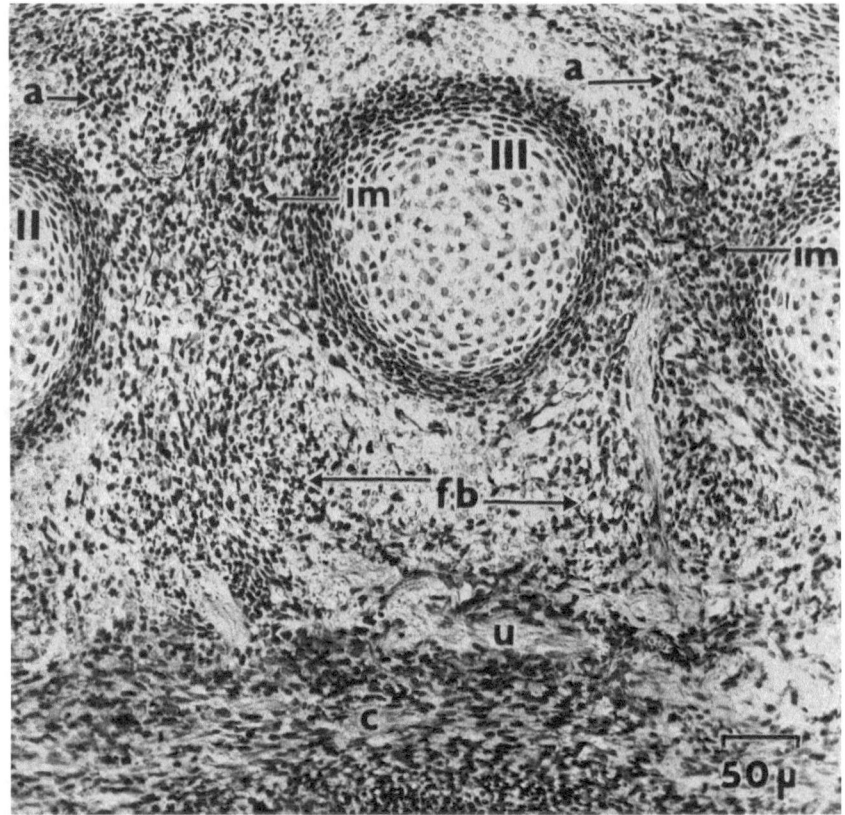

Fig. 73. Embryo 19.5 mm in C-R length, right hand, transverse section. Typical layers of primordia and their relation to the ulnar nerve (*u*) and to its perforating branch in the intermetacarpal space; *c* the contrahentes layer; *fb* layer of flexores breves profundi (i.e. the primordia of palmar interossei and of palmar portions of dorsal interossei); *im* intermetacarpal layer of primordia for the dorsal interossei; *a* accessory primordia of the dorsal interossei (interossei dorsales accessorii); *II, III* metacarpals. (Čihák, 1968b)

first dorsal interosseus, each for the corresponding part. The primordia joining into the m. interosseus dorsalis I are hence homologous with the m. flexor brevis profundus pollicis ulnaris and with the flexor brevis profundus digiti II radialis.

In all embryos between 15 and 30 mm C-R length in the second, third and fourth intermetacarpal spaces two flexores breves profundi primordia in each are found, situated on the palmar side of the space and extending dorsal into one third of the space. Further dorsally one primordium more, the third one is found (Figs. 71–73), which represents the future dorsal part of the muscle belly of the relevant dorsal interosseus. The independence of the dorsal primordia that may be homologised with the intermetacarpal muscles of lower Mammals and lower Tetrapods, is documented by the perforating branch from the ramus profundus nervi ulnaris penetrating for each of them through the intermetacarpal space and supplying the primordium (Figs. 72, 73). This branch perforates the intermeta-

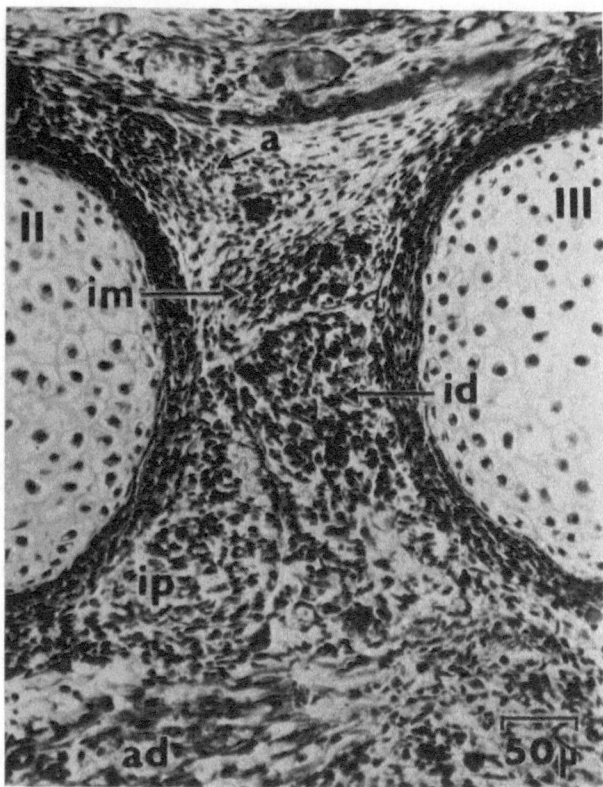

Fig. 74. Right hand of the 28 mm embryo, transverse section, second intermetacarpal space. The intermetacarpal primordium starts to fuse with one of the flexores breves profundi primordia to form the dorsal interosseus; *ip* palmar interosseus; *id* dorsal interosseus; *im* intermetacarpal primordium; *a* interosseus dorsalis accessorius. *II, III* metacarpals; *ad* adductor pollicis. (Čihák, 1963 b)

carpal space near the metacarpal base and then continues dorsally, as will be demonstrated in the description of accessory primordia of the interossei.

After attaining 25 mm C-R length the gradual fusion of the intermetacarpal primordia with members of the flexores breves profundi layer proceeds (Fig. 74) up to thorough homogeneity (Fig. 75). The fusing member of the pair of the flexores breves profundi in the relevant intermetacarpal space is that one turned towards the third finger axis. The primordia of the flexores breves profundi layer that according to the quoted migration scheme were supposed to shift as the dorsal interossei (Fig. 33) into intermetacarpal spaces, thus remain in situ, but fuse with the more dorsally situated primordia of the intermetacarpales. Hence there exists in m. interosseus dorsalis II, III and IV the same developmental duplication as in interosseus dorsalis I, differing from the first interosseus only in that the two fusing primordia are superimposed being each a member of another layer of primordia.

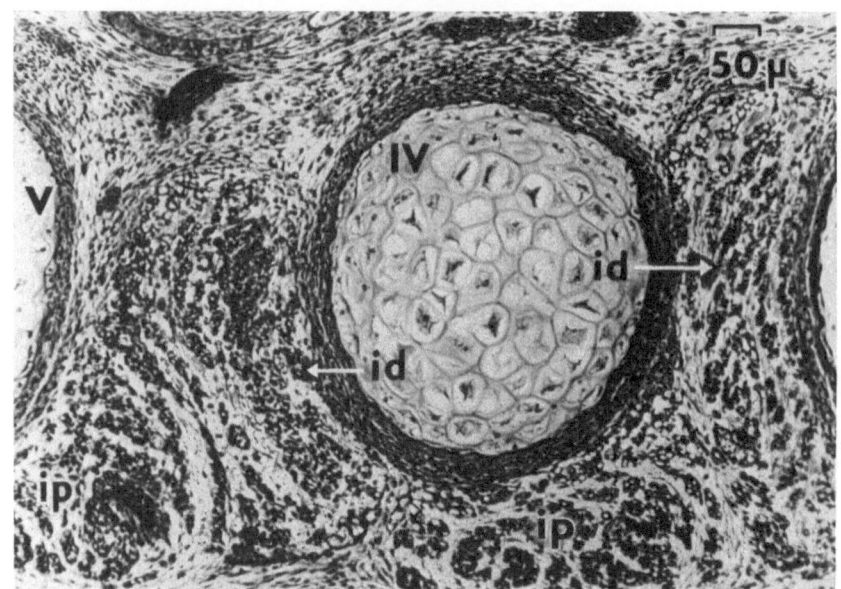

Fig. 75. Embryo 46 mm in C-R length, left hand, transverse section, 3rd and 4th intermetacarpal spaces. The fusion of the flexor brevis profundus primordium with the intermetacarpal
primordium is finished, there are only some changes in structure suggesting the originally
two parts of the dorsal interosseus

The double anlage of the second, third and fourth dorsal interossei also
appears in the insertion of these muscles, since the dorsal primordium (the intermetacarpalis) is inserted into the dorsal aponeurosis of the finger, while the palmar
primordium (the flexor brevis profundus) is partly inserted also to the shaft of
the proximal phalanx. Such duplex insertion of the dorsal interossei has been
described in adults from the functional and surgical standpoint by Kaplan (1953)
and Bunnell (1956).

The main parts of muscle bellies of the definitive interossei dorsales II–IV
originate by fusion of the two primordial layers; each of these muscles is supplied
by two nerve branches (Figs. 72, 73). The continuation of the flexores breves
profundi primordia to both margins of the hand gives rise to the primordia of
the flexor brevis and the opponens digiti minimi and to the primordia of the deep
thenar muscles, as will be described later.

The scheme of fusion of primordia into the definitive interossei and the
comparison with the pattern in phylogenetically lower Mammals is demonstrated
in Fig. 84. This scheme also summarizes the development of the contrahentes and
of other muscles of the hand, which will be described in detail later.

4. Discussion and Conclusions from Observations of Ontogenesis of the Interossei in the Human Hand

For considering homologies of the interossei primordia it proved necessary to
apply the nomenclature of comparative anatomy to the description of the morphogenesis of the human hand. This allowed the abandoning of the confusing term

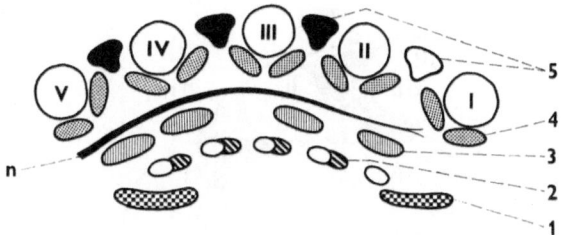

Fig. 76. Scheme of muscular layers of the hand (and foot) according to Bardeleben (1890) including the further layer of intermetacarpal (intermetatarsal) elements according to McMurrich (1903). This scheme can be imployed for the pattern of the mammalian hand in general. The fundamental features of this scheme recapitulate in the course of human onto-genesis. *1* flexores breves superficiales; *2* lumbricales; *3* layer of the contrahentes; *4* the fle-xores breves profundi in couples beneath the metacarpals or (in Primates) in intermeta-carpal spaces; *5* the intermetacarpales; *n* ulnar nerve (lateral plantar nerve in the foot). According to Čihák, 1968b, modified)

m. interosseus dorsalis which is not identical with a developmental muscle element. On the basis of this distinction it was then possible to homologise the layers of the primordia and to add to the scheme of Bardeleben (1890) one addi-tional dorsal layer of muscle primordia which also corresponds to the dorsal layer of Cunningham's division (1878a). This layer is represented by muscle primordia homologous to the muscles denoted by McMurrich (1903) as the mm. intermetacarpales (Fig. 76). From the phylogenetic viewpoint two layers of muscles participated in the development of the interossei, the mm. flexores breves profundi and the intermetacarpales.

Observations revealed that the deep palmar branch of the ulnar nerve actually formed a division between the embryonic layer of the contrahentes and the primordia of the flexores breves profundi (Fig. 76). This statement verifies the original views of Ruge (1878a) and Forster (1916).

According to Cunningham (1878a) the palmar interossei represent a layer different from that of the dorsal interossei. In Bardeleben's concept (1890) both these layers are homologous with the flexores breves profundi. As the present observations revealed, both these views were right in part. McMurrich (1903) for the first time brought the opinion that during phylogenesis the dorsal interossei originated from dorsal and palmar components. He also defined these components in the histological section of the human fetal hand. However, he employed the hand of such a long foetus that the process of fusion of the primordia could not be visible, but the comparison of his drawing with our present observations demon-strated that he rightly estimated the area of the intermetacarpal anlage. He assumed this component, however, to be present in the first dorsal interosseus where this component does not develop. This original view of McMurrich has also been supported from the aspect of comparative anatomy by Ribbing (1909, 1938) and by Forster (1916). Stjernman's (1932) homologies of the contrahentes with the palmar interossei (it was originally the view of Cunningham) and of the intermetacarpales with the dorsal interossei proved to be invalid. Howell (1936) supposed that the mammalian dorsal and palmar interossei are simple derivatives

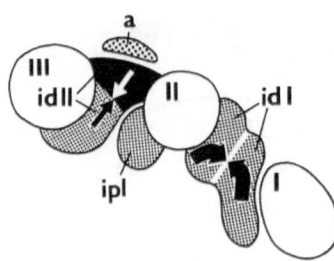

Fig. 77. Scheme of differences in the origin of the interosseus dorsalis I from the mode of origin of the other dorsal interossei. The first dorsal interosseus originates by fusion of two primordia from the flexores breves profundi layer, the interossei dorsales II, III and IV originate each by fusion of one primordium from the flexores breves profundi layer with one intermetacarpal primordium. The interosseus dorsalis accessorius (a) either remains independent (as a muscle variation) or fuses with the dorsal interosseus. The plantar interossei have each one primordium from the flexores breves profundi layer. (According to Čihák, 1968b, modified)

of the deep short flexors complex, which, e.g. in Iguana, appears in the form of deep short flexors and intermetacarpal muscles. Contrary to this view we are convinced that the present observations of ontogenesis reveal enough evidence for the mechanism of morphogenesis of the interossei, thus permitting the conclusion that the fusion of the two muscle layers is the characteristic feature of the origin of dorsal interossei in Primates. The fusion of the two layers can be observed directly in the course of human ontogenesis. The comparison of this process with corresponding muscles in Primates reveals that the same fusion proceeds from lower to higher Primates up to Man. While in Prosimians two separate layers may be found, there exist in catarrhine Monkeys already the typical interossei, of which the dorsal parts can easily be separated in a fibrous septum. The fusion of the two layers occurs in anthropoid Apes. In Man the complete fusion develops already in the course of the embryonic period, and except for the nerve of the dorsal component there remains no trace of fusion of the two muscle layers.

Baumann (1951) drew attention to the fact that during ontogenesis the dorsal interossei are each originally inserted into the dorsal aponeuroses of the two neighbouring fingers, later on reducing this insertion to one side only. He also noted that the muscle bellies and the tendons of the dorsal interossei can develop separately in a certain period of embryonic life. Although the possibility of an independent differentiation of muscle belly and the tendon is known also in other muscles, e.g. in the flexor digitorum superficialis (Dylevský, 1968a), Baumann's view can probably be explained as an interpretation of the pattern seen in an oblique section through the metacarpal region (according to illustrations in the quoted paper). The basis of this view, however, was a really observed duplication; the explanation of this problem will be attempted further in the discussion of development of the dorsal aponeurosis of fingers.

A characteristic difference in origin of the first dorsal interosseus and three further dorsal interossei (Fig. 77) has been observed. The statement that in the course of ontogenesis the mm. interossei dorsales II, III and IV each originate

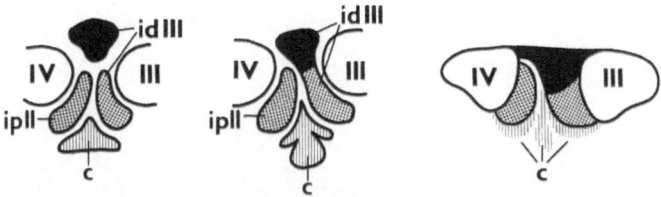

Fig. 78. Scheme of participation of the contrahentes layer rudiments (strips beneath intermetacarpal spaces—vertically shaded) in the formation of the interossei (outlined in the 3rd intermetacarpal space; same situation is in the 4th space). (According to Čihák, 1968b, modified)

by fusion of two superimposed primordia, of which the palmar one is homologous with the flexor brevis profundus and the dorsal one with the intermetacarpal muscle (Čihák, 1963b, c, 1967a), confirms for the first time from the standpoint of human ontogenesis the views of previous authors, up to now deduced from the comparative anatomy. From the comparative viewpoint Lewis (1965) reconsidered once more this problem in Primates. His results are in agreement with our observations with the only exception of the first intermetacarpal space, where Lewis (1965) finds the intermetacarpalis in lower Primates while the corresponding primordium does not develop in the human hand, in which the first dorsal interosseus originates by fusion of two neighbouring elements of the flexores breves profundi layer (Fig. 77). The rudiments of the ulnar part of the contrahentes layer also take part in the definitive formation of the interossei and of the connective tissue between them in the 3rd and 4th intermetacarpal spaces (Fig. 78). The detailed relations of deep primordia in the thumb region to neighbouring components of the flexores breves profundi layer will be demonstrated in descriptions of the developing thenar musculature.

From the comparative viewpoint the fusion of the flexores breves profundi with the intermetacarpales to form the solid dorsal interossei can be considered as a process whose completion characterizes the human hand only. Thus this developmental process is a part of the hominisation process of the hand. In this connection it is remarkable that this rearrangement concerns the very muscles controlling fine finger movements.

5. Mm. Interossei Dorsales Accessorii and their Embryonic Primordia

On the dorsal side of the intermetacarpal spaces, dorsal to the intermetacarpal primordia for the 2nd, 3rd and 4th dorsal interossei, a further primordium adjacent to the intermetacarpalis (i. e. to the dorsal component of the dorsal interosseus) can be followed from 15 mm C-R length onward. In early stages this primordium is relatively bulky and is separated from the intermetacarpal anlage by a loose mesenchyme (Fig. 43). It then flattens, from 16 mm C-R length on, and can be followed proximodistally from the dorsal side of the capitate and hamate primordia (where it is wider and flatter) up to the dorsal surface of mm. interossei dorsales II, III et IV (Figs. 73, 79, 80, 81). Toward the intermetacarpal spaces this primordium gradually joins the insertion of the intermetacarpal anlage.

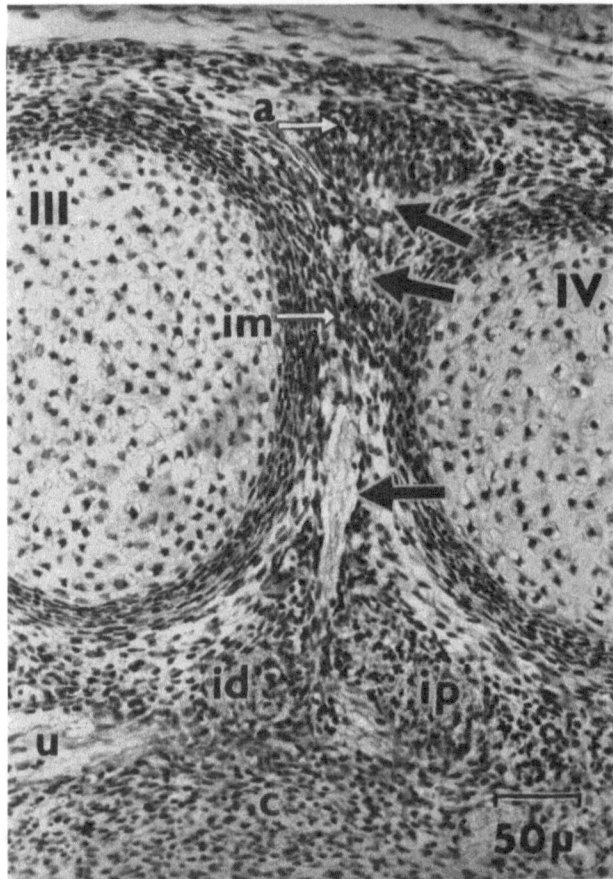

Fig. 79. Right hand of the embryo 23 mm in C-R length, transverse section. Over the 3rd intermetacarpal space the typical primordium of the interosseus dorsalis accessorius is seen (*a*), to it the supplying branch from the ulnar nerve can be followed (arrows)

⎯he accessory strip-like primordium takes part to a variable degree in the development of the entire dorsal interosseus. In the fourth intermetacarpal space it early (before 20 mm of C-R length) fuses with the 4th dorsal interosseus, with its dorsal, intermetacarpal anlage. In the second and third intermetacarpal spaces this strip persists much later. In the reconstruction (Fig. 82 B) the striking similarity of the strip with a muscular variation known as the m. extensor digitorum manus brevis is visible. But the accessory primordium cannot be classified as the extensor brevis, since in all studied embryonic series and in all controlled adult hands its nerve supply comes from the deep palmar branch of the ulnar nerve. The branch of this nerve destined for the intermetacarpal anlage (Figs. 72, 73) passes dorsally through the intermetacarpal space, comes to the dorsal side of the intermetacarpal anlage, situated between this and the accessory primordium (Fig. 79) and after supplying twigs for both of them it turns proximally and gradually divides into branches. In some of the series this perforating branch

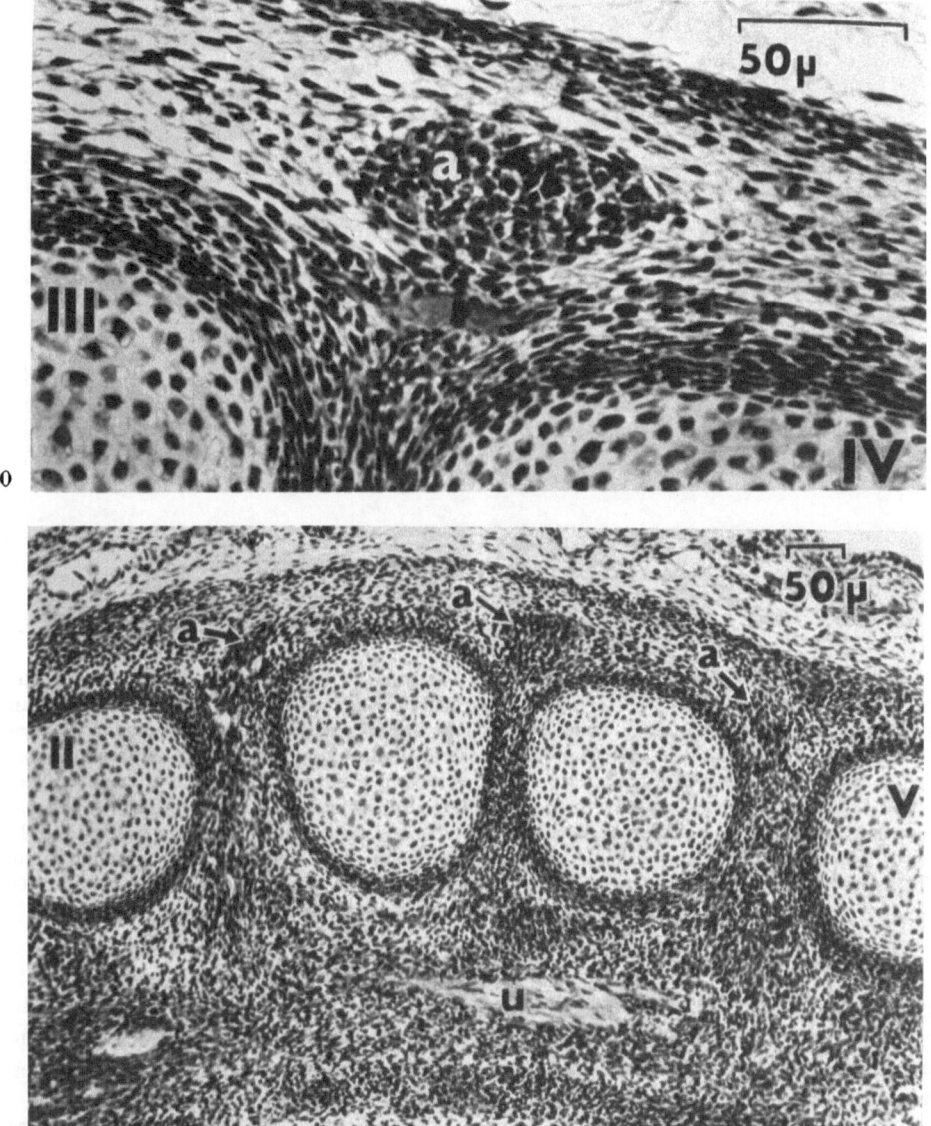

Fig. 80. Right hand of the 19 mm embryo, 3rd intermetacarpal space, transverse section. Dorsal to the space a well differentiated primordium of the interosseus dorsalis accessorius (a) is visible. The supplying branch from the ulnar nerve (with a blood vessel) can be seen beneath the primordium. *III, IV* metacarpals

Fig. 81. Embryo 18 mm in C-R length, right hand, transverse section. Primordia of the interossei dorsales accessorii (a) are well formed over the 2nd to 4th intermetacarpal spaces

first gave off the supplying twigs after its proximal turn. The terminal branches of the perforating nerve end in the region of the capsules of carpometacarpal joints. This course can be followed in serial sections in a distoproximal direction

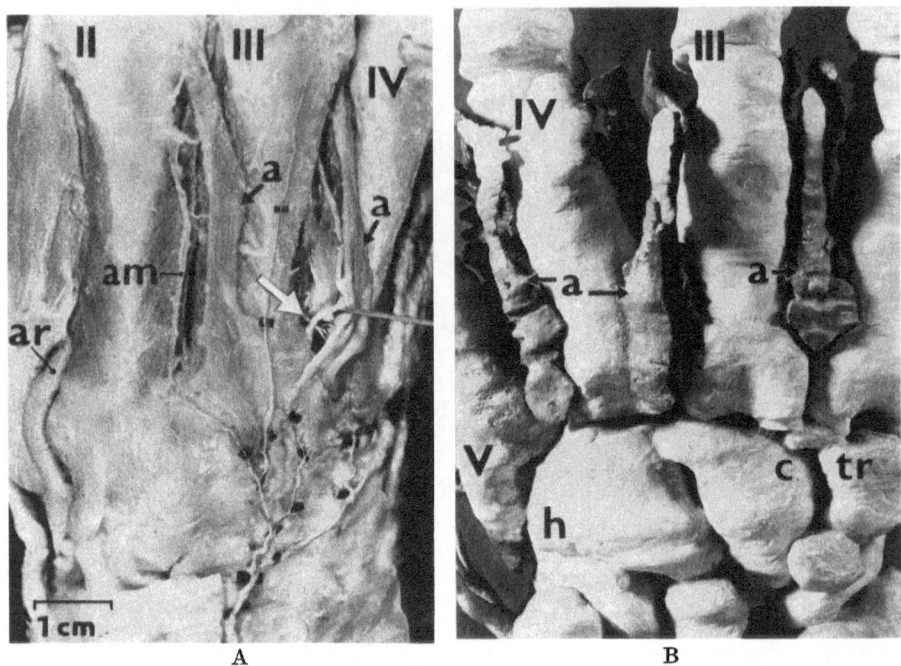

A   B

Fig. 82. A) Well developed interossei dorsales accessorii (*a*) in the adult human hand. The
preparation demonstrates the terminal branches of the nervus interosseus antebrachii
posterior (underlain with black strips), ending in the connective tissue of metacarpal peri-
osteum, of carpometacarpal articulations. These branches do not enter the interosseus dorsalis accessorius muscle. The supplying branch comes to the muscle from the intermetacarpal
space (white arrow); *am* arteria metacarpea dorsalis; *ar* arteria radialis (piercing the 1st
intermetacarpal space. B) Reconstruction of the left hand of the embryo 21 mm in C-R length,
dorsal aspect. The interossei dorsales accessorii primordia are visible in the entire length in the
2nd to 4th intermetacarpal spaces. *III–V* metacarpals; *a* primordia of the interossei dorsales
accessorii; *h* the hamatum; *c* capitatum; *tr* trapezoideum

(comp. Čihák, 1963c). Besides, the perforating nerve sends off a minute twig in
a distal direction, which reaches the metacarpophalangeal joint between the
intermetacarpal and the accessory primordia, often joined to the vasa metacarpea
dorsalia and to their concomitant nerve (that is a branch of the radial nerve).

Since the earlier literature (with the exception of Barclay-Smith 1896/97)
quoted for the muscle variations on the dorsum manus only the nerve supply by
the radial nerve, an attempt has been made at verifying whether there might
be an anastomosis (Rauber — cit. according to Barclay-Smith, 1896/97) connecting
the ulnar and radial nerves by a loop passing through the intermetacarpal space.
In a small verification series an anastomosis was found by preparation in one hand
out of eleven. But in this case also it may be accepted according to the course of
supplying branches that the accessory muscle is first supplied by the ulnar nerve
and that the anastomosis is effected by further branches, more proximal on the
dorsum manus. It was found that the branches originating from the ramus
profundus nervi radialis are distributed between the layer of the extensor indicis

proprius and the described accessory primordia—i.e. one layer further dorsally; the branches from the n. interosseus antebrachii posterior, quoted as the nerve supply of accessory elements (Kadanoff, 1958), end inside the ligamentous apparatus of wrist joints as their articular branches, but do not enter the muscles (Fig. 82 A).

Accessory muscle strips found in embryos can occur in adults on the dorsal sides of all dorsal interossei; they appear most often over the second and third (Fig. 82 A, B). The nerve supply indicates that neither the primordia observed in the embryonic period nor these muscles in adults belong to the extensors. We therefore denoted the elements the *mm. interossei dorsales accessorii* to distinguish them also in the nomenclature (with regard to their morphogenesis and nerve supply) both from the true short extensors and from the proper dorsal interossei (i.e. from the interossei composed by the flexor brevis profundus and the intermetacarpal element). In its course the interosseus dorsalis accessorius is more or less distinctly separated in embryos as well as in adults from the intermetacarpalis proper and fuses with the interosseus only near its insertion.

The interossei dorsales accessorii (spatii II et III) are frequently found in adults as rudiments of variable degree coursing on the dorsal sides of the interosseus dorsalis II and III. In the interosseus dorsalis IV the accessory element is evidently fused with the intermetacarpal component (with which it early fuses already during ontogenesis). This element is hence constant only in the embryonic period. The constancy of occurrence of the interossei dorsales accessorii in embryos, and in the 2nd and 3rd intermetacarpal spaces also in adults permits the consideration of the absence of these elements as a variation rather than their persistence.

6. Occurrence and Nerve Supply of the Interossei Dorsales Accessorii in the Hand of Adults

On the basis of findings described in the previous chapter, Dr. A. Chmelová (1963) controlled the occurrence, form variability and nerve supply of the interossei dorsales accessorii in 60 hands of adults from the material for dissections in the Department of Anatomy, Charles University, Prague. Since this study links our findings in human ontogenesis, its results will be briefly quoted here.

Accessory elements were classified into three groups according to the degree of muscle development (Fig. 83):

I. An independent muscle strip separable in its entire length from the proper dorsal interosseus, extending as a rule from the distal row of the carpal bones up to the insertion in common with the dorsal interosseus. The element is the same as in embryos in form and extent.

II. A muscle separable from the dorsal interosseus at least for half of its length.

III. Regressive forms of the accessory muscle:

a) a fibrously reduced muscle;

b) scattered solitary muscle bundles in the fascia dorsalis manus interossea;

c) a striking, strong fibrous tunnel for the dorsal interosseus, formed by the fascia dorsalis manus interossea.

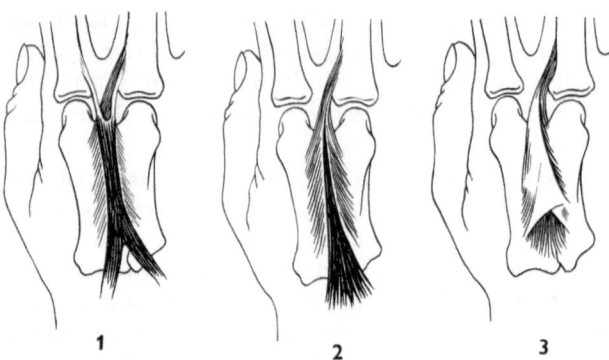

Fig. 83. Three types of shape of the interosseus dorsalis accessorius: *1* independent muscle; *2* muscle independent at least in the half of length of the intermetacarpal space; *3* fibrous changes of the muscle which reinforces the fascia dorsalis manus interossea

In the second intermetacarpal space a muscle of group I type was found in 26 hands, that of the group II in 10 hands and of the group III in 17 hands; the accessory element of the 2nd space was absent in 7 hands out of the 60 adult hands studied.

In the third intermetacarpal space a muscle of group I type was found in 14 hands, of group II in 7 hands and that of group III in 33 hands; not found in 6 hands.

In the fourth intermetacarpal space a muscle of group I type was found in 3 hands, that of group II was not found and the rudimentary muscle of group III was found in 49 hands; no accessory rudiment could be found in 8 hands.

Although the accessory primordium was not observed in the first intermetacarpal space of embryonal hands, one case of an independent muscular strip taken into the fascia dorsalis manus interossea was also found in this space in an adult.

Among the 60 hands investigated there were none in which a muscle of group I–III could not be found at least in one intermetacarpal space. The interosseus dorsalis accessorius is hence also a constant element in adults, varying, however, in the degree of development and in position in relation to intermetacarpal space.

In 30 hands the nerve supply of muscles of groups I and II was determined regardless of intermetacarpal space by preparation using the dissecting microscope. All findings were same: all muscles were supplied by branches of the ramus profundus nervi ulnaris. The branch supplying the accessory muscle most often entered the palmar surface of the dorsal interosseus distal to the supplying branch for the palmar component (of the dorsal interosseus); it then passed dorsally forming an oblique arch through the dorsal (intermetacarpal) component of the interosseus, or between the muscle and the bone metacarpal. It entered the accessory muscle in a minute hilum situated on the surface adjacent to the dorsal interosseus (Fig. 82 A). The nerve most often entered the ulnar side of the muscle, less frequently its radial side, it rarely entered in the centre of width of the muscle belly. The hilum was in about the middle of the muscle belly. The accessory muscle exceptionally found in the first intermetacarpal space was also supplied by a branch from the ramus profundus nervi ulnaris.

The branches from the n. interosseus antebrachii posterior were followed and it was found that they did not reach the accessory muscles.

An anastomosis between the ramus profundus nervi ulnaris and the nervus interosseus antebrachii posterior was found in 8 hands out of a total of 30.

1. An anastomosis was found once in the 2nd intermetacarpal space; an accessory muscle of group I type was present, but was not supplied from the anastomosis.

2. An anastomosis was found twice in the 3rd intermetacarpal space, together with muscles of group II type. In one case the muscle was entered by twigs from the ulnar nerve as well as from the nervus interosseus antebrachii posterior and from the proper arch of the anastomosis. In the second case twigs from both the ulnar and the posterior interosseus nerves entered the muscle.

3. An anastomosis was observed in the third intermetacarpal space in three hands. In all cases a reduced accessory muscle of group III type was present.

4. In two cases the anastomosis was found in the 3rd intermetacarpal space where no trace of the accessory muscle could be found.

The occurrence of the interossei dorsales accessorii in adults is hence in agreement with the regular occurrence of these primordia in embryos. The nerve supply from the ulnar nerve corresponds to findings during ontogenesis. The innervation of these muscles from the anastomosis between the ulnar nerve and the nervus interosseus antebrachii posterior can be considered an exception. Anastomosis between these two nerves is not a constant pattern and its presence is not linked with the occurrence of the accessory muscle.

The revision of accessory muscles and of their nerve supply in adults verifies that these elements, constant in embryos, are almost constant in adults and that they cannot be included among extensors.

7. Participation of Accessory Elements in the Origin of the Interossei and their Relation to the Extensores Manus Breves

Most authors considered the accessory elements on the dorsal sides of intermetacarpal spaces to belong to the extensor group and hence supplied by the radial nerve (Curnow, 1876; Testut, 1884; Le Double, 1897; Bühler, 1902; Lucien, 1909a, b, c, 1910; Fontes, 1933, 1934; Kadanoff, 1958). Barclay-Smith (1896/97) alone described the nerve supply of observed short extensors by twigs from the ulnar nerve (he evidently saw our accessory muscles). Weber and Collin (1905) took the accessory muscles to be the accessory interossei heads from their connection with the interossei. The specific view of Kadanoff (1958), claiming the fusion of reduced short extensors with the interossei, seems also to be controverted by the finding that these accessory muscles are supplied by the ulnar nerve. On comparing the various descriptions of short extensors it may be stated that two types are described: the long type of muscle originating on the distal end of the radius and coursing over the dorsum manus to the fingers, and a short type of muscle originating close to the intermetacarpal spaces. Doubtless, all short extensor types described in the literature are our interossei dorsales accessorii. In

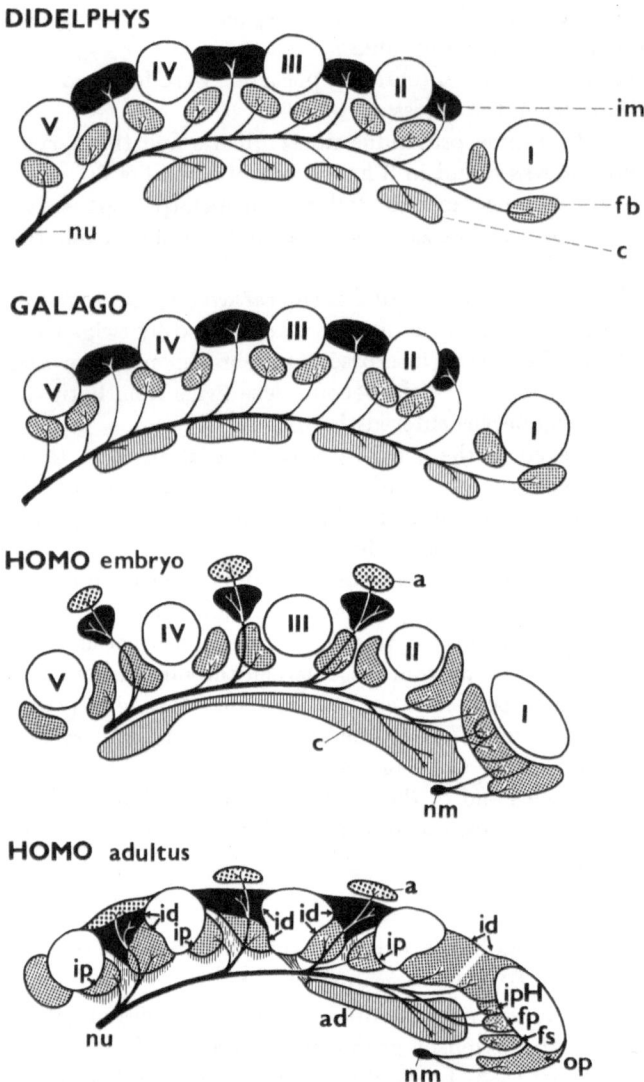

Fig. 84. Fundamental layers of muscle primordia in the comparative anatomy, in human embryo and in the adult; *c* the contrahentes layer; *fb* layer of flexores breves profundi; *im* intermetacarpal elements; *a* interossei dorsales accessorii; *id* dorsal interossei; *ip* palmar interossei; *nu* ulnar nerve; *nm* median nerve; *I*, *V* metacarpals; *ipH* the interosseus palmaris I Henlei (var.); *fp* flexor pollicis brevis, caput profundum; *fs* flexor pollicis brevis, caput superficiale; *op* the opponens pollicis; *ad* the adductor pollicis. (Partly according to Čihák, 1968 b, modified)

Kadanoff's observations (1958) also two types of short extensors were found, and it was just the short one which was presented as a proof of fusion of short extensors with the dorsal interossei.

It is necessary to add to the morphology and ontogenesis of the interossei that interosseus dorsalis I is composed of two parts, both belonging to the flexores breves profundi layer. The interossei dorsales II, III, and IV are then composed of at least two superimposed primordia each (of the flexor brevis profundus and the intermetacarpalis). In the fourth intermetacarpal space the accessory primordium (the interosseus dorsalis accessorius) almost constantly joins the interossei primordia and fuses with the dorsal interosseus. In the 2nd and 3rd intermetacarpal spaces these accessory primordia either persist as small independent muscles, or also fuse with the corresponding dorsal interossei (Fig. 84). There appears hence a further component playing the part in the morphogenesis of dorsal interossei. The manner in which such component is involved in the development of the interossei dorsales pedis will be demonstrated later.

8. Recapitulation of Observations on the Ontogenesis of the Interossei in the Human Hand

1. Three layers of muscle primordia participate in the development of the interossei of the human hand: the flexores breves profundi layer situated dorsal to the course of the ulnar nerve, the layer of intermetacarpal primordia situated in the intermetacarpal spaces dorsal to the flexores breves profundi, and the most dorsal layer of accessory primordia. The names denote the homologies of the primordia layers with the muscle layers in the hands of lower mammals.

2. The interosseus dorsalis I originates only from the flexores breves profundi layer, by fusion of two independent and independently innervated primordia, entering into the 1st intermetacarpal space from the thumb and from the 2nd finger metacarpals.

3. The interossei dorsales II, III and IV originate each by fusion of one primordium from the flexores breves profundi layer with one intermetacarpal primordium and potentially by joining the accessory dorsal primordium (especially the interosseus dorsalis IV).

4. The intermetacarpal and accessory primordia are supplied from the ulnar nerve by an independent branch piercing the intermetacarpal space in a dorsal direction.

5. The palmar interossei each correspond to one primordium of the flexores breves profundi layer.

6. Accessory primordia originate on the dorsal sides of the 2nd, 3rd and 4th intermetacarpal spatia. In their subsequent development they either fuse with the dorsal interosseus (most often in the 4th space), or they persist as the interossei dorsales accessorii muscles. They are then formed as slender muscles or their rudiments, or reduced in the form of the fascia dorsalis manus interossea strikingly thickened in the place of the accessory muscle.

7. The interossei dorsales accessorii muscles do not belong to the extensores breves; the anastomosis between the ulnar nerve and the n. interosseus antebrachii posterior, from which the accessory muscles are casually also innervated, can be formed independently of the occurrence of accessory primordia.

8. The fusion of primordia layers to form the dorsal interossei is a specific developmental pattern of the human hand, and concerns the very muscles controlling the fine movements of the fingers.

9. The Interossei Pedis in Human Ontogenesis

It has already been demonstrated in studies on the contrahentes primordia that the n. plantaris lateralis forms the boundary between superficial and deep primordia layers of the intrinsic foot musculature—like the n. ulnaris in the hand. During the study of deep hand muscle development, the primordia for the interossei manus, their interrelations and mutual fusions of primordial layers have been made clear (Čihák, 1963b, c, 1967a, 1968b, 1969c). The situation in the hand will now be compared with the arrangement, development and changes of the interossei in the course of ontogenesis of the human foot.

It was obvious already during studies of the contrahentes layer that the primary distribution of primordia layers in the foot was in accordance with that in the hand. Therefore, Bardeleben's scheme of muscle layers is employed also for the foot, where the primordia layers are accordingly denoted. Since in the developing hand intermetacarpal primordia and the accessory primordia on the dorsal sides of intermetacarpal spaces have been found besides the layers described by Bardeleben, his scheme has been supplemented by these layers in the following study. The development of the interossei of the human foot will be explained with regard to the occurrence of these intermetatarsal and accessory layers. Their existence—as will be demonstrated further—has been suggested by some of the literary data.

10. Material for Studies of the Development of the Mm. Interossei of the Human Foot

The course of development and changes in muscle primordia of the foot was followed in the layers situated dorsal to the ramus profundus nervi plantaris lateralis. The observations were carried out on histological series of 70 feet of human embryos and foetuses from 12 to 60 mm in C-R length. Most series were cut sagittally and two series parallel to the sole for control.

The C-R lengths of the employed embryos were: 12 mm, 13, 14, 15, 15.5 (2 feet), 16 (3), 16.5 (3), 17 (5), 17.5 (2), 18 (3), 19 (2), 20 (3), 21 (4), 22 (2), 23 (2), 24 (2), 25 (2), 26 (2), 27 (2), 28 (2), 29 (2), 30 (3), 31 (2), 32 (2), 33 (2), 34 (2), 35 (2), 36, 37, 38, 40 (2), 46 (2), 54 (2), 60 mm.

The staining of histological series is described on pp. 10–11.

11. Observations of the Development of the Interossei Pedis

The primordia of the interossei pedis appear on the plantar side of the metatarsals, separated from the more plantar situated contrahentes layer by the coursing lateral plantar nerve. The interossei primordia are visible as a poorly differentiated layer in embryos of 16 and 17 mm (Figs. 57, 58). Compared with the situation in the embryonic hand, they extend in a far more plantar direction, the coursing nerve remaining at a greater distance from the metatarsals. The other striking difference in comparison with the hand is that all interossei primordia in the foot are less exactly demarcated, being closely adjacent to each other. Even in embryos around 20 mm in C-R length the primordia of single interossei can hardly be identified since their margins cannot be distinguished exactly enough (Fig. 85).

As in the hand, also in the foot the primordia of the interossei originate in a number of layers. The most plantar of them corresponds to the flexores breves profundi layer of the mammalian comparative anatomy; it is the layer that reaches in the palmar direction up to the coursing lateral plantar nerve—thus attaining the demarcation against the contrahentes layer. The primordium of this layer is solid on the proximal side of the coursing lateral plantar nerve (Figs. 57, 58), distal to the nerve it divides already in small embryos (about 17 mm in C-R length) into portions for separate intermetatarsal spaces (Fig. 85). These portions correspond to the couples of primordia twins which have been observed in the hand. In the embryonic foot both twins of the couple remain undivided for a long time. Also in the human foot these twins are coupled so that they do

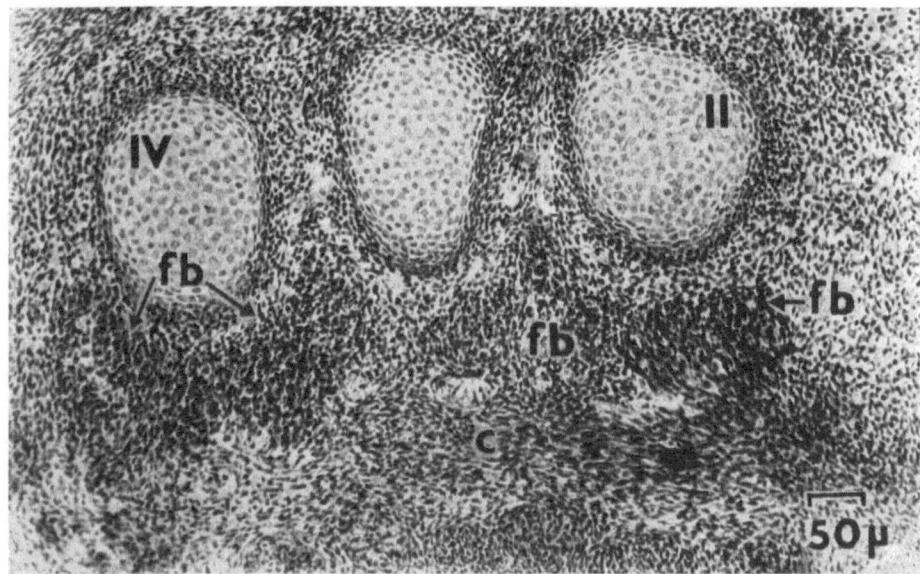

Fig. 85. Left foot of the embryo 20 mm in C-R length, transverse section. Positions of primordia for the interossei (primordia corresponding to the flexores breves profundi) (*fb*), in relation to intermetatarsal spaces and to the contrahentes layer (*c*). Intermetatarsal primordia are already fused with the flexores breves profundi forming their dorsal edges at this stage; *II, IV* the metatarsals

not relate to the metatarsals but to the palmar margins of the intermetatarsal spaces (Fig. 69). They are, however, far enough from the intermetatarsal spaces at younger stages and their volume is relatively small, e.g. in the 17 mm embryo (Fig. 89). The primordia then increase quickly and from 18 mm C-R length onward they lean against each other and reach further into the intermetatarsal spaces (Fig. 85). This, however, is made possible by the early fusion with the next dorsal layer of primordia.

The Interosseus Dorsalis I. In small embryos (between 17 and 24 mm in C-R length) the primordia from the flexores breves profundi layer extend into the first intermetatarsal space from the two sides, i.e. from the first and the second metatarsals. Both triangle-shaped primordia enter the first space (Fig. 86) ending in its dorsal part at the accessory primordium of the os intermetatarseum, which is always present in these stages as a variable rudimentary formation (comp. Figs. 24—26). The early stages of interosseus dorsalis I development are hence very similar to the situation in the hand. This pattern, however, persists only for a relatively short time; after reaching 24 mm C-R length the tibial part of the entering material becomes reduced (its fate will be demonstrated later) and the entire interosseus dorsalis I consists now only of the part entering from the second metatarsal. During subsequent development up to reaching a C-R length of 30 mm the primordium of the first dorsal interosseus remains attached to the 2nd metatarsal, not yet being linked up to the great toe metatarsal. By subsequent growth this primordium gets more bulky and then gradually

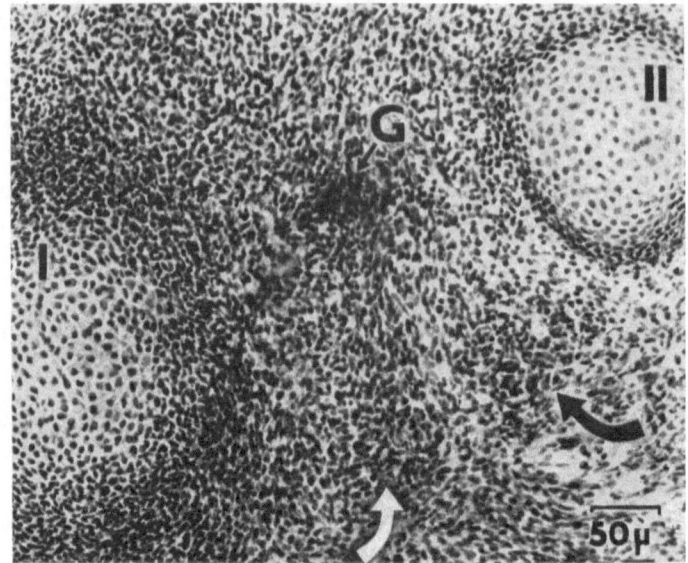

Fig. 86. Right foot of the 19 mm embryo, transverse section. Into the first intermetatarsal space the material of the flexores breves profundi layer enters from the two sides (arrows) at this stage of development. *I, II* metatarsals; *G* primordium of the os intermetatarseum Gruberi (var.)

fills in the whole 1st intermetatarsal space. The primordium of interosseus dorsalis I stands beneath the 2nd metatarsal in connection with the continuing flexores breves profundi layer (Figs. 87, 88). It involves here a further portion of the flexores breves profundi layer, which would belong (according to the scheme of other spaces) to the 2nd intermetatarsal space (Figs. 87, 88, 91, 94). The supplying nerve branch also corresponds with this situation; branching off from the ramus profundus nervi plantaris lateralis, it enters the primordia from the plantar side and divides into the two portions of the definitive muscle primordium. The joining of the 1st dorsal interosseus to the metatarsal of the great toe occurs secondarily, by the increase and expansion of the muscle, first in foetuses of about 80 mm in C-R length.

From the comparative viewpoint the interosseus dorsalis I is formed by one main component, which corresponds to the flexor brevis profundus tibialis digiti II, and by one additional, smaller, more plantar situated component, corresponding to the flexor brevis profundus fibularis digiti II (Figs. 91, 94).

The original tibial component of the early 1st interosseus primordium, which has become reduced in the course of the foregoing development, appears again after 30 mm C-R length in the form of a slender muscle primordium interposed between interosseus dorsalis I and the oblique head of the adductor hallucis, closely adjacent to the dorsal side of the oblique head of the adductor hallucis and inserted to the primordium of the metatarsophalangeal joint of the great toe. It is then of the same original position as the so-called interosseus palmaris I Henlei in the hand, and is known in the normal anatomy of foot muscles as a

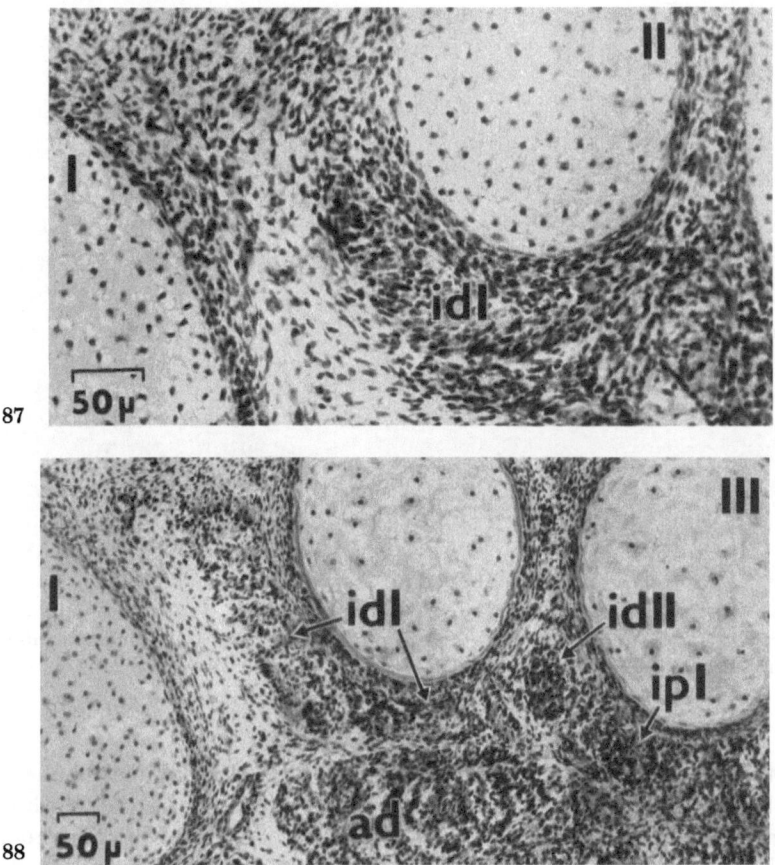

Fig. 87. Right foot of the 34 mm embryo, transverse section, first intermetatarsal space. The primordium of the first dorsal interosseus (*idI*) extends beneath the 2nd metatarsal up to the 2nd intermetatarsal space. *I, II* metatarsals

Fig. 88. Right foot of the embryo 45 mm in C-R length, transverse section. The interosseus dorsalis I extends into the 2nd intermetatarsal space and evidently contains the component of the flexores breves profundi layer for the 2nd dorsal interosseus which is then formed only by the intermetatarsal primordium; *idI, idII* dorsal interossei; *ipI* plantar interosseus; *I, III* metatarsals; *ad* the adductor hallucis

muscle variation, sometimes denoted as the interosseus palmaris I (Le Double, 1897), sometimes as the opponens hallucis (Kopsch, 1952). It follows from the development of this muscle and from its further relations concerning homology and nomenclature (as discussed in the chapter concerning the musculature of the great toe) that the most convenient name for it is *musculus interosseus plantaris hallucis*.

The mm. interossei dorsales II—IV. In the second, third and fourth intermetatarsal spaces of small embryos (about 17 mm) besides the typical well distinguishable pairs of primordia twins of the flexores breves profundi layer,

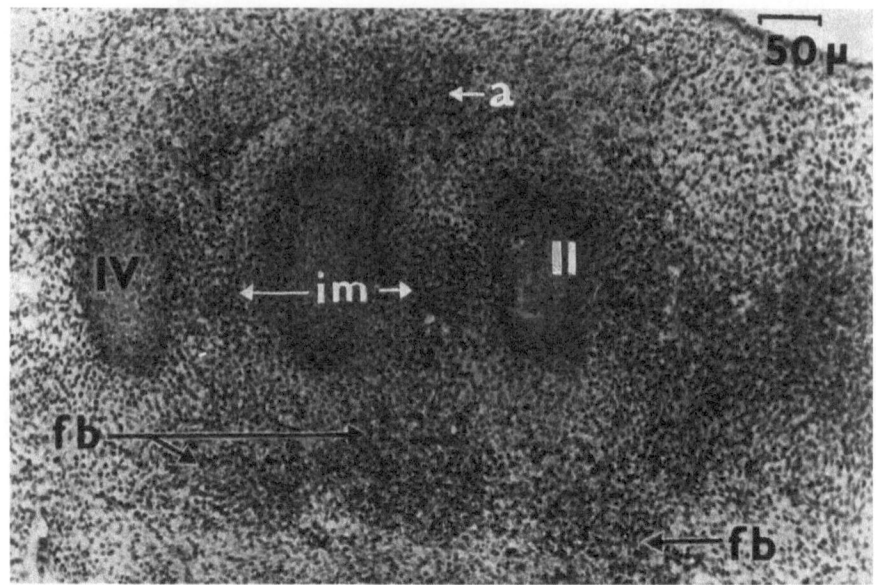

Fig. 89. Left foot of the embryo 17 mm in C-R length, transverse section. Layers of primordia of the interossei: *fb* primordia corresponding to the flexores breves profundi; *im* intermetatarsal primordia; *a* the interosseus dorsalis accessorius primordium. *II*, *IV* metatarsals

the intermetatarsal primordia (similar to the intermetacarpal ones in the hand) can still be found (Fig. 89). They are situated in the middle of the depth of the intermetatarsal spaces. From 18 mm C-R length on the primordia from the flexores breves profundi layer gradually extend into the intermetatarsal spaces and they fuse already in this stage with the intermetatarsal primordia. By this process evidence as to which part of the entire anlage of the dorsal interosseus belongs to the intermetatarsal primordium, as to the extent of the flexor brevis profundus primordium and the exact material making up the future plantar interosseus, becomes lost to a certain degree for a period of development up to 30 mm C-R length of embryo. As mentioned above in this chapter, the interossei primordia are poorly demarcated in this period of development being closely adjacent to each other. First in embryos of 30 mm the anlage of the dorsal interosseus starts to be more exactly separated from that of the plantar interosseus. In the course of later development, up to a C-R length of 60 mm, structural differences between the plantar part of the dorsal interosseus (i.e. the flexor brevis profundus primordium) and its dorsal part (i.e. the intermetatarsal primordium) are visible; a mesenchymal septum even appears between these two components. It may then be stated from this course of development that the primordia of the plantar interossei correspond solely to the flexores breves profundi layer (as they do in the hand), whilst the dorsal interossei, II—IV, each contain one plantar primordium from the flexores breves profundi layer and one dorsal intermetatarsal primordium (Fig. 91). In the second dorsal interosseus its plantar component is questionable (v. further).

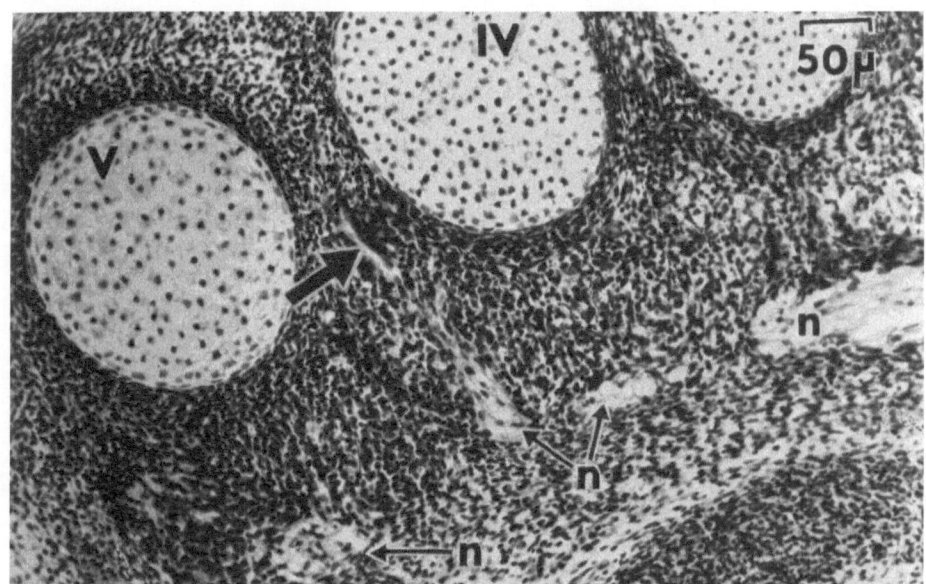

Fig. 90. Left foot of the embryo 24 mm in C-R length, transverse section. In the 4th inter-metatarsal space the nerve branch from the lateral plantar nerve perforating to dorsal is visible (arrow). It supplies the original intermetatarsal primordium and reaches up to the dorsal edge of the interosseus dorsalis primordium. *IV*, *V* the metatarsals; *n* lateral plantar nerve

Up to 40 mm C-R length of the embryo the primordia of the dorsal interossei do not extend to the dorsal sides of intermetatarsal spaces. Seen in the transverse section, their dorsal margins are not wide (as they are in the hand) but they are terminated by an acute edge (Figs. 64, 85, 91) and reach only into the middle of intermetatarsal spaces or, exceptionally, a little more dorsally. (This is a considerable difference in relation to the hand where the intermeta-carpal primordium occupies the dorsal third of the intermetacarpal space.)

The fusion of the primordia from the flexores breves profundi layer with the intermetatarsal primordia is demonstrated also by the nerve supply of the dorsal interossei. From the ramus profundus nervi plantaris lateralis a bifurcat-ing nerve enters the interosseus primordium; one twig from this bifurcation supplies the plantar primordium (the deep short flexor) the second one courses obliquely in a dorsal direction, into the intermetatarsal primordium and ends near its dorsal edge (Fig. 90). In the general arrangement of supplying nerve branches and in their connections to the dorsal sides of interossei primordia a certain difference from the hand can be observed and will be further demonstrated in the nerve supply to accessory primordia.

The described pattern appears in all embryos of corresponding age in the interossei of the 3rd and 4th intermetatarsal spaces (mm. interossei plantares II et III and mm. interossei dorsales III et IV). In the 2nd intermetatarsal space only the first plantar interosseus is typically formed; in the interosseus dorsalis II the participation of its dorsal and plantar primordium in the formation of the

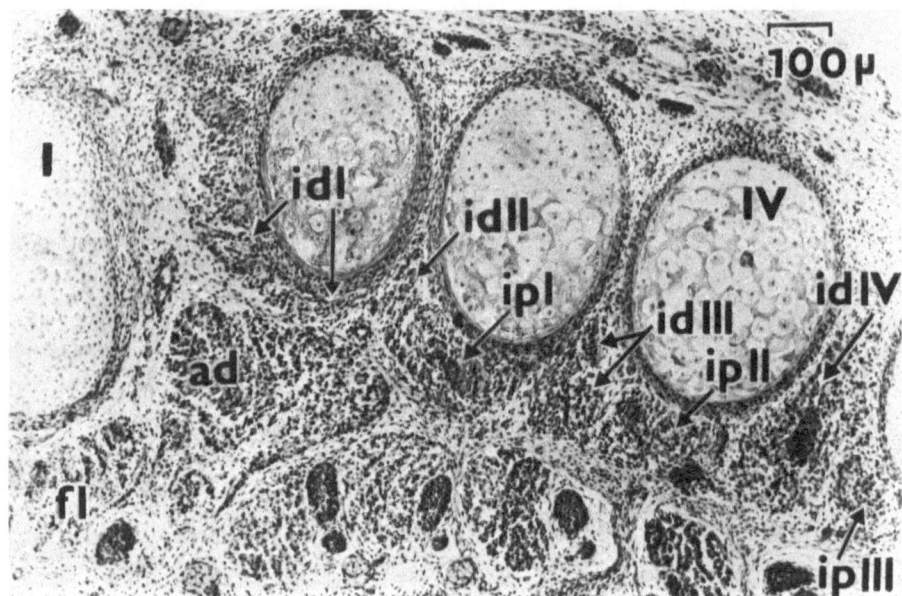

Fig. 91. Right foot of the foetus 60 mm in C-R length, transverse section. Definitive position of differentiated primordia of the interossei and of further muscles; *ipI-III* palmar interossei; *idI–IV* dorsal interossei; *ad* adductor hallucis, oblique head; *fl* flexor hallucis brevis, lateral head; *I*, *IV* metatarsals

entire muscle anlage is not well distinguishable (Fig. 91). In embryos up to 35 mm in C-R length the interosseus dorsalis I primordium extends from the 1st space, going arch-like beneath the plantar surface of the 2nd metatarsal into the margin of the 2nd intermetatarsal space up to the contact with the intermetatarsal primordium of the 2nd space. In older embryos (about 60 mm C-R length), where the mesenchymal septa are visible between the original intermetatarsal primordium and the flexor brevis profundus primordium, the duplication of primordia is found in the 3rd and 4th dorsal interossei but not in the interosseus dorsalis II. It may, therefore, be assumed that this muscle is formed only by an enlarged intermetatarsal component, the participation of the flexores breves profundi layer being either very scant or negative. It may be concluded from the distribution of primordia that the concerned material from the flexores breves profundi layer joined interosseus dorsalis I towards the other side of the 2nd metatarsal. This muscle visibly consists of two components, the more dorsal and the more plantar one (v. supra), both of them originating from the flexores breves profundi layer (Fig. 91). The view of the joining of primordia to form the interossei pedis is schematically given in Fig. 94.

12. Mm. Interossei Dorsales Accessorii Pedis and their Embryonic Primordia

In embryos of about 17 mm in C-R length, in which the layer of flexores breves profundi primordia and the layer of intermetatarsal primordia are visibly independent, further primordia are found at the level of the dorsal metatarsal

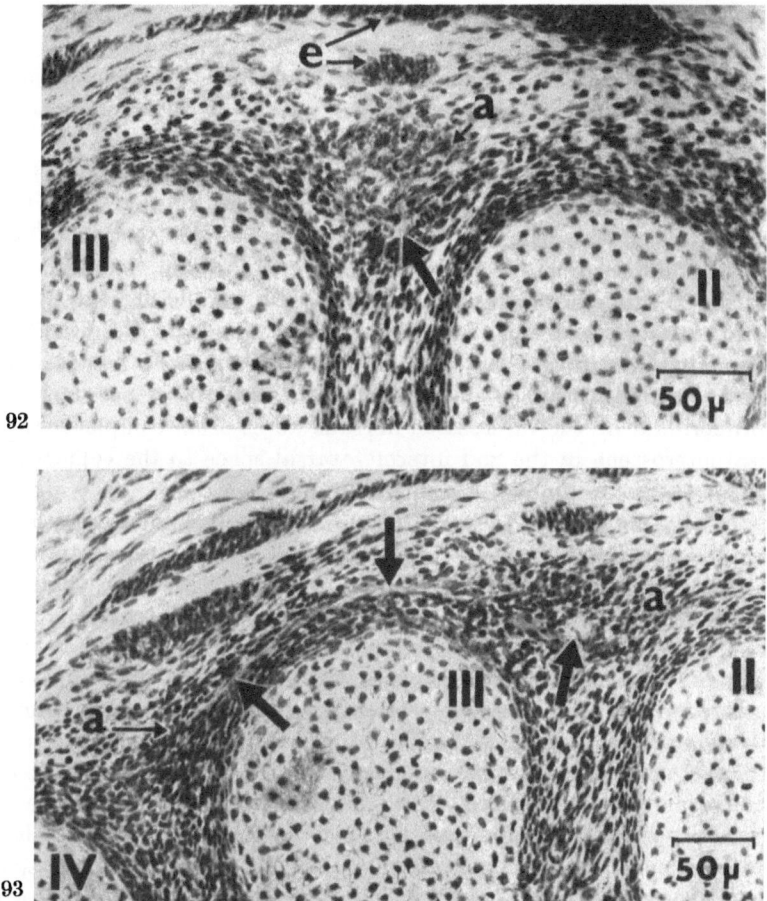

Fig. 92. Left foot of the embryo 26 mm in C-R length, transverse section, 2nd intermetatarsal space. On the dorsal side of the space the primordium of the interosseus dorsalis accessorius (*a*) is well visible. Supplying nerve in this primordium is indicated by arrows. Dorsal to the accessory primordium two layers of extensor tendons are visible. *II, III* metatarsals

Fig. 93. Same series as in Fig. 92, several sections more to distal. Accessory primordia (interossei dorsales accessorii) in the 2nd and 3rd intermetatarsal spaces. From the nerve in the primordium of the 2nd space the supplying branch passes over the 3rd metatarsal to the accessory primordium in the 3rd space (arrows); *a* accessory primordia; *II, III, IV* metatarsals

margins, situated over the 2nd and 3rd intermetatarsal spaces (Fig. 89). Comparison with the pattern of muscle primordia in the hand reveals these elements in the foot to be the interossei dorsales accessorii. In small embryos this layer of primordia is seen in the form of inexactly demarcated condensations of mesenchyme, later the typical muscle primordia are formed (Fig. 92). Their position is distinctly different from the layer of the extensor hallucis brevis and the extensor digitorum brevis (Figs. 92, 93), their pattern in transverse section distinctly reveals their appurtenance to the intermetatarsal space as its dorsal demarcation. Accessory primordia are mutually joined by the mesenchyme representing the future fascia dorsalis pedis interossea. With increasing embryo length accessory primordia are still better demarcated and they gradually assume the typical form of strip-like accessory interossei similar to those observed in the hand (v. s.).

Each accessory element has its origin near the metatarsal bases, its insertion courses distally into the developing dorsal aponeurosis of the finger together with the insertion of the proper dorsal interosseus. In the feet of embryos of our material the interosseus dorsalis accessorius primordium was nearly always formed in the 2nd intermetatarsal space (Fig. 92), completing the dorsal side of the dorsal interosseus. It has already been mentioned in the description of the interossei that the interosseus dorsalis primordium of the foot is not wide at its dorsal end, but rather edge-shaped. In the transverse section it is clear that the primordium of the interosseus dorsalis accessorius completes the form of the dorsal interosseus in the 2nd intermetatarsal space to the typical form of the dorsal interosseus as known also in the human hand.

In the third intermetatarsal space this accessory primordium is also formed quite often, in about half the cases, while in the fourth intermetatarsal space its form is only transiently suggested and the corresponding mesenchymal material there early forms the thick lamellous fascia dorsalis pedis interossea.

The nerve supply of the interossei dorsales accessorii pedis differs from the manner of innervation of corresponding muscles in the hand. Whilst in the hand these muscles are always entered by perforating branches from the ramus profundus nervi ulnaris and only exceptionally supplied from an anastomosis between the ulnar nerve and the n. interosseus antebranchii posterior, in the foot as a rule these muscles are innervated from the anastomosis between the ramus profundus nervi peronei and the ramus profundus nervi plantaris lateralis. This anastomosis normally courses only through the 2nd intermetatarsal space (a similar one is sometimes found also in the first space). It is effected by a nerve branch from the typical coursing of the nervus peroneus profundus over the first space. This nerve branch joins the perforating branch from the n. plantaris lateralis for the 2nd dorsal interosseus and the accessory muscle in the second space is directly supplied from this anastomosis. A further twig is given off from this anastomosis, coursing transversely over the third metatarsal into the accessory primordium of the third space, if this is developed (Fig. 93).

13. Discussion and Conclusions from Observations of the Ontogenesis of the Interossei in the Human Foot

In considering the muscle primordia of the interossei of the human foot it has been possible to employ (as for the hand) Bardeleben's general scheme (1890) of autopodial muscle layers. In the foot also the nerve (the lateral plantar nerve) represents the demarcation of intrinsic muscle layers (like the ulnar nerve in the hand), the interossei layers being dorsal to this nerve. It was still necessary to add further dorsal primordial layers (Fig. 76) to Bardeleben's scheme as in the scheme of layers of hand muscles.

The described observations support McMurrich's (1907, 1927) view that the material for the interossei pedis is represented by two layers of primordia, the flexores breves profundi layer and the layer of intermetatarsal primordia. The information obtained by the present study, however, is somewhat different from the concept claimed by that author. It has been stated that the intermetatarsal primordia can be found as independent elements only in very small embryos, while McMurrich (1907) strikingly outlined the dorsal sector of intermetatarsal spaces as belonging to the intermetatarsal primordia in an old fetus. It can be stated in comparison with our observations that McMurrich (1907, 1927) considered the accessory dorsal element to be the intermetatarsal primordium. The accessory element in these stages is relatively large and is situated in the 2nd and often also in the 3rd intermetatarsal space, in the position pointed out by this author for the intermetatarsal anlage. The participation of the accessory element in the formation of the dorsal interosseus is, however, inconstant. The origin of the described error consists in the simple application of the situation in the developing hand to that in the foot.

It is impossible to share the views of Lessertisseur (1958) and Jouffroy (1962) who claim that during ontogenesis and phylogenesis the interossei belong only to one layer, from which in course of development a further layer then delaminates. Our observations, on the contrary, reveal that even three primordial muscle layers can participate in the developing dorsal interossei, the flexores breves profundi layer, the layer of intermetatarsal primordia and the most dorsal layer of accessory primordia. The developmental trend, contrary to the view of these authors, can be seen in the gradual fusion of these layers, not in their delamination. This situation is the same in the hand and in the foot in Man.

While all plantar interossei in the foot are simple formations, each of them originating by a simple primordium in the flexores breves profundi layer, all dorsal interossei are combined elements and their development proceeds in a manner which varies according to components involved (Fig. 94).

1. M. interosseus dorsalis I originates by fusion of two primordia from the flexores breves profundi layer; one of them belonged originally to the 1st space (being adjacent to the 2nd metacarpal from the tibial side) and the second one belonged to the 2nd intermetatarsal space. This latter, being originally adjacent to the lateral (fibular) side of the 2nd metatarsal, joins the former primordium from the fibular and plantar side.

2. Mm. interossei dorsales II—IV originate by fusion of layers, superimposed inside the intermetatarsal space, principially in two manners:

a) In the corresponding space no accessory dorsal primordium is formed; the dorsal interosseus is composed only of the flexor brevis profundus primordium and the intermetatarsal primordium and extends dorsally only to half of the planto-dorsal depth of the intermetatarsal space. The dorsal interosseus first grows into the dorsal part of the space in later developmental stages (about 60 mm in C-R length). The participation of the plantar component from the flexores breves profundi layer in the interosseus dorsalis II is either minimal or this component is absent here, being fused with the interosseus dorsalis I.

b) In case of a well formed accessory dorsal primordium in the corresponding intermetatarsal space, the interosseus dorsalis (composed of its typical two components) fuses with it early, both filling the entire space, and the accessory primordium (being relatively very large) occupies the dorsal sector of the space.

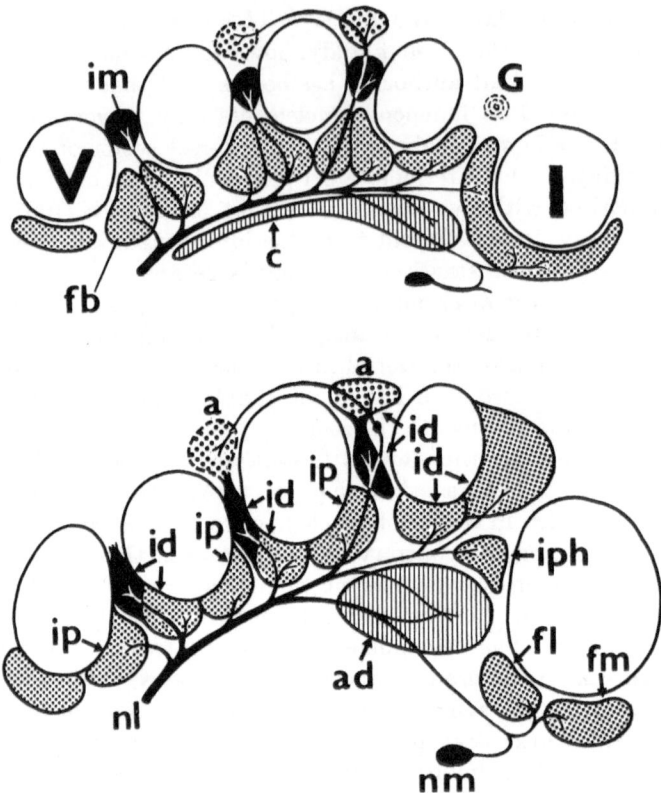

Fig. 94. Scheme of embryonic primordia layers of the intrinsic muscles in the embryonic foot (above) and of resulting muscles in adults (below); *nl* nervus plantaris lateralis; *nm* nervus plantaris medialis; *c* the contrahentes layer; *fb* the flexores breves profundi layer; *im* the intermetatarsal layer; *a* primordia of the interossei dorsales accessorii; *id, ip* dorsal and plantar interossei; *iph* the interosseus plantaris hallucis; *fl, fm* lateral and medial heads of the flexor hallucis brevis; *ad* adductor hallucis (oblique head)

The accessory primordium is at first loosely joined to the true dorsal interosseus, later on it fuses with it to a variable extent. If the accessory primordium is reduced, the thick fascia dorsalis interossea is seen in its place, as in the hand.

At least one embryonic primordium of the interosseus dorsalis accessorius is found in each foot, in the 2nd intermetatarsal space. Only exceptionally (in two feet of our material) could such a primordium not be found. Lucien (1909 a, b, c, 1910) described accessory elements in the foot in the form of rare muscle slips connecting the short extensors with the interossei, and held these connections to be occasional secondary formations. From the standpoint of ontogenesis it is impossible to consider Lucien's muscular slips the residua of the proper accessory interossei primordia, since these primordia develop in another position, joined to the intermetatarsal spaces. The development of the primordia layers suggests, however, that the observed layer of accessory primordia (completing the intermetatarsal musculature) delaminates from the deep surface of the deep extensor blastema, and is then supplied by branches from the anastomosis between palmar and dorsal nerves. The muscular slips, observed by Lucien, can be taken to be inconstant traces of the detachment of interossei dorsales accessorii primordia from the deep extensor layer. The entire layer of the interossei dorsales accessorii appears as a developmentally non-stabilized pattern.

14. Recapitulation of Observations on the Ontogenesis of the Interossei in the Human Foot

1. Three layers of muscular primordia can take part in the development of the interossei pedis: the plantar layer, corresponding to the flexores breves profundi muscles of Mammals in general, the intermediate layer of intermetatarsal primordia and the dorsal layer represented by the accessory primordia (the interossei dorsales accessorii).

2. The first dorsal interosseus is formed by one main primordium from the flexores breves profundi layer (coming from the 2nd metatarsal) and by one further adjoined primordium from the same layer, which originally belonged to the 2nd intermetatarsal space.

3. The interossei dorsales II–IV originate each by fusion of primordia, superimposed in the intermetatarsal spaces, i.e. by fusion of one primordium of the flexores breves profundi layer with the intermetatarsal anlage, already in early developmental stages (18 to 20 mm C-R length). In nearly all cases the further dorsal accessory primordium joins this complex in the 2nd intermetatarsal space and in about half of the cases in the 3rd space.

4. The plantar component (from the flexores breves profundi layer) in the 2nd dorsal interosseus is either very meagre or absent, and is joined to the 1st dorsal interosseus as its plantar material.

5. The plantar interossei correspond each to one primordium of flexores breves profundi layer.

6. The accessory components develop on the dorsal side of the 2nd and 3rd intermetatarsal spaces (only in about half of the cases in the 3rd space); they become rudimentary to various degrees and gradually fuse with the dorsal interossei.

7. The accessory primordia are always supplied by the anastomosis connecting the n. plantaris lateralis with the n. peroneus profundus. The interossei dorsales accessorii primordia develop in situ as a deep separate layer of the dorsal muscular blastema of the foot. The traces of their developmental appurtenance to the dorsal musculature can be seen in rare muscular slips in adults connecting the extensores breves of the foot with the dorsal material of some intermetatarsal spaces.

15. Comparison of Development of the Interossei in the Human Hand and Foot

In the hand and foot of Man identical and identically situated primordial layers participate in the development of the interossei. The interossei of the hand, however, differ from those of the foot in detailed pattern. The intermetatarsal primordia in the foot (contrary to the hand) appear independently only in small embryos and fuse early with the primordia of the flexores breves profundi layer to form the dorsal interossei primordia. This fusion occurs in younger embryos than the corresponding one in the hand. The joined flexor brevis profundus and intermetacarpal (intermetatarsal) primordia are differently formed in the hand and in the foot. Seen in transverse section it ends in the hand by a dorsal wide and flat surface, while in the foot it extends only in the plantar two thirds of the space and has a sharp edge. This latter is the form of the interossei observed in the hands and feet of lower Primates. In the course of ontogenesis the different form of the dorsal interossei primordia in the hand and foot is due to differently sized intermetacarpal and intermetatarsal primordia. During

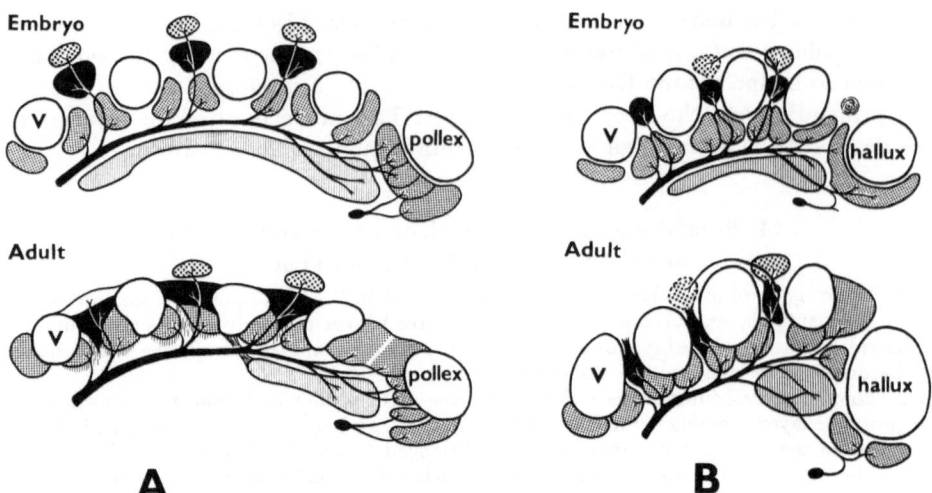

Fig. 95. Comparison of embryonic and adult hand and foot. Single layers of primordia are compared by corresponding shading. For single elements cf. the legends in Figs. 84 and 94. *A* the hand; *B* the foot. (Partly according to Čihák, 1968b, modified)

subsequent development this difference is diminished by the rapid growth of intermetatarsal primordia.

The differences between the hand and the foot, seen in the pattern of the interossei dorsales I and II, occur on the basis of the equal basic scheme of primordia due to the shifted system of their fusion into definitive muscles (cf. the scheme in Fig. 95).

Considerable difference between the hand and the foot is observed in the mode of differentiation and the nerve supply of accessory primordia. Although developing inside the dorsal margin of intermetacarpal spaces in the hand, the appurtenance of this layer to the palmar musculature is indicated by its nerve supply. The corresponding primordial layer of the foot is an evident derivative of the dorsal blastema, its appurtenance to intermetatarsal primordia being probably a secondary one, connected with the nerve supply from the anastomosis of dorsal and plantar nerves.

The comparison of the detailed participation of primordia from single layers in the origin of the interossei of the hand and the foot is indicated in the scheme in Fig. 95.

D. Development of Muscular Groups of Marginal Digits in the Hand and Foot

1. The Development of Thenar Muscles

The thenar muscles seemingly deviate from the sequence of palmar muscles known in comparative anatomy and from the previous findings in embryology. Only the deep head of the flexor pollicis brevis as a part of the flexores breves profundi layer and the adductor pollicis as derived from the contrahentes layer can be set into the scheme of palmar musculature without difficulties. If the abductor pollicis brevis is regarded as a clearly superficial palmar muscle and not as the so-called marginal element of Cunningham's (1878a) dorsal layer (so forcibly classified by this author), then according to their position in the thenar, the superficial head of the flexor pollicis brevis and together with it the opponens pollicis appear to be muscles of the intermediate layer.

The problem of the homology of the opponens pollicis is quite obscure. From the comparative-anatomical standpoint this muscle appears to be newly formed in Primates; its pattern and position as for thenar layers is also somewhat different from Man in some Anthropoids. According to Jouffroy (1962) the flexor pollicis brevis, the opponens pollicis and the abductor pollicis brevis, particularly the flexor and the opponens, are fused to such a degree that they appear as a single mass. The same author mentions that even in Man, in whom these muscles are more perfectly separated from each other, they still permit different interpretations.

Based upon previous studies demonstrating that the ontogenesis of palmar muscles follows the line of recapitulations of successive forms in the course of phylogenesis and that the study of ontogenesis permitted the clarification of the morphogenesis and homologies of all studied muscles, we attempted to obtain evidence about the development of the opponens pollicis and flexor pollicis brevis by studying their ontogenesis (Čihák, 1966b, 1969a, c). Additional information concerning ontogenesis seems to be necessary for all thenar muscles, since the fundamental studies on the development of the locomotor apparatus of the extremities (Bardeen and Lewis, 1901; Lewis, 1901/02, 1910) contain only general remarks on the differentiation of thenar muscles from one common blastema. Differentiation from the common blastema was also claimed by McMurrich (1903) for the abductor pollicis and the opponens pollicis. There are also plenty of contradictions in the comparative anatomy of Primates, especially opinions about homologies of the superficial and the deep heads of the flexor pollicis brevis and the opponens pollicis (Champneys, 1871/72; Langer, 1879; Brooks, 1886a, b, 1888; Cunningham, 1887; Hepburn, 1891/92).

The ontogenesis of thenar muscular primordia has therefore been followed in order to ascertain their homologies.

2. Material for Studies of the Development of the Thenar Muscles in the Hand

For this study 62 hands of human embryos and foetuses from 12 to 65 mm C-R length were employed, all of them studied in transverse histological series. C-R lengths of embryos and foetuses employed: 12 mm, 13.6, 14, 15 (2 hands), 15.5 (2), 16 (2), 16.5 (2), 17, 17.5 (3), 18 (4), 19 (4), 19.5 (3), 20 (4), 21 (4), 22 (2), 23 (2), 25 (4), 26 (3), 27 (2), 28 (2), 29 (2), 30 (2), 32 (2), 35 (2), 40, 45, 50, 56, 65 mm.

The staining of series is described on pp. 10–11.

3. Observations of the Development of the Thenar Muscles

The whole muscular mass of the thenar region in younger embryos can be shown as consisting of only two layers. The superficial layer is represented by the primordium of the abductor pollicis brevis, the deep one is formed by the blastema common to all the remaining thenar muscles with the exception of the

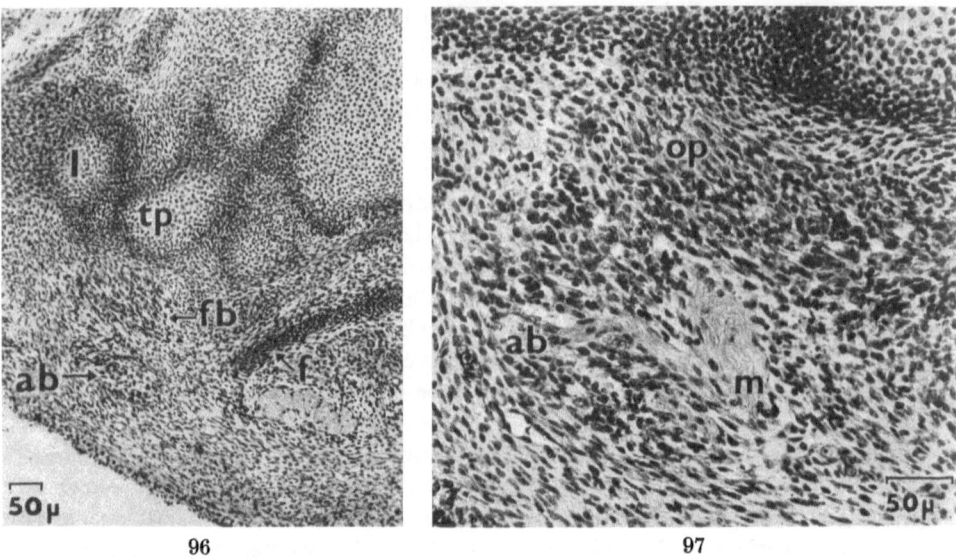

96   97

Fig. 96. Right hand of the 17 mm embryo, transverse section at the level of the distal carpal row. The muscle blastema in the thenar region differentiates into two layers of primordia. The superficial layer is the future abductor pollicis (*ab*) and the deep layer (corresponding to the flexores breves profundi *fb*) is the source of all remaining thenar muscles with the exception of the adductor pollicis; *f* primordium of tendons of the flexor digitorum profundus; *tp* trapezium; *I* first metacarpal

Fig. 97. Right hand of the 23 mm embryo, transverse section. The characteristic difference in the orientation of the cells of the two primordia layers in the thenar musculature. The division of the median nerve (*m*) for the two layers is sectioned; *ab* abductor pollicis brevis primordium; *op* region of the future opponens pollicis

adductor pollicis (Fig. 96). (The development of the adductor pollicis is described in the chapter concerning the contrahentes layer.)

The abductor pollicis differentiates in external form and cytology much earlier than the deep layer, already at the stage of 15—17 mm C-R length, while the deep thenar layer at these stages is represented only by an amorphous blastema. The abductor pollicis brevis is thus separate and independent from the very beginning of its development (Fig. 97), being sooner differentiated in form and cytology and forming the superficial layer of the thenar musculature. Its primordium is frequently found duplicated (Figs. 102, 103), the more radial and in the transverse section also the more dorsally situated part of the primordium can be connected to the abductor pollicis longus. The connection between the short and the long abductor is found in many variations, as described in detail by Kaneff (1968) according to the degree of this reduction. We did not find this connection of the two muscles from the very beginning of the differentiation of the abductor brevis, it develops as a secondary pattern in embryos after 50 mm in C-R length.

The supplying nerve branch from the median nerve entering the opponens pollicis primordium from its surface is a branch from the same nerve trunk as that innervating the abductor pollicis brevis primordium (Fig. 97). This mode of nerve supply therefore supports the impression that the anlage of the opponens pollicis belongs to the superficial thenar blastema. However, it can clearly be seen in preparations that the abductor pollicis brevis is quite different in its position and degree of differentiation (Fig. 97).

In these early embryonic stages the opponens pollicis primordium belongs neither to the superficial abductor pollicis anlage, nor is it formed as an intermediate layer between the abductor and the deep primordia. At these stages it is an inseparable part of the continuous deep blastema. This deep blastema, as a matter of fact, represents a radial continuation of the flexores breves profundi layer (Figs. 100, 101), thus representing a continuation of the basic layer for the development of the interossei.

From the beginning of its development the opponens pollicis primordium extends rather proximally, further than the primordia of the interossei. On transverse section in the borderline between the proximal and the distal carpal row the primordium of the opponens pollicis can be seen lying very close to the abductor pollicis brevis primordium (Fig. 96). It is possible to distinguish the two according to the orientation of the myoblasts, which in transverse section are seen cross-sectioned in the abductor pollicis brevis, whereas in the opponens pollicis they are sectioned mostly longitudinally (Fig. 97). The exact clue for distinguishing the two primordia is their supplying nerve branches (Fig. 97).

In the course of its subsequent development the opponens pollicis primordium changes in relation to the development of the retinaculum flexorum anlage. This developing ligament is seen in small embryos (15—16 mm) as distinctly formed on the ulnar side only, as a strip of fibroblasts attached (imperfectly, at that time) to the hamulus ossis hamati primordium. Radially, i.e. at the level of the opponens pollicis primordium, the anlage of the retinaculum flexorum terminates freely in the mesenchyme (Fig. 98); later, in older embryos, it is gradually connected with the eminentia carpi radialis (Čihák, 1966b, 1969a, c). The orientation of fibroblasts toward the opponens pollicis primordium already indicates the future origin of this muscle on the ligament (Fig. 99). The form and the degree of differentiation of the retinaculum flexorum anlage is, among others, in agreement with the development of the m. flexor digitorum superficialis, which in young embryos is a muscle situated inside the palm and in the canalis carpi, embraced by an arch-formed retinaculum flexorum anlage (Fig. 98). After the belly of the flexor digitorum superficialis primordium has ascended to the forearm (Dylevský, 1967, 1968c) and coincidently with the development of the arching of the carpal region, the shape and course of the retinaculum flexorum anlage attain their definitive pattern. Together with form changes of the retinaculum its relation to the developing palmaris longus muscle also originates and changes (Dylevský, 1969a).

Up to the stage of 28 mm in C-R length the opponens pollicis primordium develops as a typical component of the deep musculature extending by a strip as far as to the os capitatum primordium (Fig. 100). The entire deep thenar blastema embraces the thumb metacarpal from the palmar side and reaches both to its radial and ulnar surfaces (Fig. 104). The blastema is extensive, containing not only the opponens pollicis primordium, but also the flexor pollicis

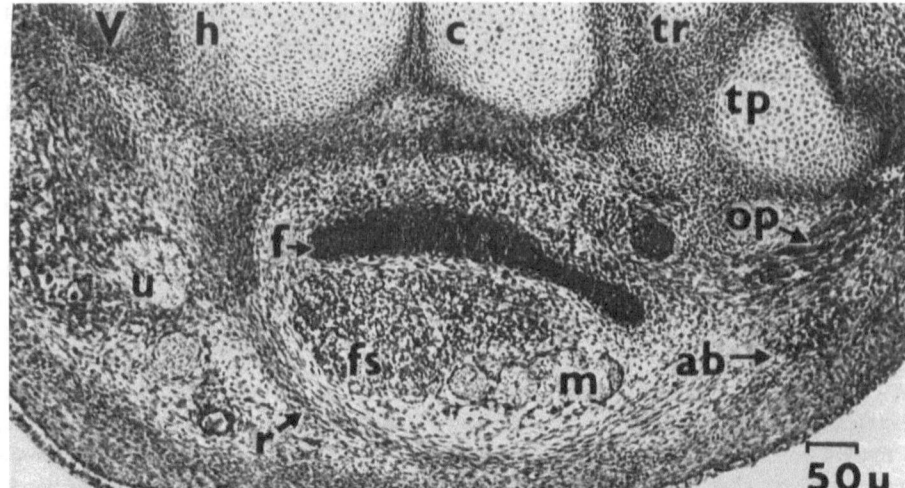

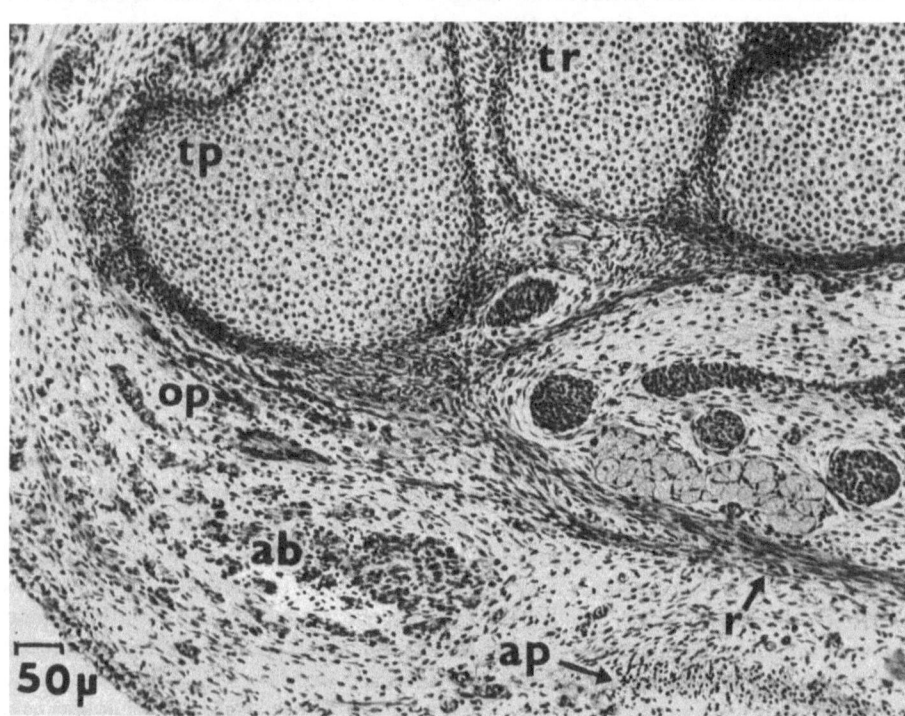

Fig. 98. Left hand of the embryo 15.5 mm in C-R length, transverse section through the distal row of the primordia of carpal bones. The developing anlage of the retinaculum flexorum is differentiated in the vicinity of the hamulus ossis hamati but does not reach to the radial carpal margin. Coursing through the palm the retinaculum anlage passes around the flexor digitorum superficialis primordium; *tp* trapezium; *tr* trapezoideum; *c* capitatum; *h* hamatum; *V* fifth metacarpal; *r* retinaculum flexorum anlage; *u* ulnar nerve; *m* median nerve; *f* primordium of tendons of the flexor digitorum profundus; *fs* primordium of the flexor digitorum superficialis; *ab* abductor pollicis brevis primordium; *op* opponens pollicis. (Čihák, 1969b)

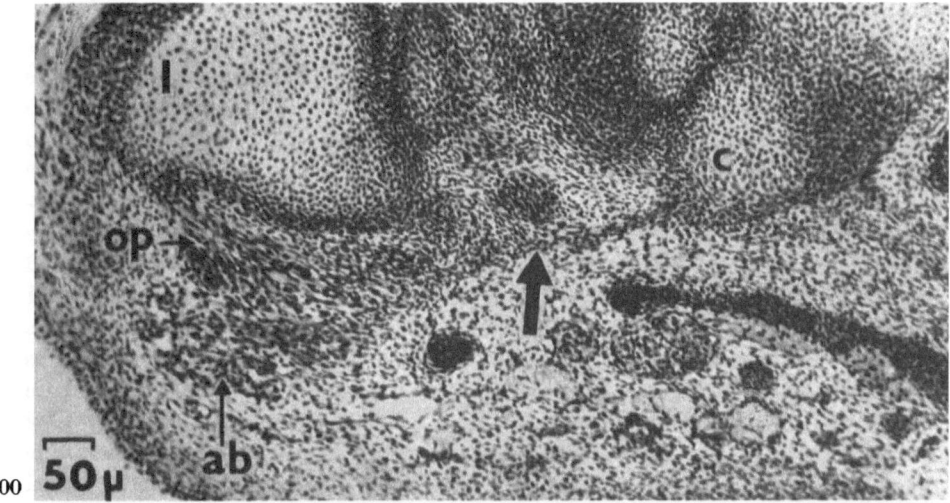

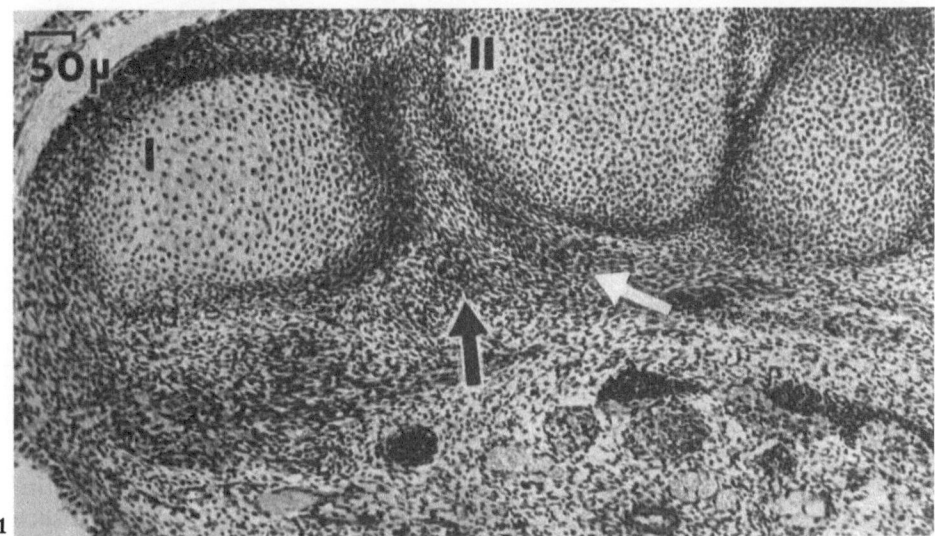

Fig. 100. Right hand of the 23 mm embryo, transverse section at the level of carpometacarpal region. The deep thenar primordium, differentiating opponens pollicis (*op*) joins the primordium of the capitate (*c*) by a mesenchymal strip (arrow); *ab* primordium of the abductor pollicis brevis; *I* first metacarpal. (Čihák, 1969b)

Fig. 101. Right hand of the 23 mm embryo, transverse section through the metacarpals near their bases. From the deep thenar primordium a part of material enters the first inter-metacarpal space as the radial component of the interosseus dorsalis I primordium (black arrow); the second component of the interosseus dorsalis I comes from the same layer (flexores breves profundi layer) but from the 2nd metacarpal (white arrow). (Čihák, 1969b)

Fig. 99. Right hand of the embryo 50 mm in C-R length, right hand, transverse section at the level of the distal carpal row. The retinaculum flexorum anlage (*r*) is differentiated already up to the radial margin of the carpus and the opponens pollicis primordium (*op*) adjoins it; *ab* the abductor pollicis brevis primordium; *ap* differentiating palmar aponeurosis; *tp* the trapezium anlage; *tr* trapezoideum. (Čihák, 1969b)

brevis, including the primordia of its deep as well as of its superficial head. The most dorsal process of the ulnar side of this blastema becomes detached in the course of early developmental stages (in embryos of about 15 mm in length) to move dorsally into the first intermetacarpal space as the radial half of the future interosseus dorsalis I (Figs. 101, 104, for comp. see the development of the interosseus dorsalis I in Figs. 70, 77). In some cases between this dorsal part and the remaining primordium a split-off remnant of cellular material can be recognized which is known in adults as a variation, the so-called m. interosseus palmaris I Henlei (Fig. 104). In the course of embryonic development individual components of the deep blastema can be identified according to ingrowing nerve branches from the ulnar and the median nerves, in later stages the primordia of single muscles are already clearly separated from one another (Fig. 102). A really distinct separation of various muscular primordia cannot be seen before the stage of 28 mm in C-R length. The positions of components and the differentiated material are indicated in Fig. 103.

In the definitively differentiated blastema (after the previous detachment of the component for the 1st dorsal interosseus and for the interosseus palmaris I Henlei) the most radially situated part represents the primordium of the opponens pollicis. In this an additional splitting into layers can sometimes be seen, so that it becomes somewhat opened from the radial side, as often observed in adults. The pocket formed by this split usually contains loose connective tissue in the adult. The original strip-like expansion of the deep blastema proceeding ulnad up to the anlage of the os capitatum (Fig. 100), becomes reduced. In the meantime the retinaculum flexorum has differentiated (see above) now reaching up to the proximity of the thenar primordium, and a part of the opponens has acquired a new origin by becoming connected to this ligament (Fig. 99). According to its ontogenesis, the origin of the opponens pollicis and the retinaculum flexorum should be regarded as a secondary junction of the muscle.

In further parts of the deep thenar blastema the primordia of both heads of the flexor pollicis brevis develop as a direct continuation of the opponens pollicis in the ulnar direction. The superficial and the deep head can be distinguished according to their position (Figs. 102—104). Each of the two heads receives its supplying nerve branch more distally than the opponens pollicis primordium. The superficial head of the flexor brevis is entered at its surface by a branch from the median nerve. The deep head receives its supplying branch from the ulnar nerve through the primordium of the oblique head of the adductor pollicis. In the course of further development the already differentiated tendon of the flexor pollicis longus shifts between the two heads of the flexor pollicis brevis. In younger embryos this tendon is situated more superficially and medially.

In addition to the changes in the shape of the entire developing thenar blastema, there also occur changes of its relation to the skeletal primordia and

Fig. 102. Right hand of the embryo 31 mm in C-R length, transverse section at the level of metacarpal bases. The deep thenar primordium (corresponding with the flexores breves profundi layer) divides into three components: the opponens pollicis primordium (*op*), the superficial head (*fs*) and the deep head (*fp*) of the flexor pollicis brevis; *f* tendon of the flexor pollicis longus; *ab* abductor pollicis brevis primordium. (Čihák, 1969 b)

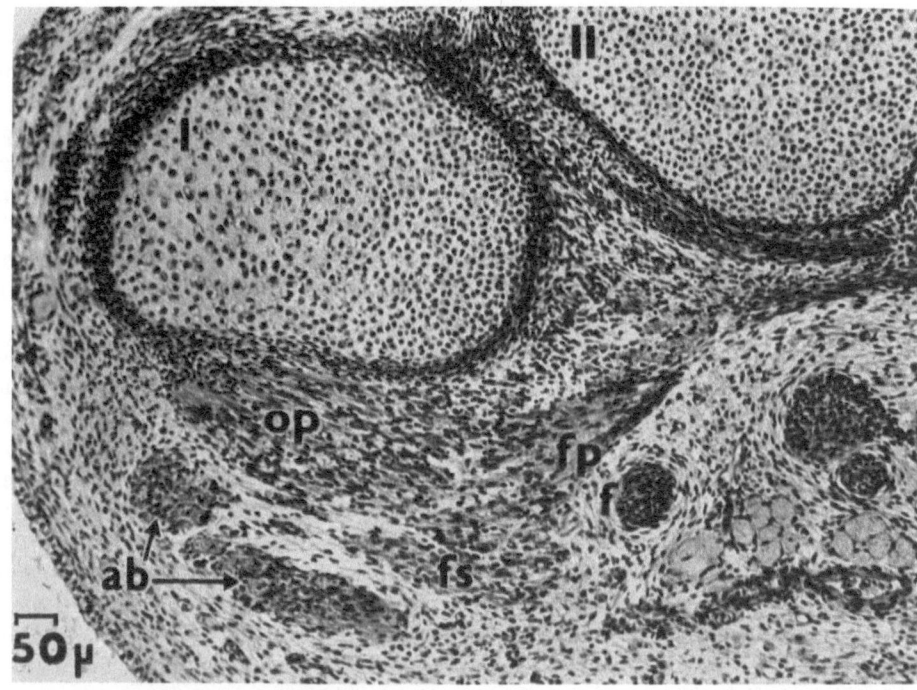

102

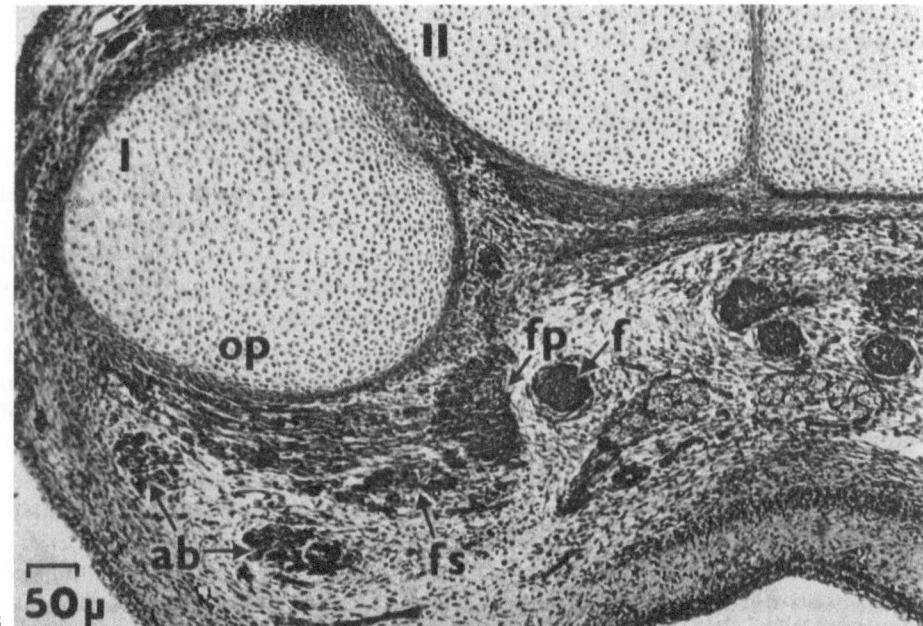

103

Fig. 103. Right hand of the 32 mm embryo, transverse section through metacarpal bases. The deep thenar primordium is definitively divided into the opponens pollicis (*op*), caput superficiale musculi flexoris pollicis brevis (*fs*) and the caput profundum musculi flexoris pollicis brevis (*fp*); *f* flexor pollicis longus tendon; *ab* abductor pollicis brevis primordium; *I, II* metacarpals. (Čihák, 1969b)

to the differentiating retinaculum flexorum. At the beginning of development, i. e. in embryos of about 15—17 mm C-R length, the entire deep thenar blastema adheres closely to the palmar surface of the first metacarpal. In further development—in embryos of 18—30 mm C-R length—the contact between the developing primordia and the perichondrium of the metacarpal anlage becomes lost. The proper insertion of the opponens pollicis is formed after the embryo has reached the C-R length of 30 mm. The attachment of the flexor pollicis brevis appears earlier, being mediated by the mesenchyme of the region of the metacarpophalangeal articulation of the thumb. No primordia of sesamoid bones can be found at that period.

By the differentiation of the two heads of the flexor brevis at the ulnar margin of the blastema common to the flexor brevis and the opponens, the primordium of the opponens pollicis looses its connection with the carpal skeleton, previously existing at the stage of the original common blastema in the form of a long strip (Fig. 100). The primordium of the opponens pollicis acquires a new connection, a new origin at the retinaculum flexorum, which has differentiated in the meantime (see above) and has also fused with the radial margin of the carpal skeleton. (Fig. 99.) By the formation of the new origin the whole mass of the opponens pollicis moves superficially, appearing secondarily as a new intermediate layer of the thenar musculature. As both heads of the flexor pollicis brevis lean against the opponens pollicis (being, in fact, derived from the original distoulnar margin of the common blastema), they are naturally attached distally to the last bundles of the opponens, i. e. in the region of the radial sesamoid bone of the thumb.

4. Discussion and Conclusions from Observations of the Ontogenesis of the Thenar

From the viewpoint of the layered pattern of the hand musculature in general it is possible to distinguish only two distinct layers of primordia in the thenar blastema: the superficial layer, represented by the abductor pollicis brevis, and the deep one which is the common primordium for the opponens pollicis and for both heads of the flexor pollicis brevis. (This complex does not include the adductor pollicis, which is derived from the contrahentes layer, representing approximately its radial half — Čihák, 1963a, b, 1967a, b, 1968a, b). From the standpoint of phylogenesis the opponens pollicis was considered a part of the deep musculature already by Howell (1936).

The frequent occurrence of aberrant bundles passing along the first metacarpal to the ulnar sesamoid bone can be explained by the late splitting off of the deep head of the flexor pollicis brevis (Brooks, 1888; Gegenbaur, 1894). These bundles were known as the so-called m. interosseus palmaris I Henlei and were often a basis for wrong interpretations of the deep head of the flexor pollicis brevis as a derivative of the adductor pollicis, or, on the contrary, of the oblique head of the adductor pollicis as a component of the flexor pollicis brevis (Brooks, 1888). As a matter of fact, these incompletely separated bundles are the source of confusion for the determination of the borderline between the deep head of the flexor brevis and the adductor pollicis by dissection, despite the fact that

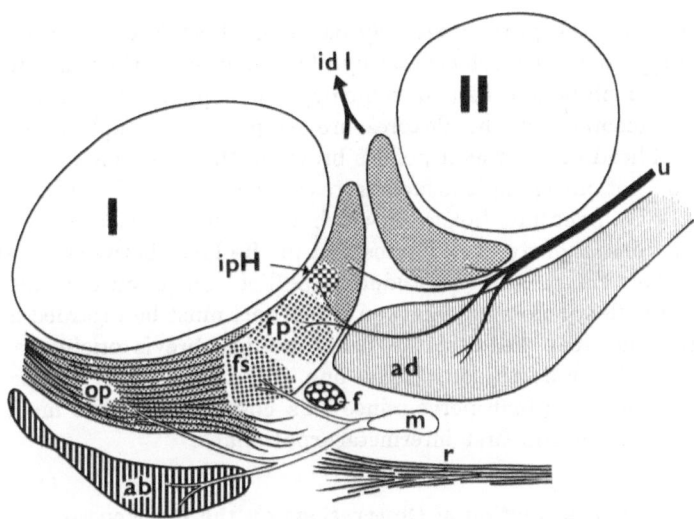

Fig. 104. Scheme of origin and of mutual relations of muscle primordia in the thenar region, outlined into the transverse section of the first intermetacarpal space. The continuous blastema surrounding the first metacarpal is homologous with the flexores breves profundi of the mammalian 1st finger in general. In the course of human ontogenesis this blastema differentiates into following primordia: *op* the opponens pollicis; *fs* superficial head of the flexor pollicis brevis; *fp* deep head of the flexor pollicis brevis; *ipH* interosseus palmaris I Henlei (var.), radial half of the interosseus dorsalis I primordium (*id I*); *ab* abductor pollicis brevis primordium; *m* median nerve; *r* the retinaculum flexorum anlage; *f* tendon of the flexor pollicis longus; *ad* adductor pollicis primordium (developing in the contrahentes layer); *u* ulnar nerve. (According to Čihák, 1969 b, modified)

the adductor develops from quite another primordium and, moreover, from another (and independent) layer of the contrahentes primordia.

The change of form connected with the secondary attachment of the opponens pollicis primordium to the developing retinaculum flexorum correlates with the alteration of shape of the entire embryonic hand, i.e. with the arcuation of the carpal region and the change in form of the eminentia carpi radialis, as well as with the change in position of the flexor digitorum superficialis belly.

Four individual muscles and one further muscular component develop from the deep thenar blastema as follows: the opponens pollicis, the superficial head of the flexor pollicis brevis, the deep head of the flexor pollicis brevis, and the variable m. interosseus palmaris I Henlei; the further, fifth component, is the radial half of the interosseus dorsalis I (Figs. 101, 104). These components differ from one another not only in their morphological differentiation, but also by the entries of nerves from the median and the ulnar nerve into different components; the branches from the ulnar nerve penetrate into the deep head of the flexor pollicis brevis and into Henle's strip through the primordium of the adductor pollicis (Fig. 104).

The origin of the opponens pollicis from the deep blastema demonstrates that this muscle is no new pattern of the Primate hand. The entire deep blastema

is homologous with the phylogenetically old deep short flexors. Thus, the opponens pollicis represents a phylogenetically old structure of the first finger. From
the viewpoint of phylogenesis and homology, the opponens pollicis is a transformed radial member of the flexores breves profundi couple of the thumb.
The superficial head of the flexor pollicis brevis is then its separated mediodistal
part. The course of ontogenesis demonstrates that it is the origin of the opponens
pollicis on the retinaculum flexorum which is to be regarded as secondary in
Man and that consequently even its position in the layer between the superficial
head of the short flexor and the abductor pollicis brevis on one side, and the
deep head of the flexor pollicis brevis on the other, must be regarded as a secondary pattern. The deep head of the flexor pollicis brevis originates from the
same primordial layer as the superficial one, differing only in its nerve supply
which comes from the ulnar nerve, since this component is the most adjacent
one to the muscles of the first intermetacarpal space.

5. Recapitulation of Observations on the Ontogenesis of the Thenar Musculature in the Human Hand

1. Two layers of muscle primordia develop in the thenar separated from the beginning
of their ontogenesis: the superficial layer giving rise to the abductor pollicis brevis, and the
deep one being the material for the opponens pollicis and for both heads of the short flexor
of thumb.

2. The adductor pollicis originates independently in the contrahentes layer.

3. The deep thenar primordia are homologous with the couple of flexores breves profundi of the thumb of lower Mammals.

4. The ulno-dorsal edge of the deep layer first separates and enters the first intermetacarpal space as the radial component of the interosseus dorsalis I.

5. In the remaining deep layer the radially situated opponens pollicis primordium and
the two heads of the flexor pollicis brevis situated ulnad to it gradually differentiate. Between
the interosseus dorsalis I, the adductor pollicis and the deep head of the flexor pollicis brevis
a variable rudimentary strip inserting to the ulnar sesamoid bone differentiates which—if
persisting—represents the so-called interosseus palmaris I Henlei (var.). This explains the
commonly employed homologisation of the deep head of the flexor pollicis brevis as the
interosseus palmaris I in the older literature.

6. The retinaculum flexorum develops relatively late and differentiates in the ulno-
radial direction; the primordium of the opponens pollicis joins it secondarily, thereby changing its position in relation to the thenar layers.

7. The tendon of the flexor pollicis longus undergoes a secondary shift from superficial
to deep between the two heads of the flexor pollicis brevis.

8. By its origin and development the opponens pollicis is homologous with the medial
component of the mm. flexores breves profundi of the thumb, it is hence a phylogenetically
old structure of thumb musculature, modified in its position and shape.

6. Ontogenesis of the Great Toe Group of Plantar Muscles in Man

In the homologies of foot muscles some contradictions appeared (similar to
the situation in the hand), particularly concerning the relation of the flexor
hallucis brevis to the oblique head of the adductor hallucis and homologies of
muscles in relation to the layers of the plantar musculature in general (Cunningham, 1878b; Brooks, 1888). There is also a controversial point concerning the
existence of the plantar interosseus of the first intermetatarsal space and its
relation to the flexor hallucis brevis (Hepburn, 1891/92), as well as the point

of the relation of the caput tibiale musculi flexoris hallucis brevis to the oblique head of the adductor hallucis (Ruge, 1878b). The situation in comparative anatomy is also made difficult by the position of muscles of the great toe which are not arranged in layers (as the thumb muscles in the hand are), but are splayed out in one layer beneath the thumb metacarpal. After explaining these points the course of ontogenesis of muscles of the great toe and the arrangement of their embryonic primordia will be compared with the general scheme of the autopodial musculature (Bardeleben, 1890) and with the development of the thumb musculature in the hand.

7. Material for Studies of the Great Toe Musculature in the Human Foot

For studying this muscle group 55 histological series of feet of human embryos and foetuses from 13 to 60 mm C-R length were employed. All feet were sectioned transversely.

C-R lengths of embryos and foetuses employed: 13 mm, 14, 15, 16 (2 feet), 16.5 (2), 17 (4), 17.5 (2), 18 (3), 19 (2), 20 (2), 21 (3), 22 (2), 23 (2), 24 (2), 25 (2), 26 (2), 27 (2), 29 (2), 30 (3), 32 (2), 33 (2), 35 (2), 37, 38, 40 (2), 46 (2), 54 (2), 60 mm.

The staining of series is described in pp. 10–11.

8. Observations of the Development of the Great Toe Group of Plantar Muscles

In small embryos (up to 18 mm C-R length) a large non-differentiated muscular blastema is visible in the great toe region, being the continuation of the deep plantar blastema to beneath the tibial margin of tarsal and metatarsal primordia (Fig. 105). At about 18 mm C-R length of embryo the superficial and the deep layer differentiate in this blastema. The superficial part represents the primordium of the future abductor hallucis (Fig. 106). As in the hand so in the foot the abductor hallucis differentiates sooner in its cytology. By its early separation, its position during the early embryonic period and by its speed of differentiation this primordium corresponds to the primordium of the abductor pollicis brevis of the hand so that their homology can be established. The primordium is supplied by an independent branch from the medial plantar nerve. However, its superficial position, as demonstrated in Fig. 106, is visible in small embryos only up to 20 mm C-R length. In subsequent developmental stages this primordium shifts quickly to the tibial margin of the foot, taking its position in the same layer as other muscular primordia of the great toe, in one row with them (Fig. 107). From the beginning of differentiation of this primordium a cytological difference between the future muscular belly and a broad insertion tendon of the future abductor is visible.

In embryos after 20 mm in C-R length the remaining part of the blastema at the great toe gradually differentiates. It has been demonstrated in relation to the development of the interossei of the foot that in the first intermetatarsal space the material of the flexores breves profundi layer is derived partly from beneath the second metatarsal (as the future interosseus dorsalis I), partly from beneath the first metatarsal, entering the space in form of the dorsal tip of the blastema (Fig. 86). The part of this material coming from beneath the first metatarsal is delayed in its development being adjacent to the oblique head of the adductor hallucis or remaining as a rudimentary strip of the denser mesenchyme in the space between the oblique head of the adductor hallucis, the first

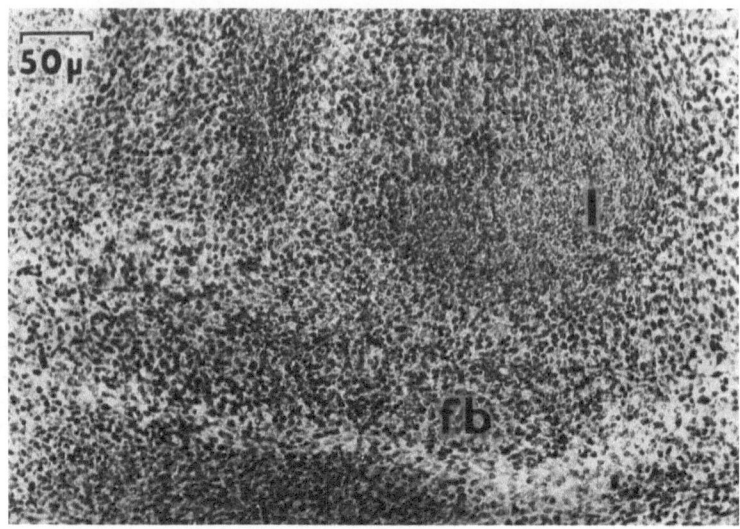

Fig. 105. Left foot of the embryo 17 mm in C-R length, transverse section at the level of metatarsal bases. The flexores breves profundi layer (*fb*) continues to beneath the 1st metatarsal anlage (*I*), to form the deep layer of primordia of the great toe muscles

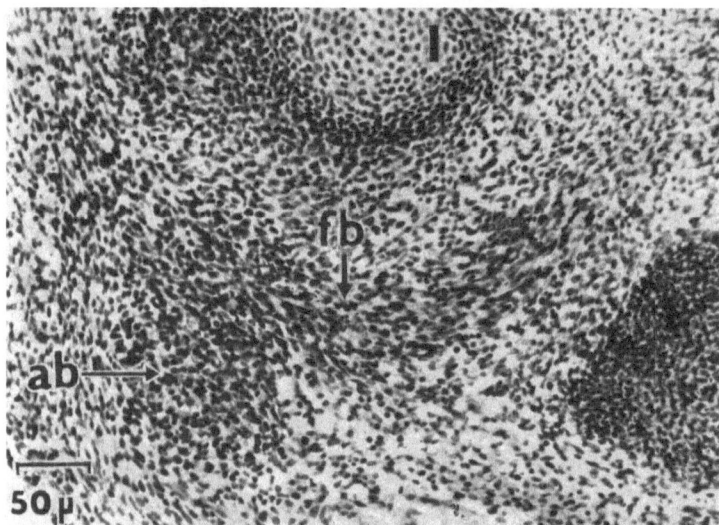

Fig. 106. Right foot of the embryo 19 mm in C-R length, transverse section. The blastema of muscles at the great toe divides into the superficial primordium of the abductor hallucis (*ab*) and the deep layer (corresponding to the flexores breves profundi *fb*)

metatarsal and the interosseus dorsalis I (Fig. 107). From 20—30 mm in C-R embryo length when the relatively large muscular primordia are closely adjacent to one another, this rudiment as a rule is hardly detectable from the oblique head of the adductor hallucis. It also inserts together with this head in the region of the future fibular sesamoid bone of the great toe (Fig. 109); it is then

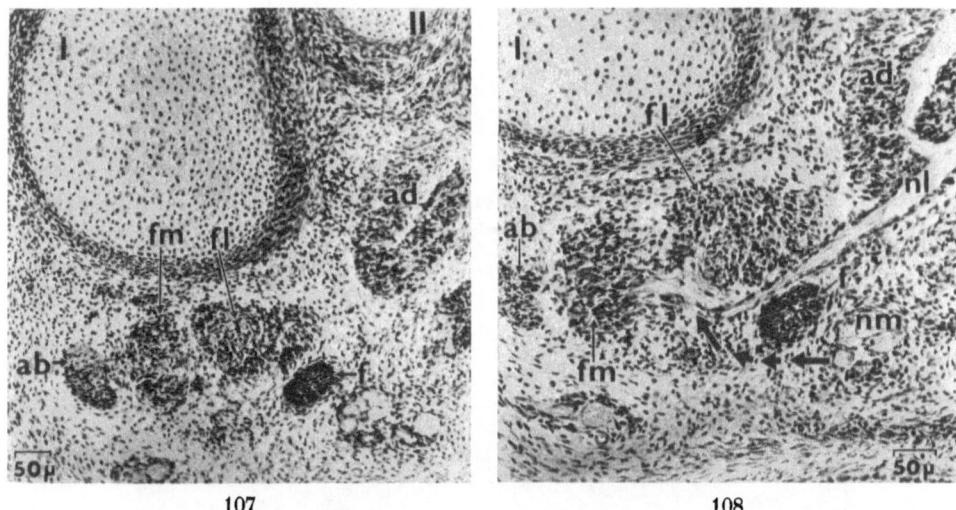

107   108

Fig. 107. Right foot of the 34 mm embryo, transverse section near metacarpal bases. The deep layer of the great toe musculature is divided into two heads of the flexor hallucis brevis, the lateral head (*fl*) and the medial head (*fm*). The abductor hallucis primordium (*ab*) stands now in one row with the two heads of the short flexor. *I, II* metatarsals; *f* flexor hallucis longus tendon; *ad* adductor hallucis (oblique head)

Fig. 108. The same series as in Fig. 107, several sections more to proximal. The nerve entry to both heads of the flexor hallucis brevis is sectioned. The perineurium of the entering nerve is interrupted at the site of division of two branches for the two heads of the flexor (arrow). To this site several sections more to proximal the anastomosis from the medial plantar nerve joins so that both flexor heads are supplied from this anastomosis (as described already by Hallopeau 1900). Abbreviations same as in Fig. 107; *nl* lateral plantar nerve; *nm* medial plantar nerve

much better visible in later developmental stages, between 50 and 60 mm C-R length. This muscle component thus represents the part of the deep blastema at the great toe metatarsal corresponding to the interosseus palmaris I Henlei (var.) in the hand, and by its position, course and insertion it also behaves as the plantar interosseus of the first intermetatarsal space. Contrary to the hand where this muscle strip mostly becomes rudimentary very early, it is constant in the foot of older foetuses; however, it is not invariably independent, it can be more or less adherent to the oblique head of the adductor hallucis or to the interosseus dorsalis I.

The remaining part of the blastema of the great toe then divides only into two side by side situated components, the future medial head and the lateral head of the flexor hallucis brevis. These two components, however, are not merely parts of the same muscle. It is visible in their development that they originate as two independent primordia (Fig. 107) and give rise to two quite independent and independently innervated muscular individuals. Both these elements course in parallel toward the metatarsal head diverging to their typical insertions in the region of the tibial and the fibular sesamoid bone of the great

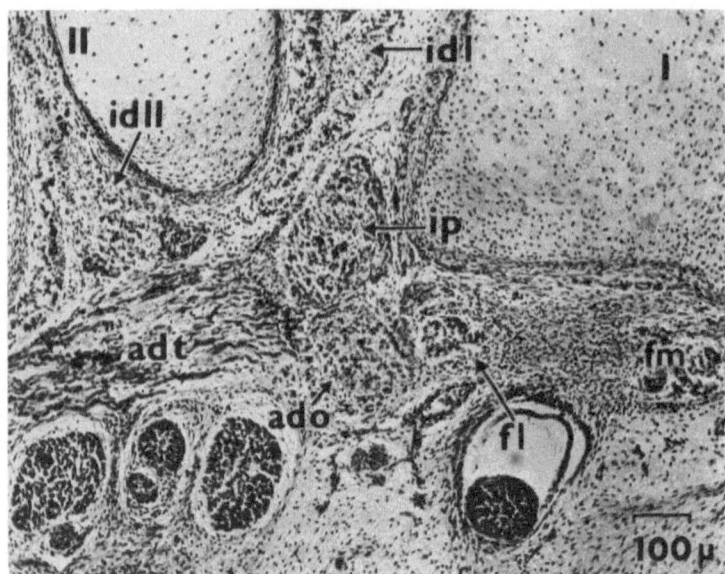

Fig. 109. Left foot of the foetus 60 mm in C-R length, transverse section near the distal end
of the first metatarsal. In addition to typical components of the musculature of the great
toe and the first intermetatarsal space the independent plantar interosseus of the first space
(*ip*) is formed. *I, II* metatarsals; *idI* first dorsal interosseus; *ado* oblique head of the adductor
hallucis; *adt* transverse head of the adductor hallucis; *fl fm* lateral and medial heads of the
flexor hallucis brevis

toe. The insertions of muscle primordia are formed already from 30 mm C-R
length onward, whilst the sesamoid bones differentiate at about 60 mm C-R
length of foetus.

In embryos from 20 mm C-R length onward then three primordia lie side
by side in one row from the tibial margin of the foot: the most tibially situated
abductor hallucis, then the two heads of the short flexor of the great toe. The
caput obliquum musculi adductoris hallucis adjoins the lateral head of the flexor
from the lateral side. Between the oblique head of the adductor and the first
metatarsal, partly adjacent to the dorsal surface of the adductor, there is the
primordium of the first intermetatarsal space palmar interosseus.

The nerve supply of the primordia of the great toe group occurs by the lateral
plantar nerve in the direction from the oblique head of the adductor hallucis
(Fig. 108), and from the medial plantar nerve in the direction from the plantar
surface. Distinguishing which primordium of the short flexors is supplied from
the medial plantar nerve and which from the lateral plantar nerve is not exact
and even impossible. Although it is assumed in textbooks that the lateral head
is supplied from the lateral plantar nerve and the medial one from the medial
plantar nerve, in fact, both heads are supplied from the anastomosis between
these two nerves, which is well visible in histological series and which occurs
immediately before nerve enters these two parts of the short flexor. This anastomosis was already known and described by Hallopeau (1900); its existence is
mentioned also by Hovelacque (1927).

The development of both components of the flexor hallucis brevis and the development of the variable component of the first space palmar interosseus then proceeds by a simple splitting of the original blastema. The earlier differentiated abductor hallucis changes its position in course of development: at the beginning it represents the superficial layer of plantar musculature being separated from the deep blastema and it secondarily joins the other primordia of the great toe muscles, forming one layer with them.

9. Discussion and Conclusions from Observations of Ontogenesis of the Great Toe Group of Human Plantar Musculature

Contrary to the thenar musculature which maintains a layered pattern in the course of ontogenesis (at least by the relation of the abductor pollicis brevis primordium to other thenar primordia), the musculature at the great toe of the foot is splayed out in a single layer, side by side in the tibiofibular direction. This difference, together with the different number of muscle individuals seems to have been the main obstacle in the comparison of the hand and the foot and to the application of the general scheme of autopodial muscle layers to the pattern of the foot.

It has been demonstrated that in the course of human ontogenesis the typical layers are also maintained in the pattern of muscle primordia in the foot, where the abductor hallucis anlage develops at the surface of the other primordia (similar to the hand). The abductor pollicis brevis and the abductor hallucis are hence homologous as the superficial component. From this standpoint Cunningham's view (1787a, b) that the abductors of the first and fifth digit in the hand and the foot are derivatives of the same layer as the dorsal interossei, cannot be upheld. The question of the appurtenance of the abductor pollicis brevis and the abductor hallucis to the typical layer of the autopodial musculature will be further discussed in the chapter concerning the superficial primordia of the hand and foot.

The further component, well comparable in the first digit musculature in the hand and the foot, is the variable accessory primordium of the palmar or the plantar interosseus in the first space. Both develop very similarly and inside comparable parts of the deep blastema. The difference between the hand and the foot is given by the pattern of the interosseus dorsalis I, which in the hand acquires the material of the deep blastema of the thumb, and the strip of Henle's muscle is only a residuum between this material and the proper deep thumb blastema, while in the foot the whole material, which enters the first space from the great toe metatarsal, changes into the first space plantar interosseus which either remains independent or adherent to the oblique head of the adductor. This slender variable strip was a source of many contradictions in the literature. It has been considered to be the deep head of the short flexor, the split off part of the adductor hallucis, the opponens hallucis (Hepburn, 1891/92; Brooks, 1888; Kopsch, 1952). If this muscular part is independent, it corresponds from the standpoint of its ontogenesis, position, shape and insertion to the interosseus plantaris. It is a typical part of the deep plantar blastema, which separates

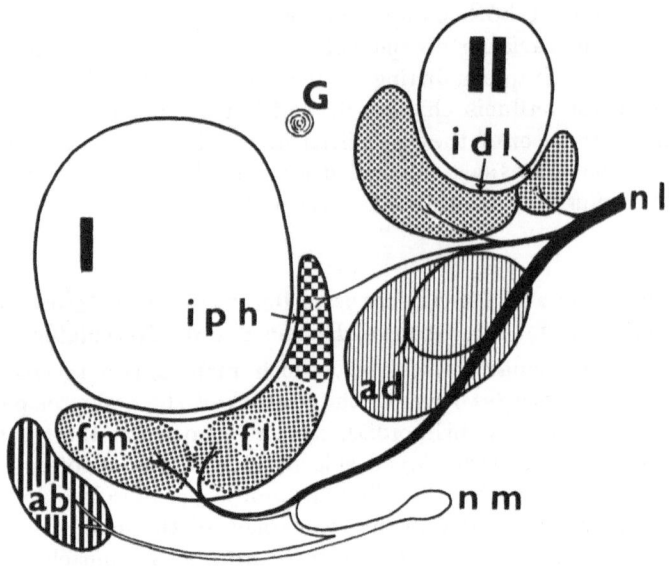

Fig. 110. Scheme of origin and mutual relations of primordia in the great toe group of plantar musculature, outlined into the schematic section (transverse) of the 1st intermetatarsal space. The continuous primordium surrounding the 1st metatarsal corresponds with the flexores breves profundi of the mammalian great toe. In the course of human ontogenesis this primordium differentiates into following muscle primordia: *fm fl* medial and lateral head of the flexor hallucis brevis; *iph* the interosseus plantaris hallucis. *I, II* metatarsals; *idI* first dorsal interosseus; *ab* abductor hallucis primordium; *ad* oblique head of the adductor hallucis; *nm, nl* medial and lateral plantar nerves (and their anastomosis); *G* transient primordium of the os intermetatarseum Gruberi

early, already after the embryo attains 18 mm of C-R length, and develops further more or less independently, either separated, or adjacent to some of the surrounding muscles. To express its position also in its name and in order not to disturb the fixed numbering of the plantar interossei, we propose for this component the term *m. interosseus plantaris hallucis*.

The comparison of the short flexor of the great toe with the muscles of the thumb in the hand is difficult since in the two cases a different number of muscles develops in the deep blastema after separation of primordia for the first space: three in the hand, two in the foot. A real homology of the two extremities is here hence invalid, the muscles, if corresponding by their function, are much more the homodynamic structures. The flexor hallucis brevis, however, among all muscles of the palm and the sole maximally maintains the original shape of the couple of muscular twins of the flexores breves profundi of lower mammals. (To this couple the whole original blastema corresponds together with parts separated into the first space.) The maintenance of the original form of the muscle couple beneath the metatarsal is, no doubt, a developmentally more original pattern than that of the rearranged thenar musculature.

The general disposition of muscle primordia in the great toe of the foot is demonstrated in the scheme in Fig. 110.

10. Recapitulation of Observations on the Ontogenesis of the Great Toe Group of Plantar Musculature

1. During ontogenesis of the foot in the region of the great toe group of the plantar musculature, first (after 18 mm C-R length) the superficial layer differentiates, forming the primordium of the abductor hallucis.

2. The layer of the deep blastema at the great toe, which is the continuation of the flexores breves profundi layer, splits and differentiates from 20 mm C-R length onward.

3. A tip of the deep layer of the blastema at the great toe metatarsal extends into the first intermetatarsal space, differentiating later into the independent muscular strip interposed between the interosseus dorsalis I and the oblique head of the adductor hallucis. By its position and insertion it is the plantar interosseus of the first space and corresponds to the interosseus palmaris I Henlei of the hand. As a correct denomination not disturbing the present nomenclatory usage the term m. interosseus plantaris hallucis is considered.

4. The remaining part of the deep blastema at the great toe metatarsal divides into two side by side situated components—the medial and the lateral heads of the flexor hallucis brevis, both having characteristic features of the independent muscle.

5. Both heads of the flexor hallucis brevis by their form and course most resemble the original couple of the flexores breves profundi of Mammals, but are not exactly homologous with them.

6. Both components of the short flexor of the great toe are innervated from the anastomosis between the n. plantaris medialis and the n. plantaris lateralis.

11. Comparison of the First Digit Musculature in the Hand and the Foot

The musculature of the first digit of the hand and the foot, seen from the developmental standpoint, is arranged according to layers of muscular primordia in which the hand and foot muscles differentiate: the adductor pollicis as well as the adductor hallucis originate in the contrahentes layer; the abductor pollicis brevis and the abductor hallucis originate in the superficial, early independent blastema, the remaining muscles of this group in the hand and in the foot are derivatives of the flexores breves profundi layer.

The following differences between the hand and the foot in the pattern of differentiation of the deep blastema (from the flexores breves profundi layer) can be distinguished:

a) The deep blastema at the thumb metacarpal in the hand takes part (contrary to the foot) in the origin of the interosseus dorsalis I.

b) In the hand only a part, in the foot the entire material expanded into the first space represents the plantar (palmar) interosseus of the first space which is a more constant formation in the foot than in the hand.

c) The remaining deep blastema in the foot differentiates into three muscles (the opponens and both heads of the flexor pollicis brevis), in the foot only into two heads of the flexor hallucis brevis. It is hence impossible to compare these muscles as single formations. Their material is merely homologous as a whole.

d) The muscles differentiated from this deep blastema in the hand undergo still further changes of their position and layer in the course of further development; in the foot the blastema only divides and the muscles remain in their original position.

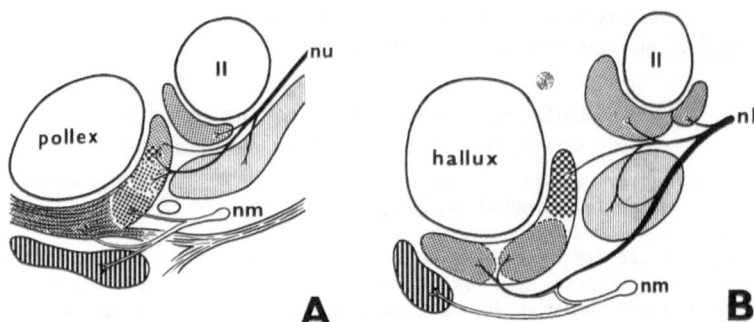

Fig. 111. Comparison of the origin and positions of primordia of the first digit musculature in the hand and foot. For detailed explanations cf. Figs. 104 and 110. *A* blastemas and differentiating primordia of muscles in the hand; *B* in the foot. (Partly from Čihák 1969b modified)

Contrary to the hand, in the foot the abductor hallucis changes its position in the course of ontogenesis shifting from its original superficial layer to the tibial margin of the remaining muscles.

The review of differences between the hand and foot is schematically given in Fig. 111.

12. The Development of the Hypothenar Muscles
Development of the Fifth Toe Group of the Plantar Musculature
(Observation and Comparison)

The muscle primordia at the fifth digit develop similarly in the hand and in the foot. The original non-differentiated mesenchymal blastema divides very early into main layers, superficial and deep. In the hand from 16 mm C-R embryo length onward, in the foot from 18 mm C-R length, the more superficially situated abductor digiti minimi separates and differentiates in its cytology. It forms a simple primordium, oval-shaped in cross section (Figs. 112, 113), which soon after its separation obtains the form of the definitive muscle. Like the abductor pollicis brevis and the abductor hallucis, the abductor digiti minimi primordium in the hand and in the foot is also differentiated sooner in its form and cytology. It differentiates as a more superficial layer evidently not belonging to the other muscles of the fifth digit (Figs. 112, 113).

The remaining muscles of the fifth digit in the hand and the foot are the derivatives of the deep layer of muscle primordia, i.e. the continuation of the flexores breves profundi layer toward the ulnar margin of the fifth metacarpal and toward the fibular margin of the fifth metatarsal. This deep layer remains undivided in the hand and in the foot for a long period. This corresponds to the fact that the entire blastema is homologous with one flexor brevis profundus digiti quinti ulnaris (fibularis) in comparative anatomy. Only after reaching 20 mm C-R length of the embryo does the blastema divide in the hand into the primordia of the flexor brevis and the opponens digiti minimi. In the foot its division is not clear. Although the opponens digiti minimi pedis is considered only as an inconstant variation in the I.N.A (1935) and is even absent in the

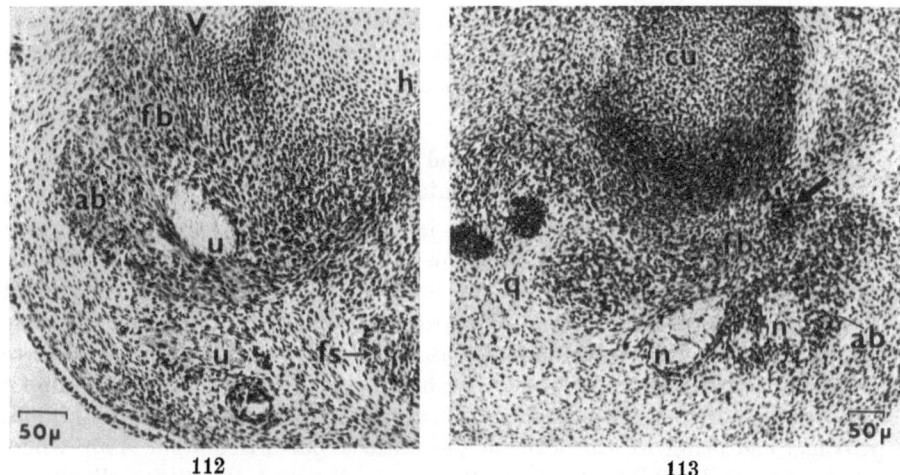

112   113

Fig. 112. Left hand of the embryo 18 mm in C-R length transverse section through the primordium of the hamatum and of the basis of the 5th metacarpal (*h*, *V*). In the section of the hypothenar primordia the superficial distinctly separated layer is better differentiated. It is the abductor digiti minimi primordium (*ab*). The deep layer, not yet differentiated in this stage, corresponds to the flexores breves profundi layer (*fb*). Between the two layers the ulnar nerve (*u*) is visible; *fs* the flexor digitorum superficialis primordium

Fig. 113. Right foot of the embryo 19 mm in C-R length, transverse section through the cuboideum (*cu*). As in the hand, also in the foot the blastema of the musculature of the 5th toe divides into the superficial layer (separated earlier and better differentiated) which is the primordium of the abductor digiti minimi (*ab*), and the deep layer corresponding to the flexores breves profundi (*fb*), where the flexor digiti minimi brevis and the opponens digiti minimi (var.) differentiate. Structural differentiation demonstrates (arrow) that there is at least the suggestion of the differentiation of the opponens digiti minimi, though this muscle is not contained in the P.N.A.; *q* the quadratus plantae primordium; *n* lateral plantar nerve

P.N.A. (1960), in the embryonic foot the subdivision of the deep blastema into the primordia of the opponens and the flexor digiti minimi brevis is always initiated after 40 mm C-R length of embryo. Both muscles, however, are better distinguishable from the inner structure of the primordia and the distribution of nerve branches than from their external form and division.

The original form of the deep blastema is semilunar in transverse section. The blastema subdivides into the more radial (tibial) and slightly palmar (plantar) situated flexor digiti minimi brevis and the more slender ulnar (fibular) situated primordium of the opponens digiti minimi, extending to the ulnar (fibular) margin of the fifth metacarpal (metatarsal).

The flexor pollicis brevis and the opponens pollicis compared with the flexor brevis digiti minimi and the opponens digiti minimi of the hand appear as symmetrically differentiated structures situated in corresponding positions at both margins of the deep palmar blastema. This symmetrical character of the marginal muscles is not present in the foot.

Seen from the phylogenetic standpoint the primordia of deep muscles of the fifth digit (flexor brevis as well as the opponens) in the hand and in the foot are homologous with the ulnar (fibular) member of the couple of flexores breves profundi of the fifth digit, whilst the abductor digiti minimi belongs to another independent layer of superficial primordia of the hand and the foot.

E. Superficial Palmar and Plantar Primordia in Human Ontogenesis

A bulky muscular blastema is found in the superficial layer of the palm and sole of small embryos. In the hand this blastema fills in the superficial palmar region subcutaneously interposed in between the trunks of the ulnar and median nerves (Fig. 114). In small embryos no other formed connective tissue structures—neither the retinaculum flexorum nor the palmar aponeurosis—are differentiated superficial to this muscular blastema (Fig. 114). Up to 19 mm of C-R embryo length this blastema does not reach proximal to the carpal region, its proximal end being at the level of the radiocarpal articulation. This whole superficial palmar blastema becomes the primordium of the flexor digitorum superficialis. Although considered by Gräfenberg (1905/06) a primordium of the short superficial palmar flexors which in later development joins with a further primordium (denoted by Gräfenberg the flexor digitorum sublimis and regarded as the antebrachial muscle), this superficial palmar primordium is actually the sole anlage of the flexor digitorum superficialis which in the course of further development differentiates proximally to the antebrachium, as shown in papers by Dylevský (1967, 1968a, c, 1969a). The nerve supply of this muscular primordium also enters from the median nerve at the level of the distal row of carpal primordia in embryos up to 20 mm in C-R length (Fig. 114). Subsequent changes of this blastema, its splitting toward the fingers and the differentiation of its tendons have been described in the above quoted papers by Dylevský. For the present considerations and conclusions concerning the development of layers of the plantar musculature, this blastema is important in the human embryo because by its origin, position and the nerve supply it is really a palmar and not the antebrachial blastema. Distal in the palm it splits into strips to single fingers, its position and developmental sequence (preceding the deep palmar mus-

Fig. 114. Right hand of the embryo 19.5 mm in C-R length, transverse section at the level of distal row of carpal primordia and the basis of the 5th metacarpal (*V*). The superficial layer of muscle primordia is demonstrated, containing the abductor pollicis brevis (*ab1*), and the abductor digiti minimi-ab5- and between them the flexor digitorum superficialis primordium (*fs*). The branch from the median nerve supplying the flexor digitorum superficialis at this level demonstrates the appurtenance of the muscle to the palmar musculature; *h* hamatum; *c* capitatum; *u* ulnar nerve; *m* median nerve. The differentiating retinaculum flexorum indicated by arrow

Fig. 115. Left hand of the 19 mm embryo, transverse section at the level of metacarpal bases, demonstrating mutual relations of superficial primordia of the hand. *I*, *V* metacarpals; *fs* flexor digitorum superficialis (its muscular slips for the fingers); *ab* abductor pollicis and abductor digiti minimi primordia; *m* median nerve; *u* ulnar nerve

Fig. 116. Right foot of the embryo 34 mm in C-R length, transverse section at the level of the tarsal distal row. Superficial primordia of the planta: *ab* abductor hallucis and abductor digiti minimi primordia; *fbr* flexor digitorum brevis; *m*, *l* medial and lateral plantar nerves; *cfI-III* the cuneiformia; *cu* cuboideum; *V* 5th metatarsal

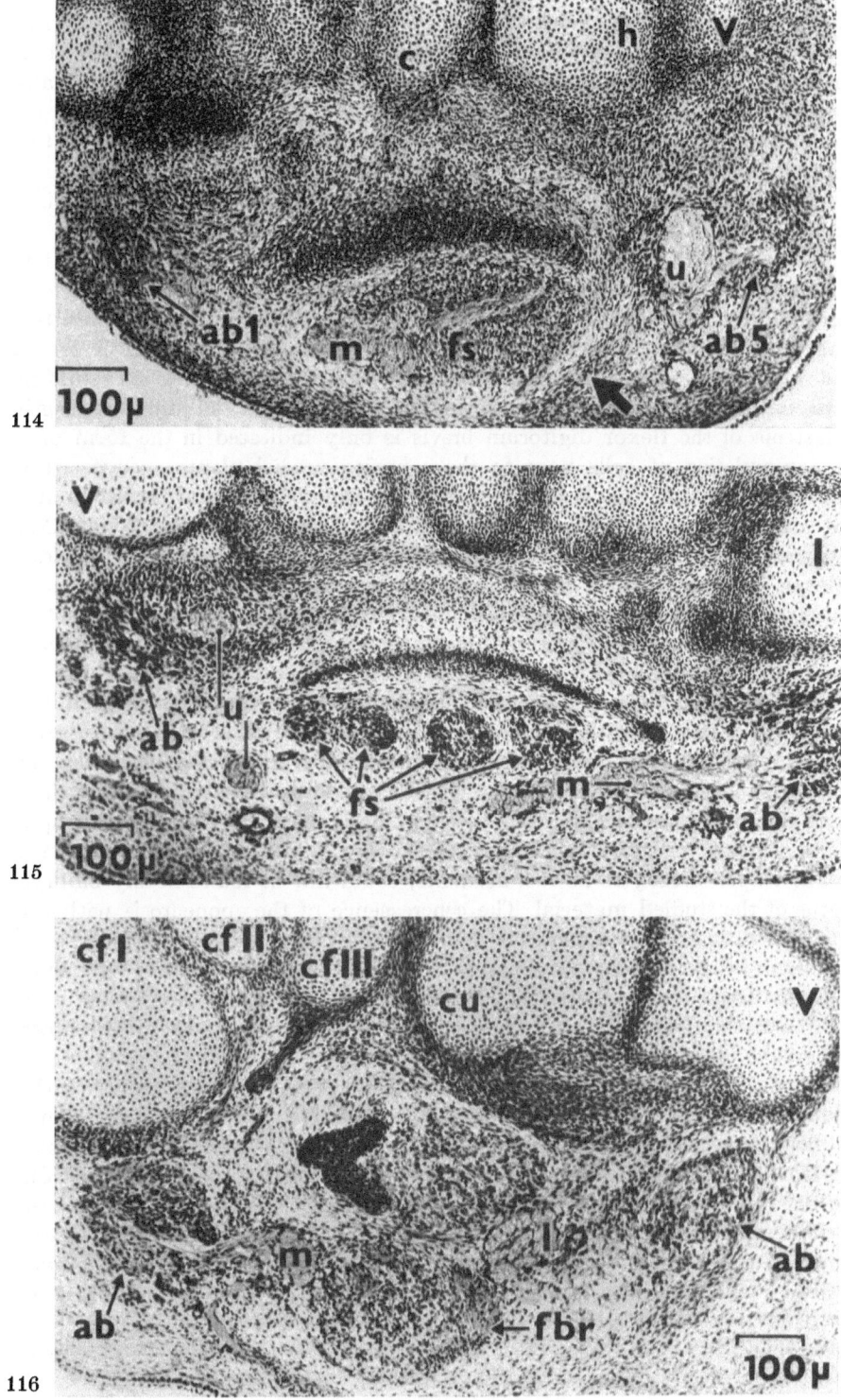

Fig. 114—116

culature) being at the same level of layers and at the same level of differentiation as the abductor pollicis brevis and the abductor digiti minimi (Figs. 114, 115). Later, from 25 mm C-R length onward, when the flexor digitorum superficialis primordium is already high in the antebrachium and in the carpal region its strips for fingers only remain, the retinaculum flexorum differentiates in the manner already described (Čihák, 1966b, 1969b, c, cf. pp. 129, 154). The retinaculum then gradually separates the primordia of the canalis carpi from the subcutaneous layer of the wrist region.

The blastema of the flexor digitorum brevis develops in the same position and in the same form in the embryonic foot. In the transverse section of the foot this primordium is similarly oval-shaped, and between the primordium and the skin of the embryonic planta no formed connective tissue structure can be found except for loose mesenchyme. In comparison with the hand there is a shift in the time of differentiation in the foot, since in embryos up to 17 mm C-R length the blastema of the flexor digitorum brevis is only indicated in the form of a small accumulation of cells near to the coursing medial plantar nerve. Only after reaching 20 mm C-R length of embryo is the primordium formed in full extent and shape of the future flexor digitorum brevis. At about 25 mm C-R length and in subsequent stages there is already a bulky muscle belly. Besides the flexor digitorum brevis primordium the superficial layer of the sole also contains the abductor hallucis and the abductor digiti minimi primordia (Fig. 116). The flexor digitorum brevis primordium flattens in the distal direction, spreads out and splits into the slips for the 2nd to 5th toe.

Unlike the hand, where later the retinaculum flexorum is formed, in the foot there is at first only the mesenchyme between the flexor digitorum brevis primordium and the skin, later in the near proximity of the skin the anlage of the plantar aponeurosis differentiates. The flexor digitorum brevis primordium remains completely separated by a layer of loose mesenchyme from the aponeurosis plantaris anlage. The connection of the flexor digitorum brevis with the plantar aponeurosis, as known in adults, could not be found in any embryo or foetus of the studied material. The concrescence of the aponeurosis with the muscle evidently appears secondarily and late. It is hence impossible to conceive of the origin of the plantar aponeurosis from the flexor digitorum brevis primordium, similarly to the invalidity of such considerations for the palmar aponeurosis and the flexor digitorum superficialis primordium, as has been shown by Dylevský (in above quoted papers).

According to the layered pattern of the hand and foot musculature, to the position of the flexor digitorum superficialis and the flexor digitorum brevis primordia in the embryonic palm and sole between the superficial abductors of marginal fingers (Figs. 114—116) and also because these superficial primordia in the hand and the foot develop a little sooner than the primordia of the deep palmar and plantar musculature, all these superficial flexors and abductors can be considered to belong to the phylogenetically old layer of the flexores breves superficiales (palmares and plantares). The comparison of these superficial layers in the hand and the foot reveals a very similar pattern of one median and two lateral primordia (Figs. 114, 116). In comparison with Bardeleben's scheme (1890) of palmar and plantar muscle layers their homology is striking.

F. The Lumbrical Muscles during Ontogenesis of the Human Hand and Foot

The lumbricales are a typical and constant layer, identical in the comparative anatomy of the hand and foot, related by origin and position to the tendons of the flexor digitorum profundus of the upper extremity and to the flexor digitorum longus of the lower extremity. Their constant occurrence and constant layer led to these muscles being included in Bardeleben's general scheme of autopodial muscles (1890) as one of the main layers in the mammalian hand and foot.

1. The Lumbricales in the Ontogenesis of the Human Hand

As already demonstrated by Gräfenberg (1905/06) the lumbrical muscles originate together with the flexor digitorum profundus tendon. In the proximal parts of the hand (in the carpal region) this tendon forms a sheet, at first straight and flat, then in older embryos (from 18 mm C-R length onward) gradually vaulting dorsally in conformity with the simultaneous vaulting of the entire carpal region. In the direction from the antebrachium toward the fingers the sheet is solid at the level of both rows of carpal primordia. At the level of the distal carpal row it starts to split up and the future tendon of the flexor pollicis longus separates radiad. From the level of the carpometacarpal articulation the sheet divides and spreads out toward the fingers. It divides into four typical tendinous strips for the fingers. At the radial margins of these developing tendons (between neighbouring tendinous strips) material remains which from the beginning is differently shaped and differentiates very early to form muscle primordia. These primordia of the lumbricales are already distinguishable at the metacarpal level in embryos of 14 mm C-R length; they then gradually differentiate in form and cytology (Fig. 117). In the course of splitting off from the common tendinous layer the lumbricales of the hand occupy the full thickness of the original sheet, and this sheet simply diverges into strips alternating in their differentiation into the tendon and the muscle (Fig. 117). In their further distal course the muscle primordia remain in the same layer as the tendons and then, toward metacarpal heads, the lumbricales first join beneath the residua of the contrahentes layer and together join the plantar side of the interossei primordia. Their tendinous insertion into the dorsal aponeurosis of fingers is visible a little later than the original differentiating muscle primordia, from 16 mm C-R length of embryo.

It has been demonstrated in the chapter concerning the development of the contrahentes layer that the material for one intermetacarpal space, i.e. the lumbricalis, contrahens, flexores breves profundi and intermetacarpalis primordia form a blastematous material pressed in between the metacarpals (Fig. 47), which then gradually separates and demarcates. In small embryos (approximately up to 22 mm C-R length) where the palmar aponeurosis is not yet clearly formed, mesenchymal slips going in more distal sectors of intermetacarpal spaces from superficial to deep and containing blood vessels perforating from the subcutaneous layer into intermetacarpal spaces, join the lumbricales primordia (Fig. 53).

The insertions of the lumbricales differentiate in typical form from 16 mm C-R length onward. As shown by Mrzena (1970) the insertions first adjoin the

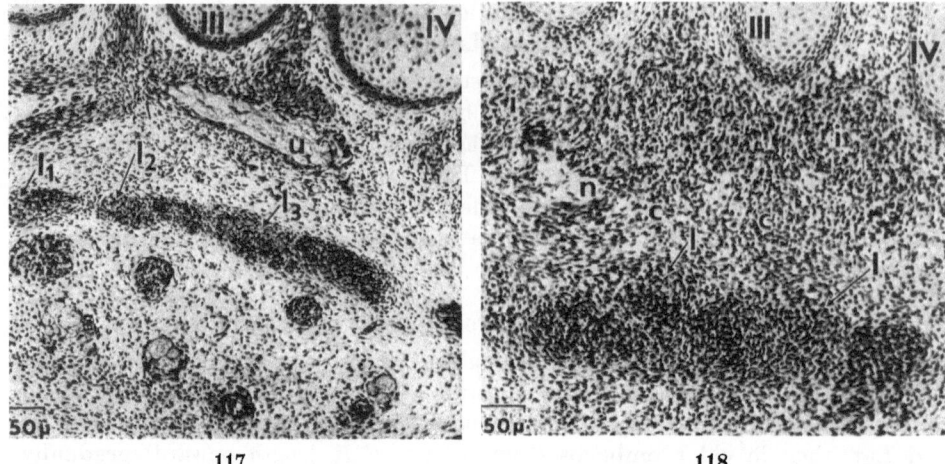

117   118

Fig. 117. Right hand of the embryo 19 mm in C-R length, transverse section demonstrating the differentiation of the originally common tendinous plate of the flexor digitorum profundus primordium into the tendons and the lumbricales primordia (l_{1-3}); *III, IV* metacarpals; *u* ulnar nerve. The differentiation of the lumbricales occurs in the entire thickness of the original plate

Fig. 118. Right foot of the 19 mm embryo, transverse section. The developing lumbricales (*l*) of the foot are not contained in the entire thickness of the original plate of flexor tendons but separate from its dorsal surface. *III, IV* metatarsals; *c* residua (strips) of the contrahentes layer; *i* interossei primordia; *n* lateral plantar nerve

palmar surfaces of the dorsal aponeuroses of the fingers and then shift to their typical insertions to the lateral margins of these aponeuroses, crossing the inser - tions of the interossei. The lumbricals are differentiated so early and they are so clearly demarcated already in small embryos that it is not probable that material from the contrahentes layer residua could fuse with them.

2. The Lumbricales in the Ontogenesis of the Human Foot

In the course of ontogenesis of the human foot the lumbricales originate and differentiate in approximately the same manner as in the hand. In embryos of 17 mm they are not yet fully differentiated. In the embryo 18 mm in C-R length the primordia of the lumbricales can be seen already as separating from the flexor digitorum longus tendon after its crossing and concrescence with the flexor hallucis longus tendon. In the transverse section, however, at first sight, it can be distinguished that the observed section is the foot, not the hand, from the fact that the lumbricales do not separate in the full thickness of the tendinous layer of the flexor digitorum longus. The lumbricales primordia in the foot separate only from the dorsal aspect of this original common sheet, which does not divide immediately after splitting off the lumbricales, and its dorsal surface remains grooved so that it is visible that the lumbricales were impressed from the dorsal side into this tendinous flexor sheet (Fig. 118). This peculiarity of the lumbricales development led Schomburg (1900) to conclude that the muscles originate independently and that they join the flexor tendons secondarily. This view cannot be supported by the present observations; it is certain, however, that the lumbricales do not differentiate in full thickness of the common sheet with the tendons, as in the hand.

The course of the lumbricales primordia in the plantar region also differs a little from the situation in the palm. The muscle primordia course obliquely toward the intermetatarsal spaces and after their separation from the tendinous sheet they adjoin the residua of the contrahentes layer so firmly that it cannot be precisely distinguished whether a part of the residua material does not fuse with the lumbricales primordia. The remaining course and insertion then differentiates quite typically, together with the interossei, into the dorsal aponeurosis of fingers. The insertion is differentiated from 22 mm C-R embryo length onward.

G. The Quadratus plantae Muscle in Human Ontogenesis

In the depth of the embryonic plantar region a relatively large muscular primordium differentiates. It is the future quadratus plantae muscle (the flexor accessorius). The beginning of its differentiation in the planta is found in embryos of about 18 mm in C-R length. The primordium is at first formed very near to the lateral plantar nerve where it begins at the level of the proximal third of the calcaneus. In small embryos it is separated in its entire length from the perichondrium of the calcaneus primordium, being adjacent to the nervus plantaris lateralis (Fig. 119). It then courses slightly obliquely in the disto-tibial direction through the planta, broadens gradually and reaches the tendons of the flexor hallucis longus and the flexor digitorum longus at the place where they cross one another. Toward the insertion to the tendons the primordium of the quadratus plantae widens in the transverse as well as in its dorsoplantar dimension. A branch from the n. plantaris lateralis, large during the embryonic period, enters this primordium (Fig. 120).

The primordium of the quadratus plantae appears quite independently in the planta. It has no relation to any of the plantar muscle layers, it is not even in contact with the skeletal primordia and its origin on the calcaneus appears relatively later, first after reaching 30 mm C-R length of embryo, when the blastema for the first time closely adjoins the perichondrium of the calcaneus anlage. The position of this primordium also differs from all other plantar musculature. If the primordia of the muscle belly and the tendon of the flexor hallucis longus are followed in the proximo-distal direction, it can be seen that the muscle belly diminishes distally being situated on the fibular side of the differentiating tendon, then it disappears in the region of the future canalis malleolaris and only a tendon remains for a short space. The quadratus plantae primordium originates in the planta exactly in continuation with the original muscle belly of the flexor hallucis longus. Hence, the quadratus plantae seems to be a separated continuation of the muscle belly of the flexor hallucis longus. The course of the entire flexor hallucis longus looks like a biceps muscle with one crural head and one plantar head. This plantar head originating in the distal continuation of the crural head adjoins the same tendon. In no case did we find a direct or non-interrupted continuation of one head into another; in small

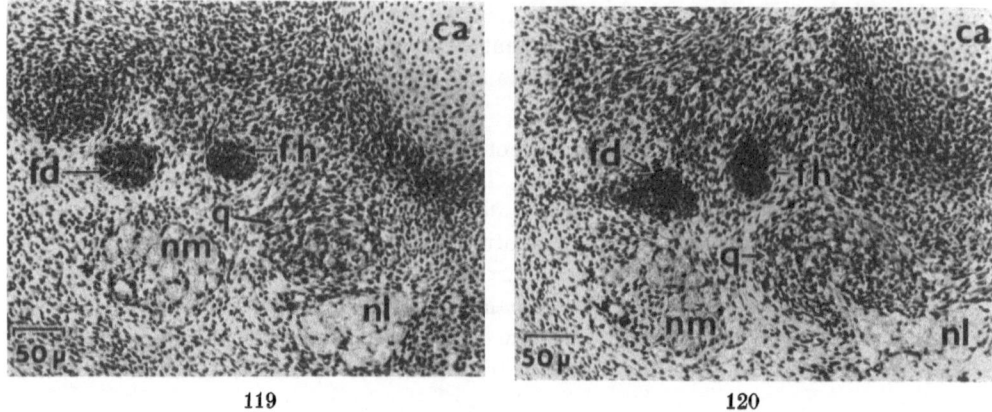

119   120

Fig. 119. Right foot of the embryo 19 mm in C-R length, transverse section of the calcaneus region, demonstrating the quadratus plantae primordium (*q*) situated close to the lateral plantar nerve (*nl*) and to the flexor hallucis longus tendon (*fh*); *ca* the calcaneus primordium; *fd* flexor digitorum longus tendon; *nm* nervus plantaris medialis

Fig. 120. In the same series as in Fig. 119 the nerve supply of the quadratus plantae primordium (*q*) from the lateral plantar nerve (*nl*) is visible. It can be also seen that the quadratus plantae primordium has no relation to the layers of primordia of the plantar musculature; *ca* calcaneus; *nm* medial plantar nerve; *fh* flexor hallucis longus tendon; *fd* flexor digitorum longus tendon

embryos, however, the distal end of the crural head remains distant to the beginning of the plantar primordium (of the quadratus plantae) only in the thickness of three or four sections of the histological series, i. e. for a distance of about 40 μ. The degree of differentiation of the quadratus plantae where in small embryos the primordium precedes the deep plantar primordia in its cytological differentiation, also maximally correlates with the level of differentiation of the crural musculature. Kopsch (1952) mentions the quadratus plantae as a downward shifted crural musculature.

In comparative anatomy this muscle is a very variable one, even within one order in some species of Mammals the quadratus plantae (m. flexor accessorius, caput plantare m. flexoris longi) appears as fully developed in the form similar to that in Man, in other species of the same order it is represented only by a slip of connective tissue (Leche, 1900). The same variability can be found also in Primates (Le Double, 1897). On comparing these facts with the situation in the course of ontogenesis it seems to be right to conclude that it is really a distal separated part of the original flexor hallucis longus primordium which after separation either differentiates normally toward a typical muscle, or becomes extinct and changes eventually into a strip of connective tissue known as a variation in Man and as a norm in a number of Mammals. The large number of variations described in Man, when the quadratus plantae receives muscular strips beginning in the depth of the posterior side of deep crural muscles (especially on the fibular side and on the fascia of the flexor hallucis longus — Le Double, 1897), also support this concept.

In connection with the quadratus plantae insertion it is also interesting to observe the manner of crossing of the two long flexor tendon primordia—the m. flexor hallucis longus and the m. flexor digitorum longus. In both muscles independent tendons first develop already in embryos of 16—17 mm in C-R length. In the place of the crossing over, the tendons first (if followed in the proximodistal direction) superimpose dorsoplantarly and they then fuse together for a short distance to form a bulky tendinous primordium representing a far larger area in transverse section than that of the original tendons. The region of the crossing-over of the two flexors is hence something more than a simple concrescence, it is a development of a tendinous formation into which the quadratus plantae is inserted and from which (after mutual crossing-over) the tendons of the flexor digitorum and the flexor hallucis course distally.

Its entire pattern in the course of ontogenesis places the quadratus plantae in connection with the flexor hallucis longus; it differentiates in a continuation of the flexor hallucis longus belly and inserts into its tendon. Only secondarily is the quadratus plantae attached to the perichondrium of the calcaneus primordium. The quadratus plantae appears as a muscle belonging to the original posterior crural deep blastema which has become a plantar muscle secondarily. (It is a situation opposite to that in the superficial palmar blastema, which is originally a palmar one and secondarily changes into the antebrachial muscle.)

H. Ontogenesis of some Connective Tissue Structures in the Hand and Foot and their Relations to Developing Muscles
1. The Aponeurosis palmaris and the Aponeurosis plantaris

In course of hand and foot ontogenesis typical connective tissue formations, known as the palmar and the plantar aponeurosis, differentiate in the subcutaneous region. They seem to be one of the typical layers of hand and foot musculature and from the ontogenetic and the phylogenetic standpoint they have also been considered to be derived from the muscle layer and muscular primordia. The layer of the so-called flexores breves superficiales (palmares, plantares) has also been associated with the development of these structures. In our series the palmar and the plantar aponeuroses, however, they appear as connective tissue structures from the beginning of their ontogenesis and in no case do they assume the form of a muscular primordium. While the palmar aponeurosis differentiates at a certain—though small—distance from the skin of the palm, the plantar aponeurosis is situated very near to the skin already in small embryos. In the course of ontogenesis in the hand the palmar aponeurosis has a complicated relation to the developing m. palmaris longus, to the retinaculum flexorum and secondarily also to the m. palmaris brevis. In all these interrelations, which are thoroughly described in the papers by Dylevský (1968b, 1969a, c), the palmar aponeurosis develops as a formation sui generis, standing all the time in addition to palmar muscle layers.

In the foot the plantar aponeurosis also remains separated from the superficial palmar primordia (m. flexor digitorum brevis) in course of the entire embryonic period which could be followed in our preparations (up to 80 mm C-R length); the connection of the plantar aponeurosis with this muscle, as

known in adults, is thus evidently a secondary one. It is contradictory to the
views claiming the plantar aponeurosis as a derivative of muscles reduced in
the course of phylogenesis or ontogenesis.

Complicated relations of the palmar as well as of the plantar aponeurosis
to their insertions, to various septa of connective tissue perforating from the
aponeurosis to the depth of the planta (originating after 50 mm C-R length of
embryo) will evidently require further observations. The clinical importance of
these structures also requires revision of many morphological points, especially
relating to the development of the palmar and plantar aponeurosis (Dylevský,
1969c).

2. The Retinaculum flexorum in the Course of Ontogenesis

In the chapter concerning the development of the thenar musculature attention has been drawn to the fact that the development of the opponens pollicis
and the change of its position in the course of ontogenesis are associated with a
gradual development of the retinaculum flexorum. The retinaculum originates
as a strip of condensed mesenchyme at the eminentia carpi ulnaris primordium,
it then differentiates and is formed radiad (Čihák, 1966b, 1969b) around the
superficial palmar primordium (the future flexor digitorum superficialis) (Fig. 98).
The retinaculum flexorum gradually differentiates up to the eminentia carpi
radialis (Fig. 99) and becomes associated with it. The typical canalis carpi develops by this process in the course of ontogenesis (in embryos of about 30 mm
C-R length). The change of the opponens pollicis position is also in accord
with these changes of proportions inside the palm. The opponens is originally
a derivative of the deep thenar primordium (part of the flexores breves profundi layer). In the course of development it adjoins the retinaculum flexorum
which by its own differentiation comes to lie close to the muscle primordium
(Fig. 99). The secondary connection of the muscle primordium with the retinaculum brings the position of the opponens pollicis nearer to the thenar surface.

The time sequence is the notable point in the development of the retinaculum
flexorum and in the origin of the canalis carpi. Whilst the development of other
connective tissue structures (fasciae, septa, connective tissue membranes etc.)
proceeds at about 50 mm C-R length of embryo and this period is typical for
the origin of connective tissue structures, the development of the retinaculum
flexorum already proceeds in embryos between 18 and 30 mm in C-R length.

3. The Dorsal Aponeurosis of the Digits in the Hand and Foot during Ontogenesis

The dorsal aponeurosis of the fingers is usually accepted in anatomy as a
sheet of thickened connective tissue including the extensor tendon. This thicken-
ing begins in adults in the region of the metacarpophalangeal joints, at the point
where the interossei and lumbricales tendons come into contact with the extensor
tendon on the dorsal side of the metacarpophalangeal articulation. Detailed studies (Baumann, 1947; Landsmeer, 1955) deal with the minute anatomy of these
"wings" of the dorsal aponeurosis and with the functional significance of single
streams of connective tissue and tendinous fibres. The entry and the extended
insertion of the lumbricales and interossei into the dorsal aponeurosis are generally
considered to be the basis of fibres which course—fan-shaped—inside the apo-

neurosis according to inserting muscles and which complete the extensor tendons to form a typical dorsal aponeurosis. Some authors also take the possibility of double-layered extensor tendons into considerations (Baumann, 1947), or claim that the fascia dorsalis manus intertendinea is involved in the formation of the dorsal aponeurosis (Landsmeer, 1955). In our material where the interossei have been studied, the pattern of the dorsal aponeurosis of the digits in the hand and foot was observed in course of ontogenesis.

The fundamental difference from the usual anatomical view can be ascertained in the pattern of the embryonic dorsal aponeurosis: this dorsal aponeurosis does not begin by insertions of the interossei at the metacarpophalangeal articulations, but in the 2nd to 4th finger it is formed far more proximally, already in the metacarpal region.

The primordium of the dorsal aponeurosis of the fingers originates in embryos of about 15 mm in C-R length and is associated with the origin and occurrence of the interossei dorsales accessorii primordia (v. s.). These interossei dorsales accessorii primordia are situated extremely dorsally at the margins of intermetacarpal spaces; they are compact in proximal thirds of intermetacarpal spaces and they diverge distally to both sides of the space. This spreading out to both sides from the intermetacarpal spaces results in these accessory primordia of neighbouring intermetacarpal spaces linking up to form a denser mesenchymal layer over the metacarpals, continuous from one space to another (Fig. 121). The extensor tendons then join this extended layer from the dorsal side. In this manner the dorsal aponeurosis of the finger in its two typical layers originates already proximally, between the proximal and middle third of metacarpal length. Such a typical double-layered pattern is visible in embryos up to 20 mm C-R length. The interossei and lumbricales then become attached to the thus formed aponeurosis, but far distal, at the metacarpal heads. The pattern of the dorsal aponeurosis is not altered in principle by the attachment of these muscles, the more distal histological sections of the series do not differ from the proximal ones where the interossei and lumbricals are not yet inserted.

In further development the connective tissue of the aponeurosis proper becomes denser and gradually obtains its architecture described in quoted publications (v. s.). The proximal part in the metacarpal region remains thinner and together with the firm joining up of the accessory primordium to the dorsal surface of the dorsal interosseus (to its intermetacarpal component) it changes into the fascia dorsalis manus interossea. In these stages this fascia freely extends over dorsal surfaces of the metacarpals and is not joined with them before 50 mm of C-R length of embryo. In embryos between 20 and 30 mm C-R length this accessory primordium spreading out over adjacent metacarpals is still visible.

It is evident that the primordium of the dorsal aponeurosis of the finger is formed more proximally; the preparations in the comparative anatomy (Dylevský, and Mrázková, 1970) and in adults also provide support for this. The proximal limitation of the aponeurosis to the region of the metacarpophalangeal articulation and to the insertions of the lumbricals and interossei are, of course, a preparation artefact, as recognized already by Landsmeer (1955), caused in adults by the separation of the dorsal aponeurosis (thickened by inserting tendons) forcibly from the connective tissue which proceeds continuously proximally into the

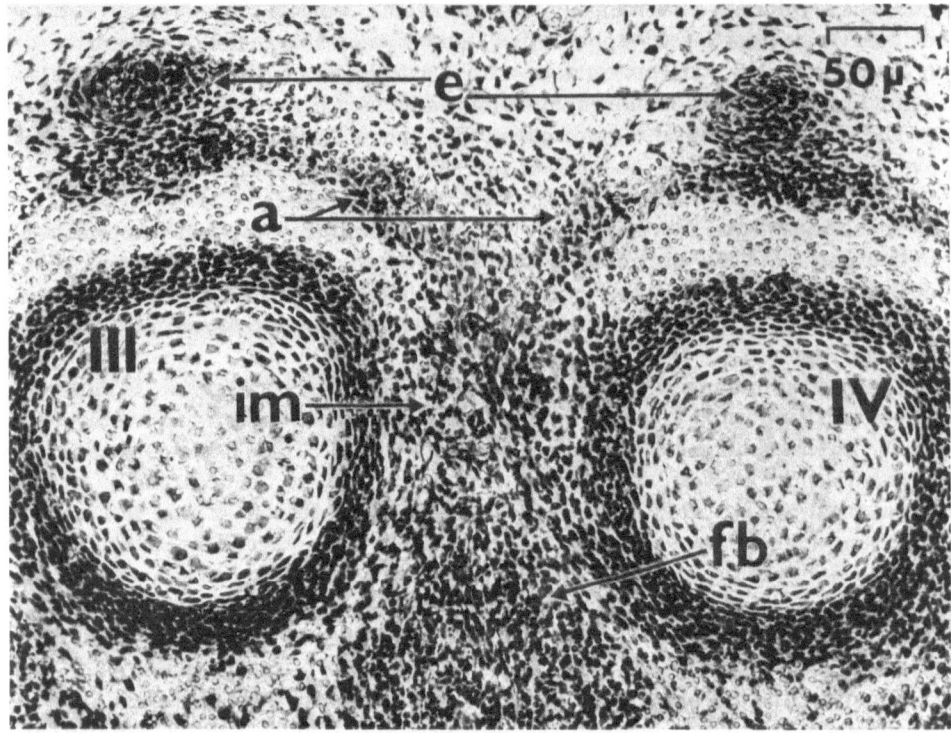

Fig. 121. Right hand of the embryo 19.5 mm in C-R length, transverse section in the half of metacarpal length. The origin of the dorsal aponeurosis is demonstrated. The expansion of insertions of the interosseus dorsalis accessorius primordia (*a*) over the dorsal side of the metacarpals is joined from dorsal by the extensor tendons (*e*). *III, IV* metacarpals; *fb* inter-ossei primordia corresponding to the flexores breves profundi layer; *im* intermetacarpal primordium

fascia dorsalis manus interossea. This proximal continuation of the dorsal apo-neurosis was observed by Landsmeer (1955) in his minute preparations and taken for the fascia dorsalis manus intertendinea. The fascia doralis manus intertendinea is, of course, involved in the structure of the dorsal aponeurosis in adults; in the quoted stages of embryonic development it is not yet formed and it can be seen in embryos that the basic layer of the dorsal aponeurosis is the fascia dorsalis manus interossea and its distal continuation.

The development of the dorsal aponeurosis of the digits of the foot proceeds in the same manner as in the hand; identical layers in identical relations to the metatarsals and to the toes take part in its origin and further embryonic develop-ment. In embryos of 18 mm C-R length the double-layered pattern is visible for the first time, it remains up to 34 mm C-R length, after this stage the dorsal aponeurosis distal on the toes firmly includes the extensor tendon.

The findings of spreading out primordia of the interossei dorsales accessorii to both sides over the two neighbouring metacarpals are, however, a basis also for the explanation of other points already observed earlier in the ontogenesis of hand muscles. It is known that there are some insertions of muscles of the intermetacarpal space, especially of the dorsal interossei, to the two neighbouring fingers in the embryonic period. Baumann (1951) presumed that one of these insertions becomes extinct in the course of ontogenesis. He also brings the observation that the tendons of insertion of the dorsal interossei are separated from the muscular bellies proper for a certain embryonic period and that they connect up in later stages. This can be explained in comparison with our series by assuming that the author observed the interosseus dorsalis accessorius primordium spreading out to both sides simultaneously with the interosseus dorsalis primordium proper, at that time far distant from the accessory primordium, in the obliquely sectioned series. Baumann (1951) observed the palmar part of the interosseus (the fused flexor brevis profundus and the intermetacarpalis primordium) separated from the dorsal part (the accessory dorsal interosseus) which is already inserted, but from his oblique series he could not recognize the two layers and took them therefore to be the separated and independently developed bellies and tendons of the interossei.

Baumann's idea (1951) concerning the reduction of tendinous insertions of the dorsal interossei can be completed by our observations that the dorsal interosseus proper has its insertion into one finger only from its very origin. This insertion of the dorsal interosseus is, however, more complicated, as shown by Salsbury (1936), Baumann (1947), Braithwaite, Channell, Moore, and Whillis (1948), Kaplan (1953), Eyler and Markee (1954), Landsmeer (1955). The dorsal interossei insert partly into the shafts of the phalanges, partly into the dorsal aponeurosis. According to our observations the component corresponding to the flexor brevis profundus inserts into the phalanx, the component corresponding to the intermetacarpalis (v. s.) has its insertion in the dorsal aponeurosis. We cannot support the view that the interossei proper are inserted at the beginning of their development to the two neighbouring fingers and that one of these insertions gets reduced. On the contrary in the embryonic period the interossei dorsales accessorii primordia are really inserted into the two sides and they enter into the fascia dorsalis manus interossea, these extensions over the metacarpals forming the primordia of the dorsal aponeuroses of fingers, already proximally in the metacarpal region. This connection is later differently reconstructed: either the entire accessory primordium is reduced to various degrees and changes into the fascia dorsalis manus interossea; in this case its insertion disappears as a formed pattern. In other cases the accessory primordium firmly joins the interosseus dorsalis, loses almost all its original connections and is inserted together with the dorsal interosseus proper (this second alternative being usual in the interossei dorsales accessorii of the foot, if formed, not only in Man but also in anthropoid Apes, e.g. in the Gorilla, as demonstrated by Straus, 1930).

In cases where the interosseus dorsalis accessorius persists as an independent and well formed muscular strip (muscles of the first group according to Chmelová, 1963 — v. s.), these muscles maintain their connection to dorsal aponeuroses of both neighbouring fingers in one third of all such observed muscles (Chmelová, 1963). In the remaining two thirds of muscles of this first group only their point of insertion with the corresponding dorsal interosseus remains. We saw no case where only one insertion of the accessory muscle and that to the finger opposite to that of the corresponding dorsal interosseus, was maintained. Baumann's observation (1951) of the reduction of interossei insertions is hence valid, but only partly, for another element—for the interosseus dorsalis accessorius, where in some these accessory elements their insertion really gets rebuilt in the quoted manner.

V. Conclusions

The development of muscles of the palm and sole as well as of muscles and tendons in the dorsum manus and pedis proceeds in course of ontogenesis *in loco*. The muscle primordia originate from the blastemas which are situated approximately in the places of definitive muscles from the beginning of their differentiation. No signs of a real migration of muscular primordia, as claimed e.g. by Ruge (1878a), are found. The positional changes of muscular primordia evidently occur only by a differential growth of the skeleton and musculature and by mutual growth differences of single muscle primordia. The actual growth, however, was not measured in this study, but evident gradual changes in the relative size of single formations were observed from stage to stage together with a gradual transition of these changes in size into changes of mutual position. These changes of position, however, are never so great as formerly implied. A gradual differentiation of a further formation can also take part in this process. Ruge (1878a), for example, described the migration of the interossei primordia from the palmar side into intermetacarpal spaces. It is true that at the beginning of development these primordia are found palmar to the intermetacarpal spaces and later also inside them (but also palmar to the spaces). In fact, no immigration of primordia into intermetacarpal spaces is here in question, but the gradual differentiation and fusion of the flexores breves profundi primordia (situated palmar from intermetacarpal spaces) with a further intermetacarpal primordium which had differentiated in the meantime inside the space.

A particular feature of the development of the skeleton and especially of the musculature in the hand and foot is the striking and consistent maintenance of the *developmental recapitulation*. We employ this term, although its significance and the manner of its employment in morphology were neither explicit in all cases, nor has it been equivocally explained (Slabý, 1962b). We employ it especially because it was found consistently in the studied material that the process of form changes of developing muscular primordia from the common blastemas up to the final forms (especially the formation of single stages and their sequence) is strikingly similar to the process of form changes found in the course of phylogenesis. This striking similarity of the developmental process seen in phylogenetic stages (e.g. from lower Mammals toward Primates) does not relate, however, only to the basic development (expressed by v. Baer's rule) where common signs develop first and then the secondary specialized ones, but this recapitulation relates to minute, sometimes quite surprising details. From this standpoint the original idea of signs of animals of various levels (Meckel, 1811, 1821) appearing in the course of embryonic development, or the idea of a developmental recapitulation as of signs of adult ancestors from the phylogenetic sequence repeating in course of phylogenesis—as after Haeckel (1866) still accepted by Sewertzoff (1927, 1931)—has played an important role in the origin of modern developmental morphology and of the concept of the phylembryogenetic modi. The objection is usually raised to the recapitulation concept that ontogenesis on one side is compared with adult organisms from phylogenesis or comparative anatomy on the other side. This objection could, however, be valid only against the original concept of recapitulation of the phylogenetic development in the course of ontogenesis, as has been simply assumed in the period of the advancement of developmental morphology. It is not well-founded to enforce this objection at the present level of knowledge in the complexity of the process of morphogenesis, heredity and of evolution in general, since only the term recapitulation remains from the original concept. It is self-evident that the term recapitulation cannot be conceived to cover the reiteration of conditions in adult species from phylogenesis. This concept was already abandonned by Križanovsky (1939) whose concept of recapitulation was not the ontogenetic repeating of signs of previous adult forms but a structure passing over from one generation to the next and repeated from its origin in each subsequent ontogenesis.

We do not want, however, to comprehend developmental recapitulation even in Kryžanowsky's concept, as an inherited structure, but we regard it as a developmental process. The term the developmental recapitulation envisages the process of form changes of a certain formation in the course of ontogenesis, i.e. *the sequence of form changes* and of mutual interrelations of formations in the course of ontogenesis which in comparison with the sequence of developmental form changes of homologous formations, deduced from single developmental levels of phylogenesis, is identical or at least maximally similar. In this comparison with phylogenesis no single species and their adult individuals are in question. (Their comparative anatomy is only the basis for the abstraction of the compared sequence of form changes and in correlation with changes in ontogenesis it is the evidence that the assessment of form changes is right.) The term developmental recapitulation is also justified because the comparison of the developmental sequence of form changes at generalized abstracted levels of phylogenetic development with identically proceeding form changes of a homologous organ during ontogenesis is at stake. It is justified not only by the formal fact that in the course of ontogenesis the sequence of changes in form is the same as in the phylogenetic past, but also by the process of ontogenesis itself. It is evident that the process of formation of a certain organ is fixed and directed genetically and is thus repeated in the course of ontogenesis of each further generation. We therefore employ the term developmental recapitulation as a brief, truthful and historically founded denomination of the morphogenetic sequence of form changes gradually developed ontophylogenetically according to the prevalent modus of addition (prolongation: Franz, 1924; anaboly: Sewertzoff, 1931).

Developmental recapitulation is linked up with the modus of addition according to Sewertzoff (1927, 1931) as well as according to Remane (1952) and Slabý (1968b). During the development of the skeleton and mainly of the musculature developmental changes at the end of the morphogenetic process occur by addition not only in Man but also at phylogenetically lower levels and in parallel lines in the development of Mammals (Dylevský, 1968d; Dylevský and Trnková, 1969). We therefore employ the term developmental recapitulation not as the term explaining the mechanism of development and its causality, but as the practical denomination of a chain of developmental changes in the course of ontogenesis which go on in an additive phylembryogenetic modus. On following these changes the idea of a general developmental trend of the observed formation is obtained by associating the phylogenetic aspect with observation in ontogenesis.

If the gradual form of development of the skeleton and muscles in the hand and foot is considered from the above mentioned standpoint in the course of ontogenesis, it may be stated that the development of both, especially of muscles, proceeds in a very conservative manner which maintains all the features of form changes which took place in the course of phylogenesis. The changes characteristic only for the human hand are realised really additively concluding morphogenesis, after the form recapitulation has been passed through.

This manner of development permits the recognition of some earlier independent and then fused together components in the course of the ontogenesis of the skeleton and musculature, and also permits an attempt at reconsidering their homologies.

During ontogenesis of the musculature e.g. the contrahentes layer in the hand and foot of Man recapitulates the characteristic primitive pattern of four strips corresponding to the four contrahentes muscles of lower mammals. Only at the conclusion of development do the features characteristic for Man proceed, i.e. the reduction of two ulnar (or fibular) strips and, moreover, in the foot the differentiation of a new component—the transverse head of the adductor hallucis.

In the course of development of the interossei characteristic layers of primordia are also recapitulated: the flexores breves profundi layer and the intermetacarpal (intermetatarsal) layer. Some of their components then gradually fuse to form a new muscle—the dorsal interosseus. This process of fusion and of the origin of a real dorsal interosseus actually recapitulates form changes of these muscles seen in phylogenesis from Prosimians to Man.

The three fundamental elements of the intermetacarpal space, i.e. two flexores breves profundi and dorsal to them the intermetacarpalis, are so fixed from the phylogenetic past (evidently even from lower developmental stages of the Sauropsids), that they recapitulate in form as primordia in the course of ontogenesis of birds (Dylevský, 1968d), as well as in the development of lower mammals outside the main stream of phylogenetic development (e.g. in the rat) as shown by Dylevský and Trnková (1969). In these cases also these elements are modified by the addition of developmental changes at the end of morphogenesis. These changes in the quoted cases are the fusion of all primordia in the intermetacarpal space to one muscle in birds, the secondary reduction of the intermetacarpalis in the rat. These examples demonstrate that the basic form and pattern of primordia as seen in the course of human ontogenesis, is really a developmentally original pattern. To this fundamental situation of layers in the intermetacarpal spaces of Man new muscular primordia develop specific for Man—the interossei dorsales accessorii—and by fusion with the other primordia again additively modify the further development of dorsal interossei, of the dorsal aponeurosis of digits etc. The mutual fusion of components of the various layers to form a qualitatively new formation—the dorsal interosseus—is a specific feature of phylogenetic and ontogenetic development of the human hand and foot.

The process of development and the homologies of further muscles in the human hand, e.g. of the opponens pollicis, of both heads of the flexor pollicis brevis, the opponens and flexor digiti minimi can also be deduced from the recapitulation of the developmentally original situation. In the development of muscles of the human foot the conservatively proceeding development also permits the recognition of the characteristic components of foot musculature phylogenetically known and their gradual developmental reconstruction. These developmental relations are given in detail in conclusions of the single chapters in the previous text.

On the basis of the course of development of muscle primordia layers in the hand and foot of Man, Bardeleben's general scheme (1890) of autopodial muscle layers can be reconsidered and completed. From the surface of the palm (planta) to the depth up to the dorsal side of the hand and foot the layers are situated as follows (Fig. 122):

1. *The flexores breves superficiales (palmares, plantares)*. To this layer three muscle primordia belong in human ontogenesis, the middle large one and two lateral ones. The middle primordium changes to form the *flexor digitorum superficialis* and by its further differentiation it proceeds to the antebrachium (Dylevský, 1967, 1968a, c); the radial primordium gives rise to the *abductor pollicis brevis*, the ulnar primordium is that of the *abductor digiti minimi*.

In the foot of human embryos three superficial primordia develop identically, a larger middle one and two smaller lateral ones. The *flexor digitorum brevis* originates from the middle primordium, the other two are primordia of the *abductor hallucis* and the *abductor digiti minimi*.

2. *The lumbricales* are the typical layer of muscles originating by differentiation of an original sheet in common with the tendinous part of the flexor digitorum profundus (flexor digitorum longus). These muscles originate in loco, already in form and situation not far different from definitive lumbricals. It is possible that during ontogenesis the lumbricales II–IV pedis receive some material from the residua of disappearing strips of the contrahentes layer.

3. *The contrahentes* (flexores breves medii, adductores digitorum, contracteurs des doigts) are the typical layer between the lumbricals [and tendons of the flexor digitorum profundus (longus)] on the palmar (plantar) side and the deep branch of the ulnar nerve (n. plantaris lateralis) on the dorsal side. In this layer, which has originally the form of four distally projecting strips to the 1st, 2nd, 4th and 5th finger, the entire *adductor pollicis* develops from two radial strips, the ulnar strips get reduced and join with the interossei.

In the foot from the tibial two contrahentes strips only the *caput obliquum of the adductor hallucis* originates; the *caput transversum* differentiates in the same layer secondarily, in its distal continuation.

4. *The flexores breves profundi* are the couples of muscles beneath the metacarpals (metatarsals) and in the palmar sectors of intermetacarpal (intermetatarsal) spaces. In lower Mammals they are arranged in couples at the metacarpals (metatarsals), in Primates in couples for intermetacarpal spaces.

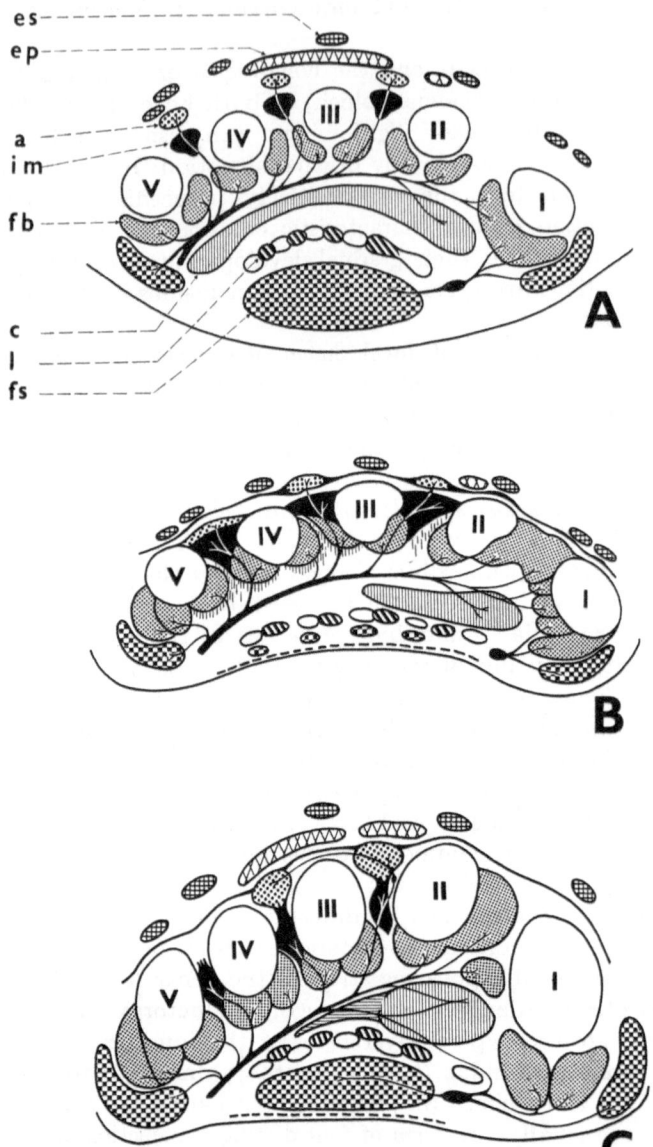

Fig. 122. Scheme of position and homologies of muscular layers of the hand and foot in:
A the general scheme, *B* the embryonic and adult human hand, *C* the embryonic and adult
human foot; corresponding layers demonstrated by shading. *I–V* metacarpals (metatarsals);
fs layer corresponding to the flexores breves superficiales (palmares et plantares), *l* lumbricales; *c* contrahentes; *fb* layer corresponding to the flexores breves profundi; *im* intermetacarpal (intermetatarsal) primordia; *a* primordia of the interossei dorsales accessorii; *ep* deep
layer of extensors; *es* superficial layer of extensors. For single muscles in the hand and foot
cf. schemes and photographs in Figs. 84, 95, 104, 110, 111. 136, 138

The following muscles originate from this layer during the ontogenesis of the human hand: the *opponens pollicis*, both heads of the *flexor pollicis brevis*, the variable *interosseus palmaris I Henlei*, two components for the *interosseus dorsalis I*, palmar *components of the interossei dorsales II–IV*, the entire *interossei palmares I–III*, in the ulnar margin of the hand the *flexor digiti minimi brevis* and the *opponens digiti minimi*. The process of development and differentiation of these muscles is described in the corresponding chapters.

During the ontogenesis of the human foot the flexores breves profundi layer gives rise to the *flexor hallucis brevis* (its tibial and fibular component), the accessory *interosseus plantaris hallucis* (in the literature also incorrectly denoted as the opponens hallucis), two components of the *interosseus dorsalis I*, *plantar parts of the interossei dorsales III et IV* (the participation of this component in the interosseus dorsalis II is uncertain and this component seems to be incorporated in the interosseus dorsalis I), all three typical *interossei plantares (I–III)* and on the fibular margin of the foot the *flexor digiti minimi brevis* and the variable *opponens digiti minimi*.

5. *The intermetacarpales* (intermetatarsales) are contained in intermetacarpal and intermetatarsal spaces. In some lower Mammals they appear as independent muscles. During the ontogenesis of the human hand and foot they appear as primordia only in the 2nd to 4th spaces. From these primordia *dorsal parts of the interossei dorsales II–IV* originate, in the foot probably the entire interosseus dorsalis II. They always have an independent innervating branch from the ulnar (fibular plantar) nerve.

6. *The interossei dorsales accessorii* belong only to the scheme of the human embryonic hand and foot since they are specific only for Man (in the foot they are also rarely found in anthropoid Apes). We do not find their homology in the comparative anatomy of the hand. They join from the dorsal side the dorsal interossei, in the hand they are found in three ulnar spaces, in the foot only in the 2nd and 3rd space. During development they either fuse firmly with the interosseus, or they maintain independence of various degrees.

7. *The extensores digitorum manus et pedis breves.* In the hand they can be found in the form of a *variable short extensor*, which differentiates in continuation with the deep extensor layer of the antebrachium. The *extensor indicis* develops in this layer. The primordia extend up to the dorsum manus, but they only rarely develop to form an accessory muscle. In the foot they form a typical layer of short extensors on the dorsum pedis—the *extensor hallucis brevis* and the *extensor digitorum brevis*. Their development is not included in this paper, since there are many relations to the extensor layer of the antebrachium, deserving special studies.

8. *The layer of tendons of the extensors.*

The described scheme is a general one and it is comparable with layers of muscles found in Mammals. Only the interossei dorsales accessorii are a special derivative of the dorsal muscular blastema in Man, being, however, completely (in the hand) or by means of an anastomosis (in the foot) supplied by nerves from the palmar (plantar) side. The relations of these elements to the extensores breves (to the deep layer of the extensor blastema in the hand) in the course of ontogenesis and in phylogenetically lower Mammals remains an open question.

11*

The time sequence in the development of the skeleton and musculature of the hand and foot proceeds in certain phases which can be characterized generally as follows:

1. *The phase of blastemas and of their fundamental layers.* It proceeds in the hand from 13 to 15 mm of C-R embryo length, in the foot from 14 to 17 mm C-R length. This phase in the course of development of the skeleton includes the formation of blastemas, which in strips of condensed mesenchyme suggest the fundamental archipterygium form with the foreshadowing of collateral rays; in the development of muscles this phase corresponds to the fundamental formation of blastematous layers.

2. *The phase of differentiation of individual primordia* inside blastematous layers and regions, proceeding in the hand between 15 and 25 mm C-R length, in the foot from 17 to 25 mm C-R length.

In this second phase single elements of the skeleton chondrify. In the development of muscles inside of blastematous layers the primordia of individual muscles differentiate.

The first two phases during development of the skeleton and musculature bear just the conspicuous character of recapitulation, since the elements of the skeleton and musculature appear at first in the pattern characteristic for phylogenetically lower levels. The two phases are very important in the course of ontogenesis for the possibility of revision and establishing of homologies. In muscle development this is the very time of appearance of independent components of primordia comparable with muscles of lower phylogenetic levels which disappear or fuse, etc. in further development. In the development of the skeleton phylogenetically extinct centralia and other elements transiently develop in this period.

3. *The phase of reconstruction* of the formed primordia, of their reduction, fusion etc., proceeding in the hand in embryos of 25–35 mm in C-R length, in the foot between 25 and 40 mm C-R embryo length.

This phase mostly represents the additive completion of the previous development, being specific for the phylogenetic level of the studied species. In the skeleton in this phase the independently chondrified components, which were comparable with the centralia, disappear, the prepollex anlage disappears, the centrale normale fuses with the scaphoideum. The fusion of primordia from various layers occurs in muscles (e.g. to form the dorsal interossei), also the extinction of primordia of the contrahentes III and IV, etc. The definitive form of bone primordia and of muscular primordia is obtained, similar to the forms of bones and muscles in adults.

4. *The phase of developing definitive forms* of the skeleton and muscles. The origin of formations of connective tissue, of the septa, fasciae, etc. This phase proceeds quickly in the period between 40 and 100 mm in C-R length of the embryo, but it continues in slight changes of proportions etc. for almost the entire embryonic period (Čihák, 1959, 1960a, 1963a).

During this phase the incongruences of articular facets in the skeleton become concordant (e.g. between the radius and carpal elements), in the foot the form of the tarsal elements is definitively formed, the angle between the distal tarsal row and the metatarsals is reduced. The muscles of the hand and foot increase relatively, the entire hand and foot flattens and is already vaulted. The fundamental form changes come to an end with the development of fasciae and septa. The fasciae and septa originate in the hand after reaching 50 mm C-R length, in the foot after 60 mm.

Within the framework of these phases of morphogenesis some muscles or other formations develop more quickly, some of them more slowly. This sequence of changes, however, is important as a whole and fully characterizes the development of forms and the rebuilding of primordia of the skeleton and musculature in the human hand and foot. Considered from the general viewpoint, the development of the studied components of the hand and foot proceeds from its very beginning in an extremely conservative manner. In form development it passes from developmentally general, primitive structures, whose form corresponds to the structures known in phylogenetically lower levels of Mammals or even of lower Tetrapods in general, up to the form of the mammalian and finally the human hand. The primitive form is here gradually replaced by the developmentally specified features. Hence in course of ontogenesis still more than in the definitive form the human hand and foot are organs in which the pattern of phylogenetically ancient signs are joined with developmentally new, specialized features, each extremity having its own special character as shown in the individual chapters.

The last point in question concerns the mutual concordance or homology of structures in the hand and foot. In general disposition and pattern the accordance is striking, e.g. in the distribution of layers of muscular primordia, in the fundamental positions of chondrified elements of the skeleton etc. In further development such coincidence becomes less apparent. The components of the skeleton are then no longer in agreement, the primordia from various layers join in different mode in the hand and in the foot, some muscles in the hand and foot cannot be mutually homologised at all (e.g. the flexor hallucis brevis with the flexor pollicis brevis), in other muscles, to the contrary, the comparison is very exact. However, the term homology is in no case adequate for the comparison of the structures of the hand and foot (also employed in past for the hand and foot as the so-called serial homology). No principial error has yet occurred by its employment, but it will be more appropriate to speak of form accordances and similarities rather than of homologies. It is better to maintain the term homology for the comparison of the hand with the hand of various levels of the system, in a conventional manner. The contemporary studies of the origin and material of the upper and lower limbs also support this idea. On the other side, the development of the hand and foot demonstrates that the similarities go further than can be considered as mere homodynamies, and that the comprehension of the structure and development of one of the extremities becomes the key for recognizing the other.

VI. Summary

The studies of the ontogenetic development of the skeleton and musculature in the human hand and foot were made on 373 histological series of hands and feet of human embryos and foetuses from 10–100 mm C-R length prepared in transverse, sagittal sections and in sections parallel with the palm and with the sole. For studies of single problems from this entire material adequate sets of 40–80 series were selected.

The review of observations and conclusions derived from it can be summarized as follows:

A. The Development of the Hand and Foot Skeleton

1. The radiale is probably included inside the distal radius end; a visible rudiment of the prepollex adjoins it at early stages of ontogenesis (from 14 to 25 mm C-R length) (Figs. 3, 4). Steiner's concept is thus supported. During human ontogenesis transient form changes of the distal radius end are visible between 19–25 mm C-R length of the embryo, suggesting this rebuilding (Figs. 4, 5).

2. The ulnare appears as homologous with the processus styloideus ulnae; this corresponds to Holmgren's and Kindahl's concept. During ontogenesis the ulnare appears in the form of a transiently bulky processus styloideus ulnae, sized and shaped as a carpal element (between 16 and 55 mm C-R length), and later it becomes reduced (Figs. 3, 4, 8–10, 14, 27).

3. The scaphoideum originates by fusion of two centralia. Their fusion proceeds from 30–50 mm C-R length of embryo. The bulkier of the two, situated at the radius, belongs to the intermedial ray and probably corresponds with the centrale radiale distale of Steiner's concept ($c\,2$ according to Holmgren and Kindahl). This is joined by the centrale normale which is homologous with the centrale ulnare distale of Steiner's concept (i. e. with the $c\,3$ according to Holmgren and Kindahl). The development of both and their fusion are visible in the course of ontogenesis (Figs. 3–6, 14, 27).

4. The lunatum corresponds to the further centrale; this corresponds to the centrale radiale proximale according to Steiner's nomenclature ($c\,1$ according to Holmgren and Kindahl). (Figs. 14, 27.)

5. The fourth centrale changes to form the triquetrum and corresponds most probably with the centrale ulnare proximale according to Steiner or with the $c\,4$ according to Holmgren and Kindahl (Figs. 14, 27).

6. The hamatum corresponds only with the carpale distale IV (Figs. 14, 27).

7. The carpale distale V originates between 13 and 15 mm C-R length of embryo (Fig. 11) and up to 17 mm C-R length it disappears; its part is evidently contained in the basis of the 5th metacarpal, corresponding with the os Vesalianum (var.). (Figs. 13, 14, 27.)

8. The intermedium persists transiently as a primordium of the so-called os triangulare, which disappears after reaching 60 mm C-R length, or persists as a variation (Figs. 8, 9, 14). A similar chondrification inside of the discus articularis ulnae corresponds to the broadened cartilage of the original ulnare (Fig. 10) and can occur together with the residuum of the intermedium in embryos up to 60 mm C-R length (Fig. 9).

9. It may be concluded from the developing carpus in Man compared with the pattern of the carpus in Reptiles, recent and fossil, that the radiale was most probably taken into the radius already in most primitive living Reptiles and even in fossil Theromorphs. The recapitulation of this developmentally long

past process is therefore less apparent in human ontogenesis than the recapitulation of the same process of ulnare rebuilding, which is evidently typical only for Mammals (Fig. 14).

10. The tibiale is included in the talus forming its main chondrifying primordium (in the corpus and the caput), visible from 16 mm C-R length of embryo (Figs. 15, 17–19).

11. The intermedium is contained in the talus, being delayed in chondrification. The region of the processus posterior corresponds to it, possibly also the os trigonum (var.). (Figs. 15, 18, 19.)

12. The fibulare is contained in the calcaneus (Figs. 15, 16, 18, 19), where it forms its distal, more medially developing part in course of ontogenesis, visible from 15 to 23 mm C-R length. The proximal calcaneus part corresponds most probably to a homologon of the pisiform of the hand, being more laterally situated and delayed in chondrification (similar to the pisiform of the hand). The relatively independent chondrification of the two calcaneus components is striking during early ontogenesis (Figs. 15, 16).

13. During the ontogenesis of the tarsus, according to some peculiarities in the chondrification process, the traces of four centralia can be found (Fig. 27).

14. One of the centralia transiently appears in the region of the processus lateralis tali (Figs. 17–19), and its separate chondrification is visible in embryos up to 20 mm in C-R length; it is the centrale tibiale proximale according to Steiner (*c1* according to Holmgren). In further development it is pushed back by the chondrification proceeding from the corpus tali into the lateral process; the centrale can then be the source of a number of accessory elements known between the talus, calcaneus, the cuboideum and the naviculare.

15. The os naviculare primordium is formed by two centralia. They are visible as independent chondrifications in embryos between 16 and 20 mm C-R length (Figs. 17–19). They correspond with the centrale tibiale distale and the centrale fibulare distale of Steiner, i.e. the *c2* and *c3* according to Holmgren. The centrale fibulare distale is not completely taken into the naviculare. Its rudiments can also become the source of accessory tarsal elements.

16. The fourth centrale corresponding to the centrale fibulare proximale according to Steiner (*c4* according to Holmgren) is transiently formed in young embryos between the distal end of the calcaneus and the cuboideum primordium (Fig. 19). In its place a rudimentary calcaneus secundarius can be found in adults.

17. The os cuboideum corresponds only with the tarsale distale IV (Fig. 27).

18. The tarsale distale V appears in early embryonic stages (up to 18 mm C-R length) in the form of a chondrifying primordium (Figs. 23, 27) which early disappears. Its part is most probably contained in the base of the 5th metatarsal and corresponds to the region of the os Vesalianum (var.).

19. In embryos of about 18 mm C-R length an indistinctly demarcated independent primordium originates in the region of the future tuberositas ossis navicularis (Figs. 20, 27). It may be considered the primordium of the os tibiale externum (var.); from the phylogenetic standpoint it appears to be the residuum of the prehallucial collateral ray. In its continuation in the same embryonic stage the independent cuneiforme I plantare develops (Fig. 22), known in adults

as a typical variation; this element is also considered in our scheme as a part of the first collateral (prehallucial) ray (Fig. 27).

20. The typical bone variation—the os intermetatarseum Gruberi—constantly originates as a well limited primordium in small embryos, persisting for a certain time; at about 25 mm C-R length of embryo it can be chondrified and at about 30 mm C-R length of embryo it disappears (Figs. 24–26). This variation seems to be split-off material of an originally bulkier and longer tarsale distale I.

21. Comparable and comparably displayed elements take part in the early developmental stages of the hand and foot. The development of the hand skeleton is characterized by the reduction of the proximal row of canonic elements and by the succession of the central elements to the radiocarpal articulation. In the foot the canonic elements all persist and the development of the tarsus is characterized by a tibiofibular narrowing, induced by fusion of canonic elements with the central elements and by joining of the rudimentary prehallucial ray to the tibial margin of the tarsus.

B. The Development of the Muscles of the Hand and Foot
1. The Development of the Contrahentes Layer

1. The contrahentes layer is generally characterized in Mammals by its position between the tendons of finger flexors and the ramus profundus nervi ulnaris (n. plantaris lateralis). In Man this layer is absent in adults. In the course of human ontogenesis, however, the layer originates and persists (up to 28 mm C-R length) to an extent similar to that in other Mammals (Figs. 34–37, 55). It originates already before reaching 14 mm C-R length of embryo.

2. A radial, ulnar and proximal part can be distinguished in the layer of the contrahentes primordia in the course of development, each of them developing in its own manner (Fig. 55).

3. The radial part of the layer gradually differentiates to form the adductor pollicis (Figs. 41, 55).

4. The ulnar part extends distal and ulnar to the course of the ulnar nerve through the palm (Fig. 55). Between 20 and 25 mm C-R length this part is divided into longitudinal slips which gradually adjoin the interossei and then fuse with them and with the mesenchyme between the interossei primordia (Figs. 48–51).

5. The reduction and fusion of strips of the ulnar part of the layer occurs through a complicated change of form of the strips. The form changes from the oval-shaped transverse section (Figs. 44, 45) to the form seen in transverse section of a stalk fixed in between the two interossei primordia of the corresponding intermetacarpal space (Figs. 48–51, 54, 55). The strip-like residua disappear in embryos of about 28 mm C-R length. It is impossible to distinguish whether the residua after fusion become the muscle tissue or only the perimysium of the interossei.

6. The proximal part of the layer connects the radial and the ulnar parts proximally to the ulnar nerve. It gradually disintegrates. Transiently, between 28 and 32 mm C-R length, this part gets denser and forms the plate comparable with the so-called contrahent-plate ("Contrahentesplatte") of anthropoid Apes (Fig. 42). Then it disappears completely. This plate is not the primordium of the fascia palmaris interossea, since that originates much later.

7. The adductor pollicis is homologous with the first and with the major part of the second contrahens of lower Mammals. The residuum in the 2nd inter-metacarpal space corresponds to the distal remnant of the m. contrahens II (Figs. 55, 56).

·8. The strip-like residua in the 3rd and 4th intermetacarpal spaces correspond to the contrahentes III and IV (of the 4th and 5th finger). (Figs. 55, 56.)

9. The temporary occurrence of the contrahentes layer in human embryos is a manifestation of a conservative manner of development, being a recapitulation of a developmentally ancient form of the layer, the persisting parts of which are finally taken into other muscles as material. The temporary appearance of the contrahent-plate is also to be considered as a display of form recapitulation.

10. In the course of ontogenesis of the human foot the contrahentes layer also appears as a blastematous layer in full extent typical for lower Mammals. It is apparent for the first time in embryos of 17 mm C-R length (Figs. 57–59).

11. During the ontogenesis of the foot the tibial and fibular parts can be distinguished in this layer according to the form and the manner of development (Figs. 59, 66). The tibial part develops to form the caput obliquum of the adductor hallucis, the strips of the fibular part remain in the stage of non-differentiated mesenchyme (Figs. 61, 62, 66) and project distally along the interossei IV and III and sometimes also beneath the 2nd intermetatarsal space (Figs. 60–62, 66).

12. In embryos of 25–30 mm in C-R length the fibular part of the layer changes into a continuous mesenchymal sheet (Fig. 62), the strips disappear. Only the caput obliquum of the adductor is differentiated (Fig. 63).

13. After reaching 30 mm C-R length of embryo the caput transversum of the adductor hallucis differentiates in the distal region of the fibular part of the layer (Fig. 64). Neither origin of the heads of the adductor join with the skeletal primordia before 50 mm C-R length (Fig. 65).

14. In the course of development of the entire layer the pattern of four contrahentes muscles recapitulates: the caput obliquum of the adductor hallucis is homologous with the first and the second contrahens. The strips in the 3rd and 4th intermetatarsal spaces are homologous with the contrahentes III et IV. The caput transversum of the adductor is not homologous with any of the typical contrahentes muscles of Mammals (Fig. 66).

15. The recapitulation of the developmentally more original forms is—contrary to the hand (Fig. 67)—only suggested and is very transient. It soon becomes superimposed by the specialized development of the bulky oblique head of the adductor, the primordia of the contrahentes III et IV are quickly reduced and the transverse head of the adductor differentiates secondarily in the distal continuation of the entire layer.

2. The Development of the Interossei in the Hand and Foot

1. Three layers of muscular primordia take part in the development of the interossei of the hand and foot. The palmar (plantar) of them corresponds to the layer of the flexores breves profundi of lower Mammals, being situated in

couples for single intermetacarpal (intermetatarsal) spaces between the ramus
profundus nervi ulnaris (n. plantaris lateralis) and the metacarpals (metatarsals).
The second layer is that of the intermetacarpal (intermetatarsal) primordia,
situated inside of the spaces, the third layer is that of the accessory primordia,
developing at the dorsal margins of spaces. The flexores breves profundi layer
and the intermetacarpal (intermetatarsal) primordia mainly take part in the
development of the interossei (Figs. 76, 77, 84, 94, 95).

2. The interosseus dorsalis I of the hand originates only in the flexores breves
profundi layer, from two primordia which enter the first intermetacarpal space
from the thumb and from the 2nd finger in embryos of 14–28 mm C-R length
(Fig. 70). Each component has its own nerve branch.

3. The interossei dorsales II, III et IV manus originate each by fusion of
one component from the flexores breves profundi layer and a further component from the intermetacarpales layer (Figs. 68, 71), which in the course of
ontogenesis from 28–40 mm C-R length gradually fuse to form a single muscle
(Figs. 74, 75, 84).

4. Each of the fusing components has its own supplying nerve branch. The
branches for intermetacarpal (intermetatarsal) primordia perforate through the
space to a considerable distance (Figs. 72, 73, 79, 90, 95).

5. The interosseus dorsalis I pedis is formed by one main primordium from
the flexores breves profundi layer and by a small adjoining primordium from
the same layer, which originally belonged to the interosseus dorsalis II (Figs. 87,
88, 91, 94).

6. The interossei dorsales pedis, III et IV, originate as in the hand by fusion
of the primordium from the flexores breves profundi layer with the intermetatarsal primordium (Figs. 85, 89, 91, 94). The intermetatarsal primordia fuse
very early with the flexores breves profundi primordia, already in embryos of
18–19 mm C-R length.

7. The interosseus dorsalis II pedis is most probably formed only by the
intermetatarsal primordium; its plantar component (the flexor brevis profundus
primordium) seems to join the interosseus dorsalis I (Figs. 87, 88, 91, 94).

8. The palmar and plantar interossei correspond each to one member of the
corresponding couple of primordia of the flexores breves profundi layer (Fig. 95).

9. At about 20 mm C-R length of the embryo a muscle differentiates from
the flexores breves profundi layer in the first space of the hand and foot. This
is variable in the hand and almost constant in the foot and interposed between
the adductor pollicis (hallucis) and the interosseus dorsalis I. Its form and position show it to be the palmar (plantar) interosseus of the first space. In the
hand it is usually denoted as the interosseus palmaris I Henlei (var.), in the foot
it was incorrectly termed the opponens hallucis; the term interosseus plantaris
hallucis is considered as the most appropriate one (Figs. 95, 109, 111).

10. All the remaining muscles of the thenar as well as of the great toe group
of the plantar musculature except for the adductor differentiate from the flexores breves profundi layer.

11. The accessory primordia originate over the dorsal surface of intermetacarpal primordia in the 2nd, 3rd and 4th intermetacarpal spaces already from

14 mm C-R length onward. They are supplied from the ulnar nerve by a branch perforating through the space for the intermetacarpal primordium (Figs. 79–81). This accessory primordium in the 4th space early fuses with the dorsal interosseus, rarely it persists; the accessory primordia in the 2nd and 3rd space remain independent to a variable degrees, forming either a typical small muscles (Fig. 82) which were often mistaken for the short extensors, or they remain as rudiments of various degrees in the fascia dorsalis manus interossea. For these muscles the term interossei dorsales accessorii is considered as the most appropriate one.

12. These accessory dorsal interossei originate from 19 mm C-R length in the foot also, most often only in the 2nd space (in about half of cases also in the 3rd space). The difference in their nerve supply, which in the foot comes from the anastomosis of dorsal and plantar nerves, is described in the text.

13. The development of the interossei dorsales II, III et IV by fusion of two superimposed layers of primordia supports from the standpoint of human ontogenesis the views held in the past only on the basis of the comparative anatomy. The participation of the interossei dorsales accessorii in the morphogenesis of the dorsal interossei and their constant occurrence is a further contribution to the knowledge of ontogenesis and of the complicated developmental pattern in the intermetacarpal (intermetatarsal) spaces. The fusion of layers of the palmar musculature (if considered from the phylogenetic standpoint) has reached its maximum in Man; it may therefore be taken to be a developmental addition, connected with the hominisation process of the hand in general.

3. The Development of the Musculature of the Marginal Digits in the Hand and Foot

1. Two blastematous layers originate in the thenar region, separated from the beginning of their development: the superficial layer from which the abductor pollicis brevis originates, and the deep one where the remaining thenar muscles (except for the adductor) originate (Fig. 96).

2. The adductor pollicis originates separately from other thenar muscles in the contrahentes layer.

3. The deep thenar primordia are homologous with the couple of flexores breves profundi of the thumb of lower Mammals (Fig. 84).

4. The ulnar and dorsal margin of the deep layer first separates (already in embryos of 14 mm C-R length) and enters the first intermetacarpal space during further development as the radial component of the interosseus dorsalis I (Figs. 70, 101, 104).

5. The remaining deep thenar blastema gradually (from 17 to 35 mm C-R length) differentiates and divides into the radiad situated opponens pollicis primordium and into side by side situated heads of the flexor pollicis brevis (Figs. 102–104). Between the interosseus dorsalis I, the adductor pollicis and the deep head of the flexor pollicis brevis a variable strip differentiates, inserting to the site of the future ulnar sesamoid bone—the so-called interosseus palmaris I Henlei (Fig. 104).

6. The retinaculum flexorum differentiates gradually from 15 mm C-R length onward in the ulno-radial direction, and the opponens pollicis primordium joins

it secondarily (Figs. 98, 99). The opponens pollicis obtains its definitive position in relation to thenar layers as a result of this junction.

7. In the course of development the flexor pollicis longus tendon gets interposed (from the surface) in between the two heads of the flexor pollicis brevis (at about 35 mm C-R length).

8. According to its origin the opponens pollicis is homologous with the radial component of the flexores breves profundi of the thumb and represents a phylogenetically ancient structure which is secondarily modified in form, position and origin on the retinaculum flexorum.

9. In the region of the great toe group of the plantar musculature, the superficial layer first differentiates (after 18 mm C-R length), forming the primordium of the abductor hallucis (Figs. 105, 106).

10. At the great toe the layer of the deep blastema, which is the continuation of the flexores breves profundi layer, splits and differentiates from 20 mm C-R length onward.

11. A tip of the deep layer of the blastema at the great toe metatarsal extends into the first intermetatarsal space and differentiates later into the independent muscular strip interposed between the interosseus dorsalis I and the oblique head of the adductor hallucis. It is the plantar interosseus of the first space by its position and insertion and corresponds to the interosseus palmaris I Henlei of the hand. The term musculus interosseus plantaris hallucis is considered as a correct denomination not disturbing the present nomenclatory usage.

12. The remaining part of the deep blastema of the great toe metatarsal divides to form the two side by side situated components (from 25 mm C-R length onward), the medial and the lateral heads of the flexor hallucis brevis (Fig. 107). The abductor hallucis changes it relative position toward the tibial margin of the foot and now stands in one layer with the other great toe muscles (Fig. 107).

13. The two heads of the flexor hallucis brevis are innervated from the ansa between the medial and lateral plantar nerve (Fig. 108).

14. The two heads of the flexor hallucis brevis most resemble the original couple of the flexores breves profundi of Mammals in form and course, but are not exactly homologous with them.

15. The musculature at the fifth digit in the hand and foot originates also in two layers (Figs. 112, 113). The superficial layer differentiates independently in the hand from 16 mm, in the foot from 18 mm C-R length, giving rise in the hand and foot to the abductor digiti minimi primordium.

16. The deep blastema of the fifth digit in the hand and foot is the continuation of the flexores breves profundi layer. It divides into the flexor and the opponens digiti minimi in the hand after 20 mm C-R length; in the foot a similar process proceeds later, after 40 mm C-R length. The division into the flexor and the opponens is incomplete in the foot, so that the anatomical nomenclature (P.N.A.) does not contain the opponens, and the I.N.A. considered the opponens digiti minimi only as a variation. Its separation, however, is always visible in embryos, at least as structural changes of the corresponding blastema region.

4. The Superficial Palmar and Superficial Plantar Primordia during Ontogenesis

1. In the superficial region of the palm and sole a bulky blastema originates, which in the hand represents the primordium of the flexor digitorum superficialis (from 14 mm C-R length onward), in the foot (from 16 mm C-R length) it is the primordium of the flexor digitorum brevis (Figs. 114, 116).

2. In the hand this primordium is up to 19 mm C-R length of embryo actually situated in the palm, then it quickly ascends toward the antebrachium and obtains the extent of the definitive muscle. Homologised as for the layer, this primordium evidently belongs together with the abductor pollicis brevis and the abductor digiti minimi primordia to the so-called flexores breves superficiales (palmares) of comparative anatomy (Figs. 114, 115).

3. The flexor digitorum brevis pedis remains separated from the developing plantar aponeurosis during all the studied developmental period.

4. In the foot also the position and the degree of differentiation of this primordium places it from the beginning of development together with the abductor hallucis and the abductor digiti minimi primordia in a common layer evidently corresponding to the flexores breves superficiales (plantares) of comparative anatomy (Fig. 116).

5. Ontogenesis of the Lumbricales in the Hand and Foot

1. The lumbricales of the hand originate in course of ontogenesis by division of a plate, originally common for the flexor digitorum profundus tendons and the lumbricales. After division, which in the hand involves the entire thickness of this plate, the lumbricals are immediately different in their cytology from the slips of future tendons (Fig. 117).

2. The lumbricales originate in situ (from 14 mm C-R length); coursing beneath the distal sectors of intermetacarpal spaces they come in contact with the residua of the contrahentes layer.

3. During early ontogenesis (before the differentiation of the palmar aponeurosis) perforating mesenchymal bundles with blood vessels from the subcutaneous region join the lumbricals in distal sectors of intermetacarpal spaces (Fig. 53).

4. The lumbricales of the foot also originate by division of the originally common plate for the tendons of the flexor hallucis longus and the lumbrical primordia.

5. The splitting off of the lumbricales does not proceed in the foot in the entire thickness of the plate, but only from its dorsal surface (in embryos 17 to 18 mm C-R length), which after this separation bears visible traces of the split-off primordia (Fig. 118). The tendinous plate itself remains undivided for a certain period.

6. In their course through the planta the primordia of the lumbricales of the foot contact the residua of strips of the contrahentes layer so firmly that the fusion of a part of the material from these contrahentes residua to lumbrical primordia cannot be excluded.

6. The Quadratus plantae during Ontogenesis

1. The quadratus plantae primordium originates from 18 mm C-R length of the embryo.

2. The first differentiation of this primordium appears in the close proximity of the coursing stem of the lateral plantar nerve.

3. The quadratus plantae primordium has no relation to any of the typical layers of muscular primordia in the planta and also at first stands in no connection to the skeleton (Figs. 119, 120), which it joins after 30 mm C-R length of embryo.

4. According to the situation of its muscle belly and its relation to the flexor hallucis longus tendon, the quadratus plantae primordium represents the continuation of the flexor hallucis longus belly into the planta. Its separation from the crural belly of the flexor represents only a distance of about 40 μ in small embryos. The term "flexor accessorius" in comparative anatomy is quite appropriate.

7. The Development of Certain Structures of Connective Tissue in the Hand and Foot

1. The aponeurosis palmaris as well as the aponeurosis plantaris are typical components of the palm and sole, characterized by their position and structure.

2. In the course of ontogenesis neither the palmar nor the plantar aponeurosis stand in relation to muscular primordia, and their development cannot be given in connection with the development of the palmar and plantar musculature.

3. Both aponeuroses differentiate from the beginning as the connective tissue; the plantar aponeurosis has a closer connection to the subcutaneous tissue of the planta.

4. The retinaculum flexorum gradually differentiates from 15 mm C-R length of embryo from the ulnar insertion radiad. (Fig. 98.) This differentiation appears as a gradual growth in the ulno-radial direction.

5. In the course of differentiation the retinaculum passes round the superficial palmar primordium, at the period when this primordium extends toward the antebrachium (Fig. 98).

6. The joining of the differentiating retinaculum flexorum to the eminentia carpi radialis influences the opponens pollicis primordium which obtains a secondary proximal insertion in the retinaculum, thus changing its position in relation to the thenar layers (Fig. 99).

7. The primordium of the dorsal aponeurosis of fingers originates in embryos of about 15 mm C-R length, in connection with the interossei dorsales accessorii primordia (v. s.).

8. The interossei dorsales accessorii primordia extend by a mesenchymal layer over neighbouring metacarpals, the tendon of the corresponding extensor joins this mesenchymal layer (which represents the primordium of the future fascia dorsalis manus interossea) from the dorsal side already at the level of metacarpal shafts (Fig. 121).

9. The aponeurosis of the finger, thus formed, is then only thickened by the insertion of the lumbricales and the interossei.

10. The primordia of the interossei dorsales accessorii insert distally and independently into the dorsal aponeurosis, to both sides, to both neighbouring fingers. The insertion is later reduced and remains only in accordance with the corresponding interosseus dorsalis.

C. Summary of General Conclusions

1. In the course of human ontogenesis the muscles of the palm and sole develop mainly in situ. No traces of shifts of blastemas, or of their layers, or traces of migration of muscular primordia were found, as assumed earlier. The changes of position can be explained either by a different rate of growth of structures or by joining of further differentiated blastematous layers to the original anlage.

2. The form development of muscles in the hand and foot, as well as the development of some parts of the skeleton of the hand and foot bear a striking character of developmental recapitulation in the course of ontogenesis.

3. In the human palm and sole following layers of muscle primordia and the following muscles developing from them can be found in the course of ontogenesis (Fig. 122):

a) The layer of the flexores breves superficiales;

the hand: the abductor pollicis brevis, the flexor digitorum superficialis, the abductor brevis digiti minimi;

the foot: the abductor hallucis, the flexor digitorum brevis, the abductor digiti minimi;

b) the lumbricales layer, approximately equal in the hand and foot;

c) the contrahentes layer, situated between long flexor tendons and the lumbricales on the palmar side and the course of the deep branch of the ulnar nerve (lateral plantar nerve) on the dorsal side:

the hand: both heads of the adductor pollicis, the residua joined with the interossei;

the foot: the oblique head of the adductor hallucis, secondarily the caput transversum of the adductor (it is not homologous with any of the typical contrahentes muscles), the residua joined to the interossei;

d) the flexores breves profundi layer, situated just dorsal to the ulnar nerve (lateral plantar nerve); it does not extend deep into the spaces;

the hand: the opponens pollicis, both heads of the flexor pollicis brevis, the interosseus palmaris I Henlei, the interosseus dorsalis I (two components), palmar portions of the interossei dorsales II, III and IV, the entire palmar interossei I–III, the flexor digiti minimi brevis and the opponens digiti minimi;

the foot: both heads of the flexor hallucis brevis, the interosseus plantaris hallucis, two components of the interosseus dorsalis I (one of them being most probably the plantar component belonging originally to the interosseus dorsalis II), the plantar portions of the interossei dorsales II, III and IV, the interossei plantares I–III, the flexor digiti minimi brevis and the opponens digiti minimi (var.);

e) the intermetacarpales (intermetatarsales) layer, differentiating inside the spaces (except for the first one);

the hand: dorsal parts of the interossei dorsales II, III and IV;

the foot: the entire interosseus dorsalis II, dorsal components of the interossei dorsales III and IV;

f) the interossei dorsales accessorii layer, situated over the dorsal margins of the intermetacarpal (intermetatarsal) spaces;

the hand: dorsal surface of the interosseus dorsalis IV, dorsal portions fused to a variable degree or variably independent muscles over the interossei dorsales II, III (sometimes IV), rarely as a variation also over the 1st dorsal interosseus;

the foot: dorsal parts of the interosseus dorsalis II, in half the cases also of the interosseus dorsalis III, or muscular slips variably independent over the interossei dorsales II and III;

g) the layer of short (deep) extensors of the hand and foot;

the hand: the extensor indicis, muscular variations as derivatives of distal parts of the deep layer of antebrachial extensors—these are not in connection with the above mentioned layer of the interossei dorsales accessorii which may imitate the short extensors; they may be distinguished according to the nerve supply;

the foot: the extensor hallucis brevis, the extensor digitorum brevis;

h) the layer of extensor tendons.

4. All quoted layers except for the layer mentioned sub f—the interossei dorsales accessorii—have their homologa in the comparative anatomy of Mammals. The layer of the interossei dorsales accessorii is, most probably, specific only for the human hand. It is the early derivative of the dorsal muscular blastema of the hand which relates to intermetacarpal (intermetatarsal) spaces and is also innervated from them, by a direct branch from the ulnar nerve in the hand, by a branched-off twig from an anastomosis between the nervus plantaris lateralis and the n. fibularis profundus in the foot.

5. The recapitulation character in the course of ontogenesis of all basic layers of hand and foot musculature (repeating in the course of ontogenesis the sequence of form changes known in the phylogenesis) permits the distinguishing of fusing components of the interossei, originating from several layers of primordia, as well as an attempt to establish homologies of most muscles in the hand and foot of Man.

Acknowledgment. The author wishes to express his gratitude to all the members of the Staff of the Department of Anatomy, Charles University Medical Faculty in Prague, who inspired the finishing of the present publication by their interest in the topic, and to all of them who with deep understanding and great enthusiasm now further elaborate many unsolved problems initiated in this publication. Sincere thanks are expressed to Mrs. Vlasta Knappová, Mrs. Alena Englichová, Mrs. Pavla Němcová and to other members of the Technical Staff of the Department for the indispensable technical assistance, especially for diligent and careful preparation of histological series and for the preparation of the photographs. It is a great pleasure to extend special thanks to Mr. Milan Med, artist and medical illustrator, for his deep interest in Anatomy and a great artistic skill with which he made all drawings, and to Miss Pavla Šubrtová who carefully adjusted and labeled the microphotographs. Thanks are due to the late Dr. Arna Rides for the linguistic revision of the text.

Since the present publication includes the summary of results of studies made during last ten years, it was necessary to employ some of the microphotographs and some redrawn schemes, published sooner. The microphotographs are made from new negatives now; they are taken from identical series ad sections, however, as the sooner published ones. The drawings are modified. The new employing of these figures was enabled by the courtesy of the Editors and the Publishers of Folia Morphologica (Praha), Prague (Figs. 34, 36–38, 41–45, 47–53, 55–67, 72, 74), of Acta Universitatis Carolinae Medica, Prague (Figs. 98–103, modified drawings in Figs. 104, 111) and of Comptes Rendus de l'Association des Anatomistes, Nancy (Fig. 73, modified schemes in Figs. 76–78, 84), this being gratefully acknowledged.

Sincere thanks are due to the Editor, Prof. Dr. T. H. Schiebler, for his interest in the topic and the kind invitation to publish this rather voluminous and thoroughly illustrated contribution in the Advances in Anatomy, Embryology and Cell Biology.

VII. References

Albrecht, P.: Sur les homodynamies qui existent entre la main et le pied des mammifères. Presse méd. Belge (1884). Cit. sec. Bardeleben (1894a).
— Ueber den morphologischen Wert überzähliger Finger und Zehen. Zbl. Chir. **13** (Beilage 24), 105–107 (1886).
Balfour, F.M.: The development of Elasmobranch fishes. J. Anat. Physiol. **10**, 377–411, 517–570, 672–688 (1876); **11**, 128–172 (1876); **11**, 406–490, 674–706 (1877); **12**, 177–216 (1878).
— On the development of the skeleton of the paired fins of Elasmobranchii, considered in relation to its bearing on the nature of limbs of the vertebrates. Proc. zool. Soc. London, Mem. edit. **1**, 714–734 (1881a).
— Handbuch der vergleichenden Embryologie (German transl.), vol. II, p. 534–558. Jena: G. Fischer 1881b.
Barclay Smith, E.: Some points in the anatomy of the dorsum of the hand, with special reference to the morphology of the extensor brevis digitorum manus. J. Anat. Physiol. **31**, 45–58 (1896/97).
Bardeen, Ch.R.: Development and variation of the nerves and the musculature of the inferior extremity and of the neighboring regions of the trunk in man. Amer. J. Anat. **6**, 259–390 (1906/07).
— Lewis, W.H.: Development of the limbs, body-wall and back in man. Amer. J. Anat. **1**, 1–35 (1901).
Bardeleben, K., v.: Das Os intermedium tarsi beim Menschen. Jena. Z. Naturw. **17** (Suppl.) (1884); Sitz.-Ber. d. Jena. Ges. f. Med. u. Naturw. 1883, 37–39 (1883a).
— Das Os intermedium tarsi der Säugetiere. Jena. Z. Naturw. **17** (Suppl.) (1884); Sitz.-Ber. d. Jena. Ges. f. Med. u. Naturw. 1883, 75–77 (1883b).
— Das Intermedium tarsi. Jena. Z. Naturw. **17** (Suppl.) (1884); Sitz.-Ber. d. Jena. Ges. f. Med. u. Naturw. 1883, 91–93 (1883c).
— Zur Entwickelung der Fußwurzel. Jena. Z. Naturw. **19** (Suppl.) (1886); Sitz.-Ber. d. Jena. Ges. f. Med. u. Naturw. 1885, 27–32 (1885a).
— Zur Morphologie des Hand- und Fußskelets. Jena. Z. Naturw. **19** (Suppl.) (1886); Sitz.-Ber. d. Jena. Ges. f. Med. u. Naturw. 1885, 84–88 (1885b).
— Ueber neue Bestandteile der Hand- und Fußwurzel der Säugethiere, sowie die normale Anlage von Rudimenten „überzähliger" Finger und Zehen beim Menschen. Jena. Z. Naturw. **19** (Suppl.) (1886); Sitz.-Ber. d. Jena. Ges. f. Med. u. Naturw. 1885, 149–164 (1885c).
— Über die Hand- und Fuß-Muskeln der Säugetiere, besonders die des Praepollex (Praehallux) und Postminimus. Anat. Anz. **5**, 439–444 (1890).
— Hand und Fuß. Verh. d. Anat. Ges. 8; Anat. Anz. **9** (Suppl.), 257–337 (1894a).
— On the bones and muscles of the mammalian hand and foot. Proc. zool. Soc. London 1894, 354–376 (1894b).
Baumann, J.A.: Valeur, variation et équivalences des muscles extenseurs, interosseux, adducteurs et abducteurs de la main et du pied, chez l'homme. Acta anat. (Basel) **4**, 10–16 (1947/48).

Baumann, J.A.: Différentiation des muscles et tendons à la main et au pied chez l'homme pendant le développement, et causes des réductions tendineuses. Acta anat. (Basel) 12, 390–395 (1951).

Baur, G.: Der Carpus der Paarhufer. Morph. Jb. 9, 599–602 (1884).

— Über das Centrale carpi der Säugethiere. Morph. Jb. 10, 455–457 (1885a).

— Zur Morphologie des Tarsus der Säugethiere. Morph. Jb. 10, 458–461 (1885b).

— Zur Morphologie des Carpus und Tarsus der Wirbeltiere. Zool. Anz. 8, 326–329 (1885c).

— Bemerkungen über den „Astragalus" und das „Intermedium tarsi" der Säugethiere. Morph. Jb. 11, 468–483 (1886).

— Neue Beiträge zur Morphologie des Carpus der Säugetiere. Anat. Anz. 4, 49–51 (1889).

Beau, A., Sommelet, J., Cayotte, J.: Recherches sur le développement de l'articulation du poignet chez l'homme. Recueil des Travaux du Laboratoire d'Anatomie de la Faculté de Médicine de Nancy, p. 27–40. Nancy: George Thomas 1952.

Born, G.: Die sechste Zehe der Anuren. Morph. Jb. 1, 435–452 (1876a).

— Zum Carpus und Tarsus der Saurier. Morph. Jb. 2, 1–25 (1876b).

— Nachträge zu „Carpus und Tarsus". Morph. Jb. 6, 49–50 (1880).

Borovanský, L., Hněvkovský, O.: Vzrůst těla a postup osifikace u hochů od narození do 19 let. (La croissance du corps et le progrès de l'ossification chez les garçons depuis la naissance jusqu'à la 19e année. — Extrait.) Česká Akademie věd a umění, Praha (1930).

Braithwaite, F., Channell, G.D., Moore, F.T., Whillis, J.: The applied anatomy of the lumbrical and interosseous muscles of the hand. Guy's Hosp. Rep. 97, 185–195 (1948).

Brash, J.C.: Neuro-vascular hila of limb muscles. Edinburgh and London: E. & S. Livingstone Ltd. 1955.

Braus, H.: Die Muskeln und Nerven der Ceratodusflosse. Ein Beitrag zur vergleichenden Morphologie der freien Gliedmaßen bei niederen Fischen und zur Archipterygiumtheorie. In: R. Semon, Zoologische Forschungsreisen in Australien und dem Malayischen Archipel I/1, 137–300 (1901).

— Die Entwicklung der Extremitäten und des Extremitätenskeletts. In: O. Hertwig, Handbuch der vergleichenden und experimentellen Entwicklungslehre der Wirbeltiere, Bd. III, 2. Teil, S. 167–338. Jena: G. Fischer 1906.

Brooks, J.: On the morphology of the intrinsic muscles of the little finger, with some observations on the ulnar head of the short flexor of the thumb. J. Anat. Physiol. 20, 645–661 (1886a).

— Variations in the nerve supply of the flexor brevis pollicis muscle. J. Anat. Physiol. 20, 641–644 (1886b).

— On the short muscles of the pollex and hallux of the anthropoid apes, with special reference to the opponens hallucis. J. Anat. Physiol. 22, 78–95 (1888).

Broom, R.: Origin of Cheiropterygium. Bull. Amer. Mus. N. H. 32, 459–464 (1913).

— The origin of the human skeleton. An introduction to human osteology. London: H. F. & G. Witherby 1930.

Brůčková, Z., Čihák, R.: Klinické a anatomické poznámky k chirurgickému léčení manus vara congenita. (Clinical and anatomical remarks concerning the surgical treatment of congenital manus vara.) Acta Chir. orthop. Traum. čech. 23, 219–223 (1956).

Bühler, A.: Beziehungen regressiver und progressiver Vorgänge zwischen tiefen Extensorenstrecker und den Musculi interossei dorsales der menschlichen Hand. Morph. Jb. 29, 563–581 (1902).

Bunnell, S.: Surgery of the hand, 3rd ed. Philadelphia-London-Montreal: J.B. Lippincott 1956.

Campbell, B.: The comparative anatomy of the dorsal interosseus muscles. Anat. Rec. 73, 115–125 (1939).

Carlsson, A.: Über die Tupaiidae und ihre Beziehungen zu den Insectivora und den Prosimiae. Acta zool. (Stockh.) 3, 227–270 (1922).

Champneys, F.: On the muscles and nerves of a Chimpanzee (Troglodytes niger) and a Cynocephalus anubis. J. Anat. Physiol. 6, 176–211 (1871/72).

Chmelová, A.: Revise výskytu tzv. krátkých extensorů ruky člověka. Předn. a abstr., VII. fakultní věd. stud. konf., Fak. všeob. lék. K. U. Praha, 28. 11. (1963). (Revision of frequence of the so-called short extensors in the human hand. Paper and Abstract, VIIth scient. confer. of students, Charles University Medical Faculty, Prague, Nov. 1963.)

Čihák, R.: Variace dorsálních svalů stehna v klinickém syndromu Genu flectum congenitum. (Variations of the dorsal muscles in the thigh in the clinical syndrome Genu flectum cong.) Čs. Morfol. 2, 1–12 (1954).
— Musculus sphincter colli v ontogenese člověka. (M. sphincter colli in der Ontogenese des Menschen.) Čs. Morf. 5, 3–15 (1957).
— Musculus pectoralis major a jeho části v ontogenese člověka. (Musculus pectoralis major und seine Komponenten in der Ontogenese des Menschen.) Čs. Morfol. 7, 174–191 (1959).
— M. pectoralis major, m. trapezius a m. latissimus dorsi v ontogenese člověka. Kand. dis., Fak. všeob. lék. K. U., Praha (1960a). (The pectoralis major, Trapezius and the Latissimus dorsi muscles in human ontogenesis. Thesis [in Czech.] typewritten. Charles Univ. Medical Faculty, Prague, 1960a.)
— The origin of interosseous muscles of human hand. Čs. Morfol. 8, 183–194 (1960b).
— M. dorsoepitrochlearis lidských fetů. Předn. na 5. celostát. konferenci čs. morfologů, Plzeň, 16. 6. (1961). (The dorsoepitrochlearis muscle in human foetuses. Paper read in the 5th Conference of Czechoslovak morphologists, June 1961.)
— M. latissimus dorsi v ontogenesi člověka. (Development of the Latissimus dorsi in human ontogenesis.) Sborn. lék. 65, 21–26 (1963a).
— The development of the dorsal interossei in the human hand. Čs. Morfol. 11, 199–208 (1963b).
— Vývoj hlubokých svalů lidské ruky. Habil. spis, 121 s., Fak. všeob. lék. K. U. Praha (1963c). (Development of deep intrinsic muscles of the human hand. Thesis [in Czech.] typewritten, 121 pp.; Charles Univ. Medical Faculty, Prague, 1963c.)
— Verwendung eines Kunststoffes zur Herstellung plastischer Rekonstruktionen nach dem Verfahren von Born. Mitteilungsblatt d. Ges. f. Exper. Med. 1966, 41–42 (1966a).
— Musculus opponens pollicis v ontogenese člověka. Předn. na IX. Morfol. kongresu Čs. anatom. spol., Bratislava, 12.–16. září (1966b). (The opponens pollicis muscle in human ontogenesis. Paper read in the IXth Morphol. congress of the Czechoslovak anatom. soc., Bratislava, Sept. 1966.)
— The developmental significance of intrinsic hand muscles. Akten des Anthropol. Kongresses Brno (Tschechoslowakei) 1965. Anthropos 19 (N. S. 11), 75–79 (1967a).
— The occurrence of mm. contrahentes and their changes during the development of the human hand. Folia morph. (Praha) 15, 197–205 (1967b).
— Mode of extinction of the contrahent muscle layer in the embryonal human hand. Folia morph. (Praha) 16, 184–194 (1968a).
— Contribution à l'ontogénèse des muscles «contrahentes» de la main humaine. C. R. Ass. Anat. 1968, 53e réun., No 141, 704–712 (1968b).
— Ontogenesis of the layer of Mm. contrahentes in the human foot. Folia morph. (Praha) 17, 432–440 (1969a).
— The opponens pollicis and the deep thenar muscles in human ontogenesis. Acta Univ. Carol. Med. (Praha) 15, 499–513 (1969b).
— Vývoj kostry a krátkých svalů lidské ruky a nohy. Dokt. dis., 301 str., Fak všeob. lék. K. U., Praha (1969c). (Development of the skeleton and the intrinsic muscles in the human hand and foot. Thesis [in Czech.] typewritten, 301 pp., Charles Univ. Medical Faculty, Prague, 1969c.)
— Eiselt, B.: Proposition for replacement of the paralysed deltoid by parts of m. pectoralis major. Acta Univ. Carol. Med. (Praha) 8, 367–381 (1962).
— — Fleischmann, M.: Reconstruction of thumb opposition by intrinsic hand muscles. Acta Univ. Carol. Med. (Praha) 9 (N. S. 6), 3–26 (1963).
— Hněvkovský, O.: Vývoj širokého svalu zádového a použití jeho složek. (Development of the Latissimus dorsi and employment of its parts.) Acta Chir. orthop. Traumat. čech. 30, 3–13 (1963).
— Popelka, S.: Částečné defekty velkého svalu prsního. (Partial defects of the pectoralis major muscle.) Acta Chir. orthop. Traum. čech. 28, 185–194 (1961).
— Puzanová, L.: Tvar a poloha pately a utváření úponové části m. quadriceps femoris v době fetální. (Form and position of the patella and architectural pattern of the quadriceps femoris in the fetal life.) Čs. Morfol. 8, 15–23 (1960).
— Vlček, E.: «Crista et fovea musculi zygomaticomandibularis» chez les Primates. L'Anthropologie 66, 503–525 (1962).

Clark, W. E. Le Gros: On the myology of the three-shrew (Tupaia minor). Proc. zool. Soc. London 1924, 461–497.
— On the anatomy of the pen-tailed tree-shrew (Ptilocercus lowii). Proc. zool. Soc. London 1926, 1179–1309.
Corner, E. M.: The morphology of the triangular cartilage of the wrist. J. Anat. Physiol. 32, 272–277 (1898).
Cunningham, D. J.: The intrinsic muscles of the hand of thylacine (Thylacinus cynocephalus), cuscus (Phalangista maculata) and phascogale (Phascogale calura). J. Anat. Physiol. 12, 434–444 (1878a).
— The intrinsic muscles of the mammalian foot. J. Anat. Physiol. 13, 1–16 (1878b).
— Challenger Reports 5, 1–192 (1882). Cit. sec. Lewis (1965).
— The flexor brevis pollicis and the flexor brevis hallucis in man. Anat. Anz. 2, 186–192 (1887).
Curnow, J.: Variations in the arrangement of the extensor muscles of the fore-arm. J. Anat. Physiol. 10, 595–601 (1876).
Davidoff, M. v.: Beiträge zur vergleichenden Anatomie der hinteren Gliedmaße der Fische. I. Morph. Jb. 5, 450–520 (1879).
— Beiträge zur vergleichenden Anatomie der hinteren Gliedmaße der Fische. II. Morph. Jb. 6, 433–468 (1880).
— Beiträge zur vergleichenden Anatomie der hinteren Gliedmaße der Fische. III. Morph. Jb. 9, 117–162 (1884).
Dean, B.: The fin-fold origin of the paired limbs in the light of the ptychopterygia of palaeozoic sharks. Anat. Anz. 11, 673–679 (1896).
— Notes on acanthodian sharks. Amer. J. Anat. 7, 209–226 (1907).
Dobson, G. E.: A monograph of the Insectivora, systematic and anatomical. Part I. including the families Erinaceidae, Centetidae and Solenodontidae. London: John van Voorst 1882.
Dohrn, A.: Studien zur Urgeschichte des Wirbelthierkörpers. VI. Die paarigen und unpaaren Flossen der Selachier. Mittheil. aus der Zool. Station zu Neapel 5, 161–195 (1884).
Dylevský, I.: Determination of age of embryos obtained by interruption of pregnancy. Folia morph. (Praha) 13, 97–103 (1965).
— Contribution to the ontogenesis of the Flexor digitorum superficialis and the Flexor digitorum profundus in man. Folia morph. (Praha) 15, 330–335 (1967).
— Tendons of the M. flexor digitorum superficialis et profundus in the ontogenesis of the human hand. Folia morph. (Praha) 16, 124–130 (1968a).
— Původ a vývoj vrstev palmární aponeurózy v ontogenezi člověka. (The origin and development of layers of the palmar aponeurosis in human ontogeny.) Sborn. lék. 70, 353–359 (1968b).
— The origin and the developmental explanation of some known variations of flexor digitorum superficialis and profundus. Anthropologie (Brno) 6, 39–44 (1968c).
— Muscles of intermetacarpal spatium in the bird wing. Development and homology. Folia morph. (Praha) 16, 277–285 (1968d).
— Ontogenesis of the M. palmaris longus in man. Folia morph. (Praha) 17, 23–28 (1969a).
— Relation between the length of long limb bones, outer dimensions of limbs and the crown-rump lenght in embrya and fetuses. Folia morph. (Praha) 17, 147–157 (1969b).
— Kritické poznámky k takzvané vývojové teorii vzniku Dupuytrenovy kontraktury. (Critical comments on the so-called developmental theory of Dupuytren's contracture.) Sborn. lék. 71, 289–296 (1969c).
— Mrázková, O.: Phylogenetic differences in pattern and composition of dorsal finger aponeurosis. Folia morph. (Praha) 18, 161–167 (1970).
— Trnková, E.: Origin and development of muscles of the intermetacarpal space in the rat limb. Folia morph. (Praha) 17, 204–212 (1969).
Eisler, P.: Die Homologie der Extremitaeten. Morphologische Studien. Sonderabdr. a. d. Abhandl. d. Naturf. Ges. Halle, Bd. XIX. Halle: Max Niemeyer 1895.
Emery, C.: Ueber die Beziehungen des Cheiropterygiums zum Ichthyopterygium. Zool. Anz. 10, 185–189 (1887).
— Zur Morphologie des Hand- und Fußskeletts. Anat. Anz. 5, 283–294 (1890).

Emery, C.: Beiträge zur Entwicklungsgeschichte und Morphologie des Hand- und Fußskeletts
der Marsupialier. In: Semon, R., Zoologische Forschungsreisen in Australien und dem
Malayischen Archipel, II, 371–400 (1897a).
— Ueber die Beziehungen des Crossopterygiums zu anderen Formen der Gliedmaßen der
Wirbeltiere. Anat. Anz. 13, 137–149 (1897b).
— Accessorische und echte Skeletstücke. Anat. Anz. 13, 600–602 (1897c).
— Die fossilen Reste von Archegosaurus und Eryops und ihre Bedeutung für die Morpho-
logie des Gliedmaßenskelets. Anat. Anz. 148, 201–208 (1897d).
— Quelques mots de réplique à Mr. A. Perrin, au sujet du carpe des Anoures. Anat. Anz.
14, 381–382 (1898).
— Hand- und Fußskelet von Echidna hystrix. In: R. Semon, Zoologische Forschungsreisen
in Australien und dem Malayischen Archipel, Bd. III/1, Teil 2, 663–676 (1901).
Eyler, D. L., Markee, J. E.: The anatomy and function of the intrinsic musculature of the
fingers. J. Bone Jt Surg. A 36, 1–9, 18 (1954).
Flower, W. H., Murie, J.: Account of the dissection of a bushwoman. J. Anat. Physiol. 1,
189–208 (1867).
Fontes, V.: Note sur le muscle manieux. C. R. Ass. Anat., 28e Réun., Lisbonne (1933),
289–294.
— Note sur le muscle manieux. Arq. Anat. Antrop. (Lisboa) 16, 139–144 (1934).
Forster, A.: Die Musculi contrahentes und interossei manus in der Säugetierreihe und beim
Menschen. Arch. f. Anat. (1916), 101–378.
Forster-Cooper, C.: In: Parker, J. T., Haswell, W. A., A text-book of zoology, 6th ed., repr.,
vol. II, p. 499–500. London: Macmillan & Co. 1951.
Franz, V.: Geschichte der Organismen. Jena: G. Fischer 1924.
Fürbringer, M.: Die Knochen und Muskeln der Extremitäten bei den schlangenähnlichen
Sauriern. Leipzig: W. Engelmann 1870.
— Morphologische Streitfragen. II. Rabl's Methode und Behandlung der Extremitätenfrage.
Morph. Jb. 30, 144–274 (1902).
Gardner, E., Gray, D. J., O'Rahilly, R.: The prenatal development of the skeleton and
joints of the human foot. J. Bone Jt Surg. A 41, 847–876 (1959).
Gegenbaur, C.: Untersuchungen zur vergleichenden Anatomie der Wirbeltiere. I. Heft. Car-
pus und Tarsus. Leipzig: Wilhelm Engelmann 1864.
— Untersuchungen zur vergleichenden Anatomie der Wirbeltiere. II. Heft. 1. Schultergürtel
der Wirbeltiere; 2. Brustflosse der Fische. Leipzig: Wilhelm Engelmann 1865.
— Über das Gliedmaßenskelet der Enaliosaurier. Jena. Z. Naturw. 5, 332–349 (1870a).
— Grundzüge der vergleichenden Anatomie. 2. Aufl. Leipzig: W. Engelmann 1870b.
— Über das Skelet der Gliedmaßen der Wirbeltiere im allgemeinen und der Hinterglied-
maßen der Selachier insbesondere. Jena. Z. Naturw. 5, 397–447 (1870c).
— Über die Modifikationen des Skeletes der Hintergliedmaßen bei den Männchen der Sela-
chier und Chimären. Jena. Z. Naturw. 5, 448–458 (1870d).
— Über das Archipterygium. Jena. Z. Naturw. 7, 131–141 (1873).
— Zur Morphologie der Gliedmaßen der Wirbeltiere. Morph. Jb. 2, 396–420 (1876).
— Zur Gliedmaßenfrage. An die Untersuchungen v. Davidoff's angeknüpfte Bemerkungen.
Morph. Jb. 5, 521–525 (1879).
— Kritische Bemerkungen über Polydactylie als Atavismus. Morph. Jb. 6, 584–596 (1880).
— Über Polydaktylie. Morph. Jb. 14, 394–406 (1888).
— Bemerkungen über den M. flexor brevis pollicis und Veränderungen der Handmuskula-
tur. Morph. Jb. 15, 483–489 (1889).
— Das Flossenskelet der Crossopterygier und das Archipterygium der Fische. Morph. Jb.
22, 119–160 (1894).
Goodrich, E. S.: Studies on the structure and development of vertebrates. London: Macmil-
lan & Co. 1930. Republication by Dover Publications Inc., New York 1958.
Gräfenberg, E.: Die Entwicklung der Knochen, Muskeln und Nerven der Hand und der für
die Bewegungen der Hand bestimmten Muskeln des Unterarms. Anat. H. 30, 1–154
(1905/06).
Gray, D. J., Gardner, E., O'Rahilly, R.: The prenatal development of the skeleton and joints
of the human hand. Amer. J. Anat. 101, 169–224 (1957).

Gregory, W. K.: Origin of the Tetrapoda. Ann. N. Y. Acad. Sci. **26**, 317–383 (1915).
— Further observations on the pectoral girdle and fin of Sauripterus Taylori Hall, a Crossopterygian fish from the upper Devonian of Pennsylvania, with special reference to the origin of the Pentadactylate extremities of Tetrapoda. Proc. Amer. phil. Soc. **75**, 673–690 (1935).
— Miner, R. W., Noble, G. K.: The carpus of Eryops. Bull. Amer. Mus. N. H. **48**, 279–288 (1923).
— Raven, H. C.: Studies on the origin and early evolution of paired fins and limbs. Ann. N. Y. Acad. Sci. **42**, 273–360 (1941).
Gruber, W.: Neues Sesambein am Fußrücken des Menschen. Abhandlungen a. d. menschl. u. vergl. Anatomie, 4. Abhandl. VII., 111–113. St. Petersburg (1852). Cit. sec. Gruber (1877), Gruber (1879).
— Ueber die beiden Arten des überzähligen Zwischenknöchelchens am Rücken des Metatarsus (Ossiculum intermetatarseum dorsale Gruber) und über den durch Anchylose eines dieser Knöchelchen entstandenen und eine Exostose am Os cuneiforme I. und Os metatarsale II. vortäuschenden Fortsatz. Virchows Arch. path. Anat. **71**, 1–13 (1877).
— Neue Fälle des Vorkommens des Ossiculum intermetatarseum dorsale articulare — Gruber — als ein Fortsatz des Cuneiforme I. in Folge von Anchylose. Beobachtungen aus d. menschlichen u. vergleichenden Anatomie, I. Heft, 17–18. Berlin: Aug. Hirschwald 1879.
— Ueber das Os centrale carpi des Menschen. Beobachtungen aus d. menschlichen u. vergleichenden Anatomie, IV. Heft. Berlin: Aug. Hirschwald 1883.
Günther, A.: Contribution to the anatomy of Hatteria (Rhynchocephalus Owen). Phil. Trans. Roy. Soc. London (1867). Cit. sec. Thilenius (1896a), sec. Rabl (1910).
— Description of Ceratodus, a genus of Ganoid fishes, recently discovered in rivers of Queensland, Australia. Phil. Trans. Roy. Soc. London (1871), 511–571.
Haeckel, E.: Generelle Morphologie der Organismen, Bd. 2, Allgemeine Entwicklungsgeschichte der Organismen, S. 300. Berlin: Georg Reimer 1866.
Hagen, W.: Die Bildung des Knorpelskelets beim menschlichen Embryo. Arch. f. Anat. u. Physiol., Anat. Abt. (1900), 1–40.
Halford, G. B.: Not like man bimanous and biped, nor yet quadrumanous, but cheiropodous. Melbourne: Wilson & MacKinnon 1863.
Hallopeau, M. P.: Note sur le nerf de l'adducteur oblique du gros orteil. B. et M. de la Soc. anatomique de Paris, 6ᵉ série, T II, 1078–1080 (1900).
Harrison, R. G.: Die Entwicklung der unpaaren und paarigen Flossen der Teleostier. Arch. mikr. Anat. **46**, 500–578 (1895).
Haswell, W. A.: On the strukture of the paired fins of Ceratodus, with remarks on the general theory of the vertebrate limb. Proc. linn. Soc. N. S. Wales **7**, 2–11 (1883).
— Studies on the Elasmobranch skeleton. Proc. linn. Soc. N. S. Wales **9**, 71–119 (1884).
Henckel, K. O.: Beiträge zur Entwicklung der Primatenhand. III. Über die Entwicklung des Discus articularis des distalen Radio-Ulnargelenks beim Menschen. Morph. Jb. **68**, 293–300 (1931).
Henke, W., Reyher, C.: Studien über die Entwickelung der Extremitäten des Menschen, insbesondere der Gelenkflächen. S.-B. Akad. Wiss. Wien, math.-nat. Kl. **70**, 217–273 (1874).
Hepburn, D.: The comparative anatomy of the muscles and nerves of the superior and inferior extremities of the anthropoid apes. J. Anat. Physiol. **26**, 149–186, 324–356 (1891/92).
Hněvkovský, O., Čihák, R.: Muskelvariationen bei Genu flectum congenitum. Z. Orthop. **88**, 371–381 (1957).
— — Musculus sternocleidomandibularis u člověka. Vzácný případ spojený s achodroplasií a s myositis ossificans progressiva congenita. (Sternocleidomandibularis muscle in man; Rare case associated with Achondroplasia and congenital progressive Myositis Ossificans.) Acta Chir. orthop. Traum. čech. **34**, 12–22 (1967).
Holmgren, N.: On the origin of the tetrapod limb. Acta zool. (Stockh.) **14**, 185–295 (1933).
— Contribution to the question of the origin of the tetrapod limb. Acta zool. (Stockh.) **20**, 89–124 (1939).

Holmgren, N.: On the tetrapod limb problem — again. Acta zool. (Stockh.) 30, 485–508 (1949).
— An embryological analysis of the mammalian carpus and its bearing upon the question of the origin of the tetrapod limb. Acta zool. (Stockh.) 33, 1–115 (1952).
Hořejší, J.: Ontogenesis of external deltoid muscle formation in man. Acta Univ. Carol. Med. (Praha) 13, 81–91 (1967).
Howell, A.B.: Phylogeny of the distal musculature of the pectoral appendage. J. Morph. 60, 287–315 (1936).
Huxley, T. H.: Handbuch der Anatomie der Wirbeltiere. (German transl.), S. 34–35. Breslau: J. U. Kern's Verlag 1873.
— Contributions to morphology. Ichthyopsida. No 1. On Ceratodus Forsteri, with observations on the classification of fishes. Proc. zool. Soc. London 1876, 24–58.
Jones, F. Wood: The principles of anatomy as seen in the hand, 2nd ed., Reprint. London: Ballière, Tindall and Cox 1944.
— Structure and function as seen in the foot, 2nd ed., Reprint. London: Ballière, Tindall and Cox 1949.
Jouffroy, F.K.: La musculature des membres chez les Lémuriens de Madagascar. Mammalia 26, Suppl. 2 (1962).
— Lessertisseur, J.: Réflexions sur les muscles contracteurs des doigts et des orteils (contrahentes digitorum) chez les Primates. Ann. Sci. Nat. Zool. 12e Sér. 1, 211–235 (1959).
Kadanoff, D.: Über die Erscheinungen des Umbildungsprozesses der Finger- und Zehenstrecker beim Menschen. Morph. Jb. 99, 613–661 (1958).
Kajava, I.: Die kurzen Muskeln und die langen Beugemuskeln der Säugetierhand. I. Monotremata und Marsupialia. Anat. H. 42, 1–194 (1911).
Kaneff, A.: Zur Differenzierung des M. abductor pollicis biventer beim Menschen. Morph. Jb. 112, 289–303 (1968).
— Čihák, R.: Die Umbildung des M. extensor digitorum lateralis in der Phylogenese und in der menschlichen Ontogenese. Acta anat. (Basel) 77, 583–604 (1970).
Kaplan, E.B.: Functional and surgical anatomy of the hand. London: J.B. Lippincott 1953.
Keith, A.: Human embryology and morphology, 6th ed., Reprint. London: E. Arnold & Co. 1949.
Kindahl, M.: Die Entwicklung des Carpus und Tarsus bei Elephantulus myurus Johnstoni. Z. mikr.-anat. Forsch. 50, 173–189 (1941a).
— Untersuchungen einiger Entwicklungsstadien der Hand und des Fußes von Erinaceus europaeus. Z. mikr.-anat. Forsch. 50, 458–464 (1941b).
— Beitrag zur Kenntnis der Entwicklung des Extremitätenskelets bei Centetes ecaudatus und Ericulus setosus. Z. mikr.-anat. Forsch. 51, 322–333 (1942a).
— Einige Mitteilungen über die Entwicklung der Hand und des Fußes bei Talpa europaea L. Z. mikr.-anat. Forsch. 52, 267–273 (1942b).
— On the development of the hand and the foot of Tarsius and Microcebus myoxinus. Acta zool. (Stockh.) 25, 49–58 (1944a).
— Die embryonale Entwicklung der Hand und des Fußes bei Felis ocreata domestica L. Z. mikr.-anat. Forsch. 54, 555–564 (1944b).
— The embryonic development of the hand and the foot of Eremitalpa (Chrysochloris) granti (Broom). Acta zool. (Stockh.) 30, 133–152 (1949).
Klaatsch, H.: Die Brustflosse der Crossopterygier. Ein Beitrag zur Anwendung der Archipterygium-Theorie auf die Gliedmaßen der Landwirbeltiere. Festschrift zum siebenzigsten Geburtstage von Carl Gegenbaur. Bd. I, S. 259–392. Leipzig: Wilhelm Engelmann 1896.
Kohlbrugge, I.H.F.: Muskeln und periphere Nerven der Primaten mit besonderer Berücksichtigung ihrer Anomalien. Eine vergleichend-anatomische und anthropologische Untersuchung. Verh. Kon. Akad. Wet. Amsterdam (Tweede sectie), Deel V, No 6, 41–246 (1897).
Kollmann, J.: Handskelett und Hyperdaktylie. Verh. d. Anat. Ges. 2; Anat. Anz. 3, 515–530 (1888).
Kopsch, F.: In: Rauber-Kopsch: Lehrbuch und Atlas der Anatomie des Menschen, 18. Aufl., Bd. I, S. 607. Leipzig: G. Thieme 1952.

Kryžanowsky, S. G.: Das Rekapitulationsprinzip und die Bedingungen der historischen Auf-
fassung der Ontogenese. Acta zool. (Stockh.) **20**, 1–87 (1939).

Landsmeer, J. M. F.: The anatomy of the dorsal aponeurosis of the human finger and its
functional significance. Anat. Rec. **104**, 31–44 (1949).

— Anatomical and functional investigations on the articulation of the human fingers. Acta
anat. (Basel), Suppl. 24 (Suppl. 2 ad Vol. 25) (1955).

Langer, C.: Die Muskulatur der Extremitäten des Orang als Grundlage einer vergleichend-
myologischen Untersuchung. S.-B. Akad. Wiss. Wien, math.-nat. Kl. **79**, III. Abt.,
177–222 (1879).

Lanz, T. v., Wachsmuth, W.: Praktische Anatomie, I, 4: Bein und Statik. Berlin: Springer
1938.

Lazarus, S. P.: Zur Morphologie des Fußskelettes. Morph. Jb. **24**, 1–166 (1896).

Leboucq, H.: Recherches sur la morphologie du carpe chez les mammifères. Arch. Biol.
(Liège) **5**, 35–102 (1884).

— Sur la morphologie du carpe et du tarse. Anat. Anz. **1**, 17–21 (1886).

Leche, W.: Mammalia, Musculatur. Bronn's Klassen und Ordnungen des Tierreiches, VI, 5.
Leipzig: C. F. Winter'sche Verlagshandlung 1900.

Le Double, A. F.: Traité des variations du système musculaire de l'homme. Paris: Schleicher
Frères Éd. 1897.

Legueu et Juvara: Les aponévroses de la paume de la main. Bull. Soc. Anat. Paris (1892).
Cit. sec. Testut et Latarjet (1948), sec. Paturet (1951).

Lessertisseur, J.: Doit-on distinguer deux plans de muscles interosseux à la main et au pied
des Primates? Ann. Sci. nat. Zool. **11**, 77–103 (1958).

Lewis, O. J.: The evolution of the mm. interossei in the primate hand. Anat. Rec. **153**,
275–288 (1965).

— Hamshere, R. J., Bucknill, T. M.: The anatomy of the wrist joint. J. Anat. (Lond.) **106**,
539–552 (1970).

Lewis, W. H.: The development of the arm in man. Amer. J. Anat. **1**, 145–184 (1901/02).

— Die Entwicklung des Muskelsystems. In: Keibel, F., Mall, F. P.: Handbuch der Entwicklungsgeschichte des Menschen, Bd. I, 12. Kap., S. 457–526. Leipzig: S. Hirzel 1910.

Lucien, M.: Développement du ligament dorsal du carpe chez l'homme. C. R. Ass. Anat. **8**,
97–101 (1906).

— Note sur le développement du ligament annulaire antérieur du carpe chez l'homme.
C. R. Soc. Biol. (Paris) **62**, 169–171 (1907).

— Le muscle court extenseur du cinquième orteil chez l'homme. C. R. Soc. Biol. (Paris)
67, 67–68 (1909a).

— L'indépendance des faisceaux constitutifs du muscle pédieux. C. R. Soc. Biol. (Paris) **67**,
376–377 (1909b).

— Le pédieux et les muscles interosseux dorsaux chez l'homme. Considérations sur le développement du muscle pédieux. Bibl. anat. (Basel) **19**, 229–237 (1909c).

— Les chefs accessoires du muscle court extenseur des orteils chez l'homme. Bibl. anat.
(Basel) **20**, 147–156 (1910).

Lunda, O., Čihák, R.: Klinický význam m. extensor digitorum manus brevis a podobných
variací. (Clinical significance of musculus extensor digitorum manus brevis and similar
variations.) Rozhl. Chir. **46**, 652–658 (1967).

Marti, T.: Die Skelettvarietäten des Fußes, ihre klinische und unfallmedizinische Bedeutung.
Bern: Hans Huber 1947.

McMurrich, J. P.: The phylogeny of the palmar musculature. Amer. J. Anat. **2**, 463–500
(1903).

— The phylogeny of the plantar musculature. Amer. J. Anat. **6**, 407–437 (1907).

— The Evolution of the Human Foot. Amer. J. Phys. Anthropol. **10**, 165–171 (1927).

Meckel, J. F.: Entwurf einer Darstellung der zwischen dem Embryozustand der höhern
Thiere und dem permanenten der niedern Statt findenden Parallele. In: Meckel, J. F.:
Beiträge zur vergleichenden Anatomie, Bd. II, 1. Heft, Kap. I, II, S. 1–123. Carl Hein-
rich Reclam, Leipzig 1811.

— System der vergleichenden Anatomie. Erster Teil, Allgemeine Anatomie, S. 396–416.
Halle: Regnersche Buchhandl. 1821.

Mivart, St. G.: Notes on the Fins of Elasmobranchs, with Considerations on the Nature and Homologues of Vertebrate Limbs. Trans. zool. Soc. London 10, 439–484 (1879).

Mollier, S.: Die paarigen Extremitäten der Wirbeltiere. I. Das Ichthyopterygium. Anat. H. 3, 1–160 (1893).

— Die paarigen Extremitäten der Wirbeltiere. II. Das Cheiropterygium. Anat. H. 5, 433–529 (1895).

— Die paarigen Extremitäten der Wirbeltiere. III. Die Entwicklung der paarigen Flossen des Stöhrs. Anat. H. 8, 1–71 (1897).

Mrzena, V.: Mm. lumbricales v ontogenese člověka. Předn. na stud. věd. konf. Lék. fak. Univ. P. J. Šafaříka, Košice, listopad (1970). (The lumbrical muscles in human ontogenesis. Paper read in the Scient. confer. of Students, Faculty of Med., P. J. Šafařík Univ., Košice, Nov. 1970).

Olivier, G.: Formation du squelette des membres chez l'homme. Paris: Vigot Frères Édit. 1962.

O'Rahilly, R.: A survey of carpal and tarsal anomalies. J. Bone Jt Surg. A 35, 626–642 (1953).

— The prenatal development of the human centrale. Anat. Rec. 118, 334 (1954).

— Developmental deviations in the Carpus and Tarsus. Clin. Orthop. 10, 9–18 (1957).

— Gray, D. J., Gardner, E.: Chondrification in the hands and feet of staged human embryos. Contr. Embryol. Carneg. Instn 36, 185–192 (1957).

Osburn, R. C.: Observations on the paired limbs of vertebrates. Amer. J. Anat. 7, 171–194 (1907).

Paturet, G.: Traité d'anatomie humaine, T. II. Paris: Masson & Cie. 1951.

Pfitzner, W.: Bemerkungen zum Aufbau des menschlichen Carpus. Verh. d. Anat. Ges. 7; Anat. Anz. 8 (Suppl.), 186–193 (1893).

— Beiträge zur Kenntnis des menschlichen Extremitätenskelets. VII. Die Variationen im Aufbau des Fußskelets. Morph. Arbeiten 6, 245–527 (1896).

— Beiträge zur Kenntnis des menschlichen Extremitätenskelets. VIII. Die morphologischen Elemente des menschlichen Handskelets. Abschn. I.: Allgemeiner Theil. Z. Morph. Anthrop. 2, 77–157 (1900); Abschn. II.: Specieller Theil. Z. Morph. Anthrop. 2, 365–678 (1900).

Primrose: The anatomy of the Orang-Utang. Trans. Canad. Inst. 6 (1899); cit. sec. Wood-Jones (1944), sec. Forster (1916).

Rabl, C.: Gedanken und Studien über den Ursprung der Extremitäten. Z. wiss. Zool. 70, 474–558 (1901).

— Bausteine zu einer Theorie der Extremitäten der Wirbeltiere. Leipzig: Wilhelm Engelmann 1910.

Rajtová, V.: The development of the skeleton in the Guinea-pig. II. The morphogenesis of the carpus in the Guinea-pig. (Cavia porcellus). Folia morph. (Praha) 15, 132–139 (1967).

— Development of the Skeleton in the Guinea pig IV. Morphogenesis of the Tarsus in the Guinea pig (Cavia porcellus). Folia morph. (Praha) 16, 162–170 (1968).

Raven, H. C.: Comparative anatomy of the sole of the foot. Amer. Mus., Nov. No 871, 1–9 (1936).

Remane, A.: Die Grundlagen des natürlichen Systems, der vergleichenden Anatomie und der Phylogenetik. Leipzig: Akadem. Verlagsges., Geest & Portig K.-G. 1952.

Retterer, E.: Contribution au développement du squelette des extremités chez les mammifères. J. Anat. (Paris) 20, 467–614 (1884).

Ribbing, L.: Die Unterschenkel- und Fußmuskulatur der Tetrapoden und ihr Verhalten zu der entsprechenden Arm- und Handmuskulatur. Acta Univ. Lund. (N.S.) Afd. 2, 5, No 5, 1–158 (1909).

— Die Muskeln und Nerven der Extremitäten. In: Bolk, Göppert, Kallius, Lubosch, Handbuch der vergleichenden Anatomie der Wirbeltiere, Bd. V. Berlin-Wien: Urban & Schwarzenberg 1938.

Romer, A. S.: Osteology of the reptiles. Chicago-Illinois: The University of Chicago Press 1956.

— Price, L. W.: Review of the Pelycosauria. Geol. Soc. of Amer. Special Papers, Nr 28. Published by the Society, Dec. 6 (1940).

Rosenberg, E.: Über die Entwicklung der Wirbelsäule und das Centrale carpi des Menschen. Morph. Jb. 1, 83–197 (1876).

Rosenberg, E.: Über einige Entwicklungsstadien des Handskelets der Emys lutaria Marsili. Morph. Jb. 18, 1–34 (1891/92).

Ruge, G.: Entwicklungsvorgänge an der Muskulatur des menschlichen Fußes. Morph. Jb. 4 (Suppl.), 117–152 (1878a).

— Zur vergleichenden Anatomie der tiefen Muskeln in der Fußsohle. Morph. Jb. 4, 644–659 (1878b).

Salsbury, C.R.: The interosseous muscles of the hand. J. Anat. (Lond.) 71, 395–403 (1937).

Schauinsland, H.: Weitere Beiträge zur Entwicklungsgeschichte der Hatteria. Skelettsystem, schalleitender Apparat, Hirnnerven etc. Arch. mikr. Anat. 56, 747–867 (1900).

— Beiträge zur Entwicklungsgeschichte und Anatomie der Wirbeltiere I. Sphenodon, Callorhyncus, Chamaeleo. Zoologica 16, H. 39, 1–98 (1903).

Schmalhausen, J.J.: Die Entwicklung des Skelettes der hinteren Extremitäten der anuren Amphibien. Anat. Anz. 33, 337–344 (1908).

— Die Entwicklung des Extremitätenskelettes von Salamandrella Kayserlingii. Anat. Anz. 37, 431–446 (1910).

Schmidt-Ehrenberg, E.Ch.: Die Embryogenese des Extremitätenskelettes der Säugetiere. Ein Beitrag zur Frage der Entwicklung der Tetrapodengliedmaßen. Rev. suisse Zool. 49, 33–131 (1942).

Schomburg (1900): cit. sec. Gräfenberg (1905/06).

Schulin, K.: Über die Entwicklung und weitere Ausbildung der Gelenke des menschlichen Körpers. Arch. Anat. Physiol., Anat. Abt. (1879), 240–274.

Schwalbe, G.: Über das Intermetatarseum. Ein Beitrag zur Entstehungsgeschichte des menschlichen Fußes. Z. Morph. Anthrop. 20, 1–50 (1917).

Semon, R.: Die Entwickelung der paarigen Flossen des Ceratodus forsteri. In: R. Semon, Zoologische Forschungsreisen in Australien und dem Malayischen Archipel. I/1, S. 59–111. Jena: G. Fischer 1898.

Senior, H.D.: The chondrification of the human hand and foot skeleton. Anat. Rec. 42, 35 (1929).

Sewertzoff, A.N.: Die Entwicklung der pentadaktylen Extremität der Wirbeltiere. Anat. Anz. 25, 472–494 (1904).

— Über die Beziehungen zwischen der Ontogenese und der Phylogenese der Tiere. Jena. Z. Naturw. 63, (H. 1), 51–180 (1927).

— Morphologische Gesetzmäßigkeiten der Evolution. Jena: G. Fischer 1931.

Slabý, O.: Morfogenese a evoluční morfologie karpu ovce. (Morphogenesis and evolutionary morphology of the carpus of the sheep.) Čs. morfol. 6, 301–322 (1958a).

— Morfologický význam proximální a centrální řady karpálních elementů ve světle novějších teorií o vývoji autopodia savců. (Morphologic interpretation of the proximal and central rows of carpal elements in Man in the light of newer theories about the development of the autopodium in Mammals.) Čs. morfol. 6, 184–203 (1958b).

— Problém vývojových anomalií autopodia ve vztahu k morfologickým problémům této oblasti končetin. (The problem of developmental anomalies of the carpus and tarsus in relation to the morphologic problems of this region.) Acta Chir. orthop. Traum. čech. 25, 296–301 (1958c).

— Fylembryogenese neopodia končetin člověka. (Phylembryogenesis of the neopodium of the extremities in man.) Plzeňský lék. Sborn. 10, 229–240 (1959).

— Několik úvah o praepollexu a postminimu. (Some aspects concerning the problems of praepollex and postminimus.) Plzeňský lék. Sborn. 11, 121–131 (1960).

— Morfogenesa autopodia našich jelenovitých savců. (The morphogenesis of the autopodium of our Cervidae.) Čs. morfol. 10, 94–106 (1962a).

— Princip rekapitulace jako metoda embryologického bádání o historickém vývoji živočichů. (The principle of recapitulation as method of embryologic research of the historical development of animals.) Plzeňský lék. Sborn. 18, 5–15 (1962b).

— Vývoj a morfologická interpretace karpu Procavia capensis Pall. (Development and morphologic interpretation of the carpus in Procavia capensis Pall.) Čs. morfol. 11, 305–313 (1963a).

Slabý, O.: Příspěvek k řešení problému carpale 5 u kopytníků (carpale 5 během morfogenese končetiny u Moschiola memminna). (Contribution to the problem of carpale in Ungulates [carpale 5 during the morphogenesis of the extremity in Moschiola memminna].) Čs. morfol. 11, 314–316 (1963b).

— Morfogenese karpu vepře domácího (Sus scropha dom.) ze srovnávacího hlediska. (Morphogenesis of the carpus of the pig [Sus scropha dom.] from the comparative point of view.) Čs. morfol. 12, 363–372 (1964a).

— Několik komparativně morfologických poznámek k vývoji karpu u Bos taurus. (Several comparatively morphological aspects concerning the development of the carpus in Bos taurus.) Plzeňský lék. Sborn. 24, 43–50 (1964b).

— Problém vývojově specialisovaných struktur řešený na karpu kopytníků. (The problem of morphogenesis of the developmentally specialised structures presented in the carpus of Ungulata.) Plzeňský lék. Sborn. 28, 39–48 (1967a).

— Die Morphogenese und phylogenetische Morphologie des Carpus der Paarhufer. Rozpravy Čsl. Akad. věd., ř.mat.-přír. 77/7. Praha: Academia 1967b.

— Vývojové anomálie kostry končetin člověka a jejich vztah k fylogenesi. (Die Entwicklungsanomalien des menschlichen Extremitätenskelettes und deren Beziehung zu der Phylogenese.) Studie ČSAV, No 4. Praha: Academia 1968a.

— Wege und Gesetzmäßigkeiten der Evolution in bezug auf die phylogenetische Entwicklung der Extremitäten. Acta Univ. Carolinae Medica — Monographia XXXV. Prague: Charles Univ. 1968b.

Steiner, H.: Hand und Fuß der Amphibien; ein Beitrag zur Extremitätenfrage. Anat. Anz. 53, 513–542 (1921).

— Die ontogenetische und phylogenetische Entwicklung des Vogelflügelskelettes. Acta zool. (Stockh.) 3, 307–360 (1922a).

— Über die embryonale Hand- und Fuß-Skelett-Anlage bei den Crocodiliern, sowie über ihre Beziehungen zur Vogel-Flügelanlage und zur ursprünglichen Tetrapoden-Extremität. Rev. suisse Zool. 41, 383–396 (1934).

— Der ursprüngliche Aufbau des Extremitätenskelettes der Tetrapoden. Verhandl. Schweiz. Naturf. Ges. Bern, Teil II (1922b); cit. sec. Steiner (1934), (1935).

— Beiträge zur Gliedmaßentheorie: Die Entwicklung des Cheiropterygium aus dem Ichthyopterygium. Rev. suisse Zool. 42, 715–729 (1935).

— Der Aufbau des Säugetier-Carpus und -Tarsus nach neueren embryologischen Untersuchungen. Rev. suisse Zool. 49, 217–223 (1942).

Štěrba, O.: Das Homologon des M. subclavius beim Pferd (Equus caballus L.) Anat. Anz. 120, 41–46 (1967a).

— Srovnávací anatomie m. trapezii a jeho morfogenese u prasete. (Comparative anatomy of the trapezius muscle and its morphogenesis in the pig. Thesis [in Czech] typewritten). Diss. VŠZ., Brno (1965).

— The morphogenesis of M. trapezius and M. sternocleidomastoideus in the pig (Sus scropha f. dom. L.). Sb. VŠZ., Brno, ř. B, 36, 489–498 (1967b).

— Pectoral muscles of some Insectivores. Zool. listy 17, 149–156 (1968a).

— Comparative anatomy of M. trapezius and sternocleidomastoideus. Acta Sc. Nat. Brno 2 (N.S.), Fasc. 9, 1–27 (1968b).

— Berg, R.: Zur Morphogenese des M. trapezius bei der Katze. Anat. Anz. 112, 221–226 (1963).

Stieda, L.: Der Talus und das Os trigonum Bardeleben's beim Menschen. Anat. Anz. 4, 305–319, 336–351 (1889).

— Über die Homologie der Brust- und Becken-Gliedmaßen des Menschen und der Wirbeltiere. Anat. H. 8, 591–704 (1897).

Stjernman, R.O.G.: Vergleichend-anatomische Studien über die Extremitäten-Muskulatur bei Tapirus indicus. Acta Univ. Lund. (N.S.) Avd. 2, 28, No 5, 1–154 (1932).

Straus, W.L., Jr.: The foot musculature of the highland Gorilla (Gorilla beringei). Quart. Rev. Biol. 5, 261–317 (1930).

Streeter, G.L.: Chondrification in the hand and foot. Carnegie. Inst. Wash. Year Book No 28, 8 (1929).

Streeter, G. L.: Developmental horizons in human embryos. Description of age groups XI, 13 to 20 somites and age group XII, 21 to 29 somites. Contr. Embryol. Carneg. Instn 30, 211–245 (1942).
— Developmental horizons in human embryos. Description of age groups XIII, embryos about 4 or 5 millimeters long, and age group XIV, period of identation of the lens vesicle. Contr. Embryol. Carneg. Instn 31, 27–63 (1945).
— Developmental horizons in human embryos. Description of age groups XV, XVI, XVII and XVIII, being the third issue of a survey of the Carnegie Collection. Contr. Embryol. Carneg. Instn 32, 133–203 (1948).
— Developmental horizons in human embryos (fourth issue). A review of the histogenesis of cartilage and bone. Contr. Embryol. Carneg. Instn 33, 149–167 (1949).
— Developmental horizons in human embryos. Description of age groups XIX, XX, XXI, XXII and XXIII, being the fifth issue of a survey of the Carnegie Collection. Contr. Embryol. Carneg. Instn 34, 165–196 (1951).
Sunderland, S.: The innervation of the first dorsal interosseous muscle of the hand. Anat. Rec. 95, 7–10 (1946).
Testut, L.: Les anomalies musculaires chez l'homme expliquées par l'anatomie comparée; leur importance en anthropologie. Paris: G. Masson 1884.
— Latarjet, A.: Traité d'anatomie humaine, 9e éd., T. I, p. 1103–1104. Paris: G. Doin & Cie. 1948.
Thacher, J. K.: Median and paired fins, a contribution to the history of vertebrate limbs. Trans. Connect. Acad. 3, 281–310 (1877/78).
— Ventral fins of ganoids. Trans. Connect. Acad. 4, 233–242 (1878).
Thane, G. D. (1883); cit. sec. Lewis (1965).
Thilenius, G.: Die „überzähligen" Carpuselemente menschlicher Embryonen. Anat. Anz. 9, 665–671 (1894).
— Untersuchungen über die morphologische Bedeutung accessorischer Elemente am menschlichen Carpus (und Tarsus). Morph. Arbeiten 5, 462–554 (1896a).
— Das Os intermedium antebrachii des Menschen. Morph. Arbeiten 5, 1–16 (1896b).
— Accessorische und echte Skeletstücke. Anat. Anz. 13, 483–490 (1897).
Thompson, D'Arcy, W.: On the hind limb of Ichthyosaurus and on the morphology of vertebrate limbs. J. Anat. Physiol. 20, 532–535 (1886).
Tokmakoff, A. S.: Zur Anatomie des „Os intermetatarseum Gruberi". Anat. Anz. 66, 334–341 (1928).
Tornier, G.: Die Phylogenese des terminalen Segmentes der Säugetier-Hintergliedmaßen. Morph. Jb. 14, 223–328 (1888).
— Die Phylogenese des terminalen Segmentes der Säugetier-Hintergliedmaßen II. Morph. Jb. 16, 401–483 (1890).
Trnková, E., Dylevský, I.: Musculi contrahentes in the ontogenesis of the rat limb. Folia morph. (Praha) 17, 213–218 (1969).
Versluys, J.: Das Skelet. In: Ihle, J. E. W., van Kampen, P. N., Nierstrasz, H. F., Versluys, J., Vergleichende Anatomie der Wirbeltiere. Berlin: Springer 1927.
Vialleton, L.: Membres et ceintures des Vertébrés Tétrapodes. Critique morphologique du transformisme. Paris: O. & G. Doin 1924.
Virchow, H.: Das vorn und hinten gefurchte erste Keilbein am Fuße des Menschen. Verh. Anat. Ges., 31; Anat. Anz. 55, (Suppl.), 79–86 (1922).
Watson, D. M. S.: On the primitive tetrapod limb. Anat. Anz. 44, 24–27 (1913).
— The evolution of the tetrapod shoulder girdle and fore limb. J. Anat. (Lond.) 52, 1–63 (1917).
Weber, A., Collin, R.: Observation de chefs accessoires des interosseux dorsaux de la main chez l'homme. Bibl. anat. (Basel) 14, 183–189 (1905).
Weber, M.: Die Säugetiere. Einführung in die Anatomie und Systematik der recenten und fossilen Mammalia, Bd. I., Anatomischer Teil. 2. Aufl. Jena: G. Fischer 1927.
Westoll, T. S.: The origin of the primitive tetrapod limb. Proc. roy. Soc. 131, 373–393 (1943).
Wiedersheim, R.: Die ältesten Formen des Carpus und Tarsus der heutigen Amphibien. Morph. Jb. 2, 421–433 (1876).

Wiedersheim, R.: Nachträgliche Bemerkungen zu meinem Aufsatze: „Die ältesten Formen des Carpus und Tarsus der heutigen Amphibien". Morph. Jb. 3, 152–154 (1877).
— Über die Vermehrung des Os centrale im Carpus und Tarsus des Axolotls. Morph. Jb. 6, 581–582 (1880).
— Das Gliedmaßenskelett der Wirbeltiere mit besonderer Berücksichtigung des Schulter- und Beckengürtels bei Fischen, Amphibien und Reptilien. Jena: G. Fischer 1892.
— Grundriß der vergleichenden Anatomie der Wirbelthiere, 3. Aufl., S. 132–141. Jena: G. Fischer 1893.
— Vergleichende Anatomie der Wirbeltiere, 6. Aufl. Jena: G. Fischer 1906.
— Einführung in die vergleichende Anatomie der Wirbeltiere. Jena: G. Fischer 1907.
Windle, B.C.A.: On the embryology of the mammalian muscular system. I. The short muscles of the human hand. Trans. roy. Irish Acad. 28, 211–244 (1883).
Young, A.H.: The intrinsic muscles of the Marsupial hand. J. Anat. Physiol. 14, 149–165 (1880).

Subject Index